THROMBOSIS

Animal and Clinical Models

ADVANCES IN EXPERIMENTAL MEDICINE AND BIOLOGY

Recent Volumes in this Series

Volume 96
HORMONE RECEPTORS
Edited by David M. Klachko, Leonard R. Forte, and John M. Franz

Volume 97
PHARMACOLOGICAL INTERVENTION IN THE AGING PROCESS
Edited by Jay Roberts, Richard C. Adelman, and Vincent J. Cristofalo

Volume 98
IMMUNOBIOLOGY OF PROTEINS AND PEPTIDES • I
Edited by M. Z. Atassi and A. B. Stavitsky

Volume 99
THE REGULATION OF RESPIRATION DURING SLEEP AND ANESTHESIA
Edited by Robert S. Fitzgerald, Henry Gautier, and Sukhamay Lahiri

Volume 100
MYELINATION AND DEMYELINATION
Edited by Jorma Palo

Volume 101
ENZYMES OF LIPID METABOLISM
Edited by Shimon Gatt, Louis Freysz, and Paul Mandel

Volume 102
THROMBOSIS: Animal and Clinical Models
Edited by H. James Day, Basil A. Molony, Edward E. Nishizawa, and Ronald H. Rynbrandt

Volume 103
HOMEOSTASIS OF PHOSPHATE AND OTHER MINERALS
Edited by Shaul G. Massry, Eberhard Ritz, and Aurelio Rapado

Volume 104
THE THROMBOTIC PROCESS IN ATHEROGENESIS
Edited by A. Bleakley Chandler, Karl Eurenius, Gardner C. McMillan, Curtis B. Nelson, Colin J. Schwartz, and Stanford Wessler

Volume 105
NUTRITIONAL IMPROVEMENT OF FOOD PROTEINS
Edited by Mendel Friedman

Volume 106
GASTROINTESTINAL HORMONES AND PATHOLOGY OF THE DIGESTIVE SYSTEM
Edited by Morton Grossman, V. Speranza, N. Basso, and E. Lezoche

THROMBOSIS

Animal and Clinical Models

Edited by

H. James Day

Temple University
Philadelphia, Pennsylvania

and

Basil A. Molony, Edward E. Nishizawa,
and Ronald H. Rynbrandt

The Upjohn Company
Kalamazoo, Michigan

PLENUM PRESS • NEW YORK AND LONDON

Library of Congress Cataloging in Publication Data

Brook Lodge Conference on Thrombosis, 1977.
Thrombosis: animal and clinical models.

(Advances in experimental medicine and biology; v. 102)
Proceedings of the conference held at Augusta, Michigan, October 10–11, 1977.
Includes index.
1. Thrombosis–Congresses. 2. Diseases–Animal models–Congresses. I. Day, H. James. II. Title. III. Series [DNLM: 1. Thrombosis–Congresses. 2. Blood platelets–Physiology. W1 AD559 v. 102/QZ170 B871t 1977]
RC691.5.B76 1977 616.1'35 78-7219
ISBN 0-306-40009-X

Proceedings of the Brook Lodge Conference
on Thrombosis, held at Augusta, Michigan,
October 10–11, 1977

A Division of Plenum Publishing Corporation
227 West 17th Street, New York, N.Y. 10011

Printed in the United States of America

Preface

In 1976 a delegation from The Upjohn Company contacted one of us (H.J.D.) and proposed the idea for a workshop on animal and human models in thrombosis research. The reasons for choosing this subject were the rapid proliferation of animal and human models, the growing demand for interpretation of the data generated by numerous studies, and the increasing emphasis on the platelet-vessel wall interaction. It was agreed that a critical review of this field was needed. The Upjohn Company, which is involved in designing therapies for intervention in thrombosis, felt it worthwhile to sponsor the Workshop to gather and share with others working in this field as much information as possible on the suitability of different animal and human models.

The 2-day Brook Lodge Conference on Animal and Human Models in Thrombosis Research was held October 10-11, 1977, at Augusta, Michigan. We are indebted to The Upjohn Company, Kalamazoo, Michigan, for providing the means and facilities. We wish to express our appreciation to the many people who helped make the Workshop possible, including David I. Weisblat, Vice-President of Pharmaceutical Research and Development, and William E. Dulin, Manager of Diabetes and Atherosclerosis Research, The Upjohn Company.

This book contains papers presented by the participants, summaries of discussions following presentation of the papers, and transcripts of open discussion sessions. The book like the Workshop reflects the work and cooperation of many people. We thank especially five people from The Upjohn Company: Diana Schellenberg, Product Research Scientific Editing, who coordinated preparation of the book; Cindy L. Shattuck, Diabetes and Atherosclerosis Research, who performed most of the heroic task of typing the book; Suzanne K. Moyer, Product Research Scientific Editing, who assisted with the editing; and Diane L. Kozloski, Diabetes and Atherosclerosis Research, and Rose Losinski, Product Research, who provided secretarial assistance.

The Editors

H. J. Day, M.D.

B. A. Molony, M.D.

E. E. Nishizawa, Ph.D.

R. H. Rynbrandt, Ph.D.

Contents

SESSION II

ANIMAL MODELS
R.H. Rynbrandt, Chairman

SESSION III

CLINICAL MODELS
B.A. Molony, Chairman

THROMBOSIS
Animal and Clinical Models

INTRODUCTION TO THE BROOK LODGE WORKSHOP ON ANIMAL AND HUMAN MODELS IN THROMBOSIS RESEARCH

H. James Day, M.D.

Department of Medicine, Section of Hematology, Temple University Health Sciences Center, Philadelphia, PA

Remarkable progress has been made in the field of thrombosis research in the past decade. The platelet has been shown to have an important part not only in hemostasis but also in the pathogenesis of thromboembolic disorders. Much has been learned about platelet-vessel wall interactions and such factors as lipids and prostaglandins in promoting hemostasis and possibly thrombosis. That more should be learned about the initial reactions — those involving platelets and the vessel wall — in the genesis of a thrombus seems particularly important because their regulation can offer new opportunities to prevent thromboembolic disease.

There is also increasing recognition of the significance of the platelet-vessel wall interaction in the genesis of arteriosclerosis. Understanding this interaction may lead to development of therapeutic agents to reverse or prevent this important public health problem.

The list of thromboembolic complications is long and some of the conditions seem only remotely related. In order to design adequate therapy, we must understand the underlying disease process, and in order to understand the disease, we must develop better animal and human models.

Someone has said, "You have to be crazy to use animal models to study human disease, but you're crazy if you don't because of the insight you can get from animal work." This points to both the necessity to use animal models for human pathology and the dilemmas in interpretation which these models present.

The limitations of any model for a disease process include the fact that it may pertain to only one aspect. This may be because the total process is too complex to model in entirety, or because we believe we are modeling the most relevant component. With thrombosis, the manifestations may be so different from one person to another that no global model is adequate.

Thus, while the prospect of effective antithrombotic therapy hovers enticingly on the horizon, the limitations of present models for the disease have impeded evaluation of these agents. In the mid-1970s, a need was felt to review and discuss in a workshop format what was known about animal and human models in thrombosis, and the result was the Brook Lodge Conference in October 1977. The presentations covered six major areas of emphasis: the role of platelets in thrombosis and atherosclerosis; platelet-vessel wall interaction; increased platelet activities; material secreted by platelets; animal models now being used in thrombosis research; and human models — present and future — which may shed light on the disease process and on the usefulness of various antithrombotic therapies.

Session I

PLATELETS IN THROMBOSIS AND ATHEROSCLEROSIS

E. E. Nishizawa, Chairman

PLATELETS AND THROMBOSIS IN THE DEVELOPMENT OF ATHEROSCLEROSIS AND ITS COMPLICATIONS*

J. F. Mustard, M.D.,Ph.D., M. A. Packham, Ph.D., and R. L. Kinlough-Rathbone, M.D., Ph.D.

Department of Pathology, McMaster University, Hamilton, Ontario, Canada, and Department of Biochemistry, University of Toronto, Toronto, Ontario, Canada

ABSTRACT

Platelets, blood flow, and endothelial injury are among the factors that determine the sites at which atherosclerosis develops. Smooth muscle cells in the vessel wall proliferate in response to endothelial injury; and in addition, endothelial injury plays a role in the development of mural and occlusive thrombi in major arteries and thereby contributes to the development of clinical complications of atherosclerosis. Factors that cause endothelial injury therefore appear to be involved both in the development of atherosclerosis and in its thromboembolic complications. Platelets appear to have a key role in both processes. In animal experiments, platelets that adhere to the subendothelium release a factor which stimulates smooth muscle cell proliferation. In addition, platelets that interact with the damaged vessel wall release factors that result in further accumulation of platelets at an injury site, and also accelerate the coagulation process. Recently it has been shown that repeated endothelial injury produces a surface on the vessel wall that is more thrombogenic than that produced by a single injury, and also results in the accumulation of proteoglycans in the vessel wall. Proteoglycans may trap lipoproteins and thus promote their accumulation at sites of endothelial injury. Injury itself leads to increased permeability of the vessel wall to plasma proteins.

*Supported by grants MT 1309 and MT 2629 from the Medical Research Council of Canada.

Our increased understanding of the pathways involved in these processes has made it possible to examine the effects of smoking, diet, and drugs on the process. Smoking and diet may damage the endothelium, thereby influencing the development of atherosclerosis and its thromboembolic complications. There are three possible ways of detecting changes in the endothelium: 1) by measuring platelet survival, because in some animals damage to the endothelium is associated with shortened platelet survival; 2) by assaying materials released from the platelets into the circulation; and 3) by examining the blood for platelets that have undergone a release reaction. The detection of altered platelets could be used as an indicator of vessel injury or thromboembolism.

A number of drugs that modify platelet function are now being tested for their effects on these reactions. In animals, drugs such as aspirin or sulfinpyrazone do not appear to inhibit platelet adherence to the subendothelium or release of constituents from platelets adhering to collagen. Thus, it is not surprising that these drugs seem to have little effect on the proliferative response of the vessel wall to endothelial injury. Nevertheless, other effects of these drugs may be important in modifying the thromboembolic complications of vessel wall damage. The results of clinical trials now underway may indicate whether modifying platelet function can significantly influence the clinical complications of atherosclerosis.

INTRODUCTION

The distinguishing features of atherosclerosis (1-4) include the following:

1) It begins as an intimal lesion.

2) The lesions are focal and initially mainly distributed around vessel orifices and branches.

3) The intimal thickenings are rich in smooth muscle cells, connective tissue, and proteoglycans.

4) The intimal thickenings often contain increased amounts of lipid, particularly low density lipoprotein, cholesteryl ester, and, in advanced lesions, cholesterol crystals.

5) The sites of predilection for early atherosclerosis are areas of increased endothelial permeability.

6) Advanced atherosclerotic lesions often have thrombi associated with their surface, and histological and morphological evidence indicates that incorporation of thrombus material into the

vessel wall has contributed to the intimal thickening.

The extent of atherosclerosis has been shown experimentally to be modified both by vessel wall injury (5,6) and by feeding fats which increase serum lipids (7). Smoking, elevated serum cholesterol and high blood pressure appear to predispose man to complications of atherosclerosis. Evidence accumulated over the last 50 years shows that the principal factors governing the localized proliferation of smooth muscle cells and the development of atherosclerotic lesions are endothelial injury, blood flow, and interactions of the formed elements of the blood and lipoproteins (particularly LDL) with the wall (1,2,4,6).

ENDOTHELIAL INJURY

When the endothelium is injured, the vessel wall becomes more permeable to plasma proteins (8,9,10), and formed elements, particularly platelets, can interact with the collagen in the subendothelium (11). Some white blood cells also accumulate (10). When platelets interact with the subendothelium they release their constituents among which is the mitogen that stimulates smooth muscle cell proliferation (12,13). In experimental animals, endothelial injury causes smooth muscle cell proliferation in the intima (6,14, 15). This can be prevented in rabbits if the animals are made thrombocytopenic before the endothelial injury (16,17). These observations indicate that platelets may have a dominant role in this initial response in the rabbit. It is not yet certain whether there are a number of other sources of mitogens that stimulate smooth muscle cell proliferation following endothelial injury, but macrophages (18) have a mitogen similar to that found in platelets.

Because platelets play a major role in the smooth muscle cell proliferation that occurs in response to endothelial injury, factors influencing the interaction of platelets with the damaged vessel wall must be considered. Experiments in rabbits have shown that following a single balloon catheter injury, platelets rapidly accumulate on the subendothelium (19,20). Most of the platelets in the initial layer that forms on the damaged surface appear to remain on the wall and are not replaced by fresh platelets to any significant extent (20). Therefore the major mitogenic stimulus probably occurs immediately after the platelets adhere to the wall. If animals are made thrombocytopenic several hours after their aortas are injured with a balloon catheter, smooth muscle cell proliferation is not affected (21). If the wall is injured a second time after an interval of a few weeks, the injured vessel is more thrombogenic and platelet fibrin thrombi form on the surface (22).

Experiments with rabbits have shown that a single aortic injury with a balloon catheter does not have any detectable effect on platelet survival (20). This is hardly surprising because no more than 0.25% of the circulating platelets interact with completely denuded aorta (20). In monkeys, however, removal of the aortic endothelium with a balloon catheter has been found to shorten platelet survival (23). Although there is no clear explanation for this difference, it could be that in monkeys there is more extensive thrombosis on the surface of the damaged aorta. Platelets may be permanently lost from the circulation when they are trapped in fibrin-containing thrombi in which fibrin does not rapidly undergo dissolution. Limited evidence for this concept comes from experiments in which a cannula inserted into the aorta of rabbits formed large platelet-fibrin thrombi and caused a reduction in platelet survival (24).

Because endothelial injury also increases the permeability of the vessel wall to plasma constituents, plasma proteins and lipoproteins accumulate at such sites (25). Thus if any of these proteins or other factors that accumulate further modify the vessel wall response to injury, their effects would be greatest at the sites of injury. Low density lipoproteins have been found to enhance smooth muscle cell proliferation in the presence of plasma factors and platelet mitogen (26). Furthermore, low density lipoproteins (LDL) are metabolized by smooth muscle cells (27). It appears that when smooth muscle cells are forced to take up LDL in excess of their cholesterol requirements, they accumulate cholesteryl esters and develop morphological characteristics similar to those of smooth muscle cells in atherosclerotic lesions (28). Theoretically accumulation of LDL in the lesion could be a factor contributing to overloading of smooth muscle cells. LDL accumulation in the vessel wall may be due to increased proteoglycan formation as a result of vessel injury (29,30). Low density lipoproteins can bind to proteoglycans (31) and this could trap LDL at injury sites in the wall.

The sites of predilection for atherosclerosis are around vessel orifices and branches (4). Examination of these sites in normal animals (8,32,33) and young humans (34) killed in accidents has shown that the endothelium is often abnormal and, in some areas, the endothelium appears to have been lost. Accumulation of formed elements, particularly platelets, white blood cells, and platelet-fibrin thrombi, has been observed at these sites. In addition, the endothelium around such sites in animals shows an enhanced ability to incorporate tritiated thymidine (35-37), which indicates that endothelial cell turnover is increased. The explanation for the endothelial alteration in these regions has not been established, but an important determinant of these endothelial changes could be the influence of hemodynamic forces (38,39) either by themselves or in conjunction with blood-borne injurious substances.

Factors in addition to hemodynamic forces proposed as injurious to the endothelium include products from cigarette smoking, viruses and bacteria, antigen-antibody complexes, lipoproteins, epinephrine, and homocystine (4,40). The effects of some of these agents on the endothelium are maximized in areas of disturbed flow; this has been demonstrated with antigen-antibody complexes in serum sickness in animals (41).

Repeated Vessel Wall Injury

If the endothelium is repeatedly injured, further platelet interaction with the wall can occur following each injury. Following a second endothelial injury, the vessel wall is more thrombogenic than after the initial injury (22). Moore and his colleagues have observed that if the endothelium is repeatedly injured, extensive atherosclerotic lesions are produced; these have the morphological characteristics of atherosclerotic lesions (6,42), i.e., fatty streaks, fibrous plaques and raised lipid-rich lesions, cholesterol clefts, and foam cells. The mechanism by which repeated injury leads to these changes is not clear. Initially it was thought that the sites where the endothelium was lost and did not regenerate would be areas continuously exposed to plasma and platelets and hence would be most affected. However, maximum lipid accumulation has been observed at sites where the endothelium has regenerated and then presumably been lost with each of the repeated injuries (43,44). These observations indicate that at these sites the clearance and/or metabolism of the lipid that accumulates is more important than the permeability of the wall to the lipoproteins (45). The subendothelium beneath the regenerated endothelium may have different properties and react differently to platelets when it is repeatedly re-covered and re-exposed than it does at sites where the endothelium has not re-grown.

Experimentally it can be shown that 1 day after a single injury, the de-endothelialized vessel wall is much less reactive to platelets than the denuded vessel wall immediately following balloon injury (20). To understand the sequence of events that occurs, detailed knowledge is required of the vessel wall constituents and of the response of subendothelial surfaces to repeated injury. Proteoglycan accumulation may be increased at such sites and promote lipid accumulation, or the subendothelial surface may be more thrombogenic.

Hyperlipidemia and Vessel Injury

Vessel injury associated with hyperlipidemia can lead to more extensive atherosclerosis than either stimulus alone (7,46). In experiments with rats in which arteries were subjected to extensive injury, hyperlipidemia had only a small effect on the development of the lesions (47). However, with less severe vessel wall injury such as that associated with serum sickness in rabbits, the extent of the lesions is much greater if the animals are fed a hypercholesterolemic diet than if they are fed a normal diet which is low in fat (48). In a study of the relationship between hyperlipidemia and endothelial injury, Bjorkerud and Bondjers (45) concluded that endothelial injury has a greater effect on the development of atherosclerotic lesions than the degree of hypercholesterolemia. Thus, with slight endothelial injury, hypercholesterolemia would be expected to have a greater effect on the development of the lesions than with repeated endothelial injury. The observation that there appears to be decreased clearance of LDL at points of repeated endothelial loss and regeneration (30,45) indicates that proteoglycans may play a role in this accumulation. Increased proteoglycan accumulation has been observed in the intima at sites of repeated injury (30). Since LDL can bind to proteoglycans, this may be the explanation for its accumulation at such sites.

In addition to the effect of LDL on smooth muscle cells and the accumulation of cholesterol in the vessel wall, elevated serum lipids may injure the endothelium (23). The nature of the lipid and the mechanism by which it injures the endothelium are not known.

VESSEL INJURY AND THROMBOSIS

Vessel injury in areas of disturbed flow can lead to accumulation of formed elements on the surface and the formation of platelet thrombi and/or platelet-fibrin thrombi (49). The extent of thrombus formation is related to the balance between the factors promoting the accumulation of the blood constituents and the factors leading to their dissolution.

When the endothelium of an artery is injured or removed, platelets come into contact with subendothelial structures and adhere to the basement membrane, collagen, and microfibrils (11,49). Blood flow and the forces generated by red cells in flowing blood play a significant part in causing the platelets to come in contact with the vessel wall (50). When platelets interact with collagen, they release the contents of their granules. These granules are the amine storage granules (which contain serotonin, ADP, and a number of other substances), lysosomal granules, and at least one other type of granule which probably contains the antiheparin factor (platelet factor 4), proteoglycan, and possibly β-thromboglobulin (40,51). Although platelets can apparently adhere to microfibrils and to basement membrane, these surfaces have not been demonstrated to cause the release of platelet granule contents (11,52). When platelets come in contact with collagen the arachidonate pathway is activated and the short-lived intermediates of the pathway, the prostaglandin endoperoxides (PGG_2 and PGH_2) and thromboxane A_2, are formed (53-55). Both the released ADP and the intermediates of the arachidonate pathway cause platelets to change from discs to spheres with pseudopods, and to adhere to each other and to platelets that are adherent to the vessel wall.

Exposed collagen in the damaged vessel wall can activate factor XII (56) of the coagulation pathway, and when the endothelium is injured, tissue thromboplastin becomes available (57). When platelets are exposed to ADP, they may activate factor XII (58). Thus, an injury site and the platelet mass that forms can promote the initiation and/or acceleration of coagulation.

When platelets interact to form an aggregate, the membrane phospholipoprotein (platelet factor 3) which is necessary for key steps in the coagulation sequence becomes available (59). One consequence of these events is initiation of thrombin formation in and around the platelet mass. Thrombin causes platelets to change shape and adhere to each other, and to discharge their granule contents (including ADP); and thrombin also activates the pathway leading to the formation of the prostaglandin endoperoxides (PGH_2 and PGG_2) and thromboxane A_2 (60,61). Thrombin appears to activate a phospholipase A_2 that frees arachidonate from position 2 of the platelet membrane phospholipids, phosphatidyl choline, and phosphatidyl inositol (61). The released ADP and the products formed from arachidonate cause more platelets to change shape and adhere to each other and to the platelets adherent to the vessel wall.

Thrombin also catalyses the conversion of fibrinogen to fibrin, and the polymerizing fibrin adheres to the platelet mass and stabilizes it (62). Fibrin formation is necessary if the platelet aggregate is to persist, because without fibrin, platelet aggregates that have been induced to form by the action of ADP, thrombin, and the intermediates of the arachidonate pathway readily deaggregate (63,64) and can be washed away by flowing blood. In the venous circulation there can be regions of stasis where thrombin can cause extensive fibrin formation; red cells, trapped among the fibrin strands, form a red thrombus.

When fibrin is fully polymerized and the thrombin associated with it has been inactivated, platelets will not adhere to it (62). Thus, fully polymerized fibrin around a thrombus probably inhibits further growth of the thrombus. A question that has not yet been answered is how long the platelets that adhere to the damaged vessel wall retain the surface characteristics that are required for more platelets to adhere to them.

Platelets in a thrombus form a material (HETE) that is chemotactic for polymorphonuclear leukocytes (65). They also produce a factor which interacts with the fifth component of complement to form a chemotactic material (66).

At an injury site on a vessel wall, activators of plasminogen may be released and cause increased fibrinolytic activity around the thrombus (67). Activation of factor XII also promotes activation of plasminogen to plasmin (68,69). If lysis of the fibrin holding the platelet aggregate together occurs at a rate greater than fibrin formation, the thrombus could readily break up and the platelets could return to the circulation.

Blood flow patterns affect the size of a thrombus that forms in flowing blood in arteries. When blood flow is disturbed, thrombus formation is greater than in regions where flow is not disturbed (70-72). Flow separation in areas of disturbed flow causes platelets (but not red cells) to become trapped in vortices; there they may remain long enough to facilitate their interaction with each other and with platelet-stimulating materials that may be present in the region of disturbed flow (73). Platelets appear to interact with the surface of the vessel wall more readily in vortices. Occlusive thrombi seldom occur in the arterial system except in areas where flow is disturbed, such as at a stenosis.

Direct observation of thrombus formation in the microcirculation (74) has shown that although thrombi form rapidly at sites of vessel injury, they tend to embolize, and the fragments are swept away by the flowing blood. The thrombus usually re-forms and again undergoes dissolution. However, the number of times thrombus reformation can occur appears to be limited. Baumgartner (75) has observed that removal of the endothelium of the rabbit aorta results in immediate formation of thrombi on the subendothelial surface when the aorta is perfused. However, if the injured wall is examined 40 minutes after removal of the endothelium, only a thin layer of adherent platelets remains. Thus, a mural thrombus can form at an injury site on a damaged vessel, remain there for a short time, and embolize into the distal microcirculation. In healthy animals, most of these platelet and platelet-fibrin emboli rapidly break up with return of the platelets to the circulation (40).

In normal rabbits, a single injury to the endothelium in large arteries appears to lead to formation of a monolayer of platelets on the injured surface; this monolayer is gradually lost over the next few days. The surface provided by the monolayer of platelets and the exposed subendothelial surface after the platelets are lost from it are no longer very reactive to platelets, even though the surface has not been re-endothelialized.

Since thrombi can undergo dissolution, it is probable that platelets that have been exposed to ADP, thrombin, and thromboxane A_2 will return to the circulation. Platelets that have been exposed to thrombin (63,64) or ADP survive normally. Therefore it may be possible to detect platelets that have taken part in thrombus formation in the circulation. An estimate of the extent of thrombus formation may be obtained by measuring materials released from platelets such as platelet factor 4 (PF4) or β-thromboglobulin (76-78), or by estimating the proportion of degranulated platelets in the circulation (79). β-thromboglobulin has a longer half-life in the circulation than PF4; see the discussion by Dr. Kaplan at this workshop [pages 105 to 120]. This makes β-thromboglobulin the more attractive of the two measures for detecting the platelet release reaction *in vivo*. Platelets that are trapped in a thrombus or an embolus that does not break up are lost from the circulation but the released material should be detectable in the circulation. In some intravascular reactions, such as those associated with immune reactions, degranulated platelets have been found in the circulation (80).

THROMBOSIS AND ATHEROSCLEROSIS

Thrombosis and the Evolution of Atherosclerotic Plaques

Thrombosis contributes to the development of atherosclerosis through organization of the thrombi and incorporation of the thrombus material into the vessel wall (81-83). In advanced atherosclerosis, this appears to be an important mechanism in clearly marked narrowing of arteries (84). The development of extensive narrowing of the lumen of major coronary arteries is a principal factor in the development of clinical manifestations of atherosclerosis.

Thrombosis and the Complications of Atherosclerosis

Thrombosis could cause complications of atherosclerosis through at least two mechanisms: mural thrombi that embolize into the distal microcirculation, and occlusive thrombi that block blood flow to that part of the organ distal to the obstruction. Occlusive thrombi are associated with myocardial infarction both in humans and in experimental animals (85). They also tend to occur in association with advanced atherosclerosis where stenosis or narrowing of the lumen is sufficient to lead to flow disturbances. The argument that occlusive thrombi occur *after* an infarct is interesting and may be valid in some circumstances. However, the bulk of the morphological evidence shows that infarcts subtend the site of obstruction (85). The observation that coronary artery thrombi will take up radioactive fibrinogen after the infarct has occurred (86) can be explained on the basis that both the platelet and fibrinogen contents of a thrombus are continuously turning over (87,88).

In experimental animals, mural thrombi in the coronary arteries do not cause full thickness infarcts, but produce focal subendocardial lesions (89). These are believed to be due to platelet and platelet-fibrin emboli from the mural thrombi lodging in the microcirculation of the myocardium. This pattern of myocardial injury is very similar to that found in sudden death associated with myocardial ischemia (90). Attempts have been made to show that sudden death in man is produced by disturbances of the microcirculation caused by platelet-fibrin emboli from mural thrombi in the main branches of the coronary arteries. There is some morphological evidence from human autopsy studies that platelet-fibrin emboli are increased in the myocardial microcirculation in association with sudden death (91,92) due to coronary artery disease.

Lipids, Thrombosis, and Atherosclerosis

In addition to the effects of LDL on smooth muscle cells in the development of atherosclerotic lesions, there are other mechanisms by which lipids may cause or modify endothelial injury and contribute to the development of atherosclerosis and its thromboembolic complications.

Saturated fatty acids of chain lengths greater than fourteen carbons have been reported to promote experimental thrombosis in rats (93,94). Unsaturated fatty acids (94), particularly linoleic acid, have been reported either to have little effect or to inhibit thrombus formation. Dietary linoleic acid in man has been found to make platelets less sensitive to aggregation (95) and aggregating agents (96). In contrast, dietary arachidonic acid, which gives rise in platelets to the aggregating agents PGG_2, PGH_2, and thromboxane A_2, made human platelets more sensitive to aggregating agents (97). Addition of di-homo-γ-linolenic acid to human diets made platelets less sensitive to aggregating agents and decreased the ability of platelets to adhere to collagen (98). This fatty acid is a precursor of PGE_1, which is a strong inhibitor of platelet aggregation and platelet adherence to collagen.

In both humans and animals, diets rich in saturated fat shorten platelet survival (23,99,100). In addition to its effects on platelets, dietary fat has also been reported to modify blood coagulation (101). Hypercholesterolemia has been observed to injure the endothelium (23,102). The effect of lipids, particularly cholesterol and LDL, on the response of smooth muscle cells to injury has been discussed earlier. The role of diet in influencing serum cholesterol and LDL levels is well described in a number of articles.

PLATELET CHANGES AND PREDICTING ATHEROSCLEROSIS

There is considerable interest in developing methods to detect altered platelet function that may be the result of the clinical manifestations of atherosclerosis or may contribute to the development of atherosclerosis. Among the methods used to detect altered platelets are: 1) *in vitro* tests of platelet aggregation; 2) *in vivo* tests of platelet aggregation; 3) detection of altered platelets; 4) detection of material released from platelets; and 5) measurement of platelet survival.

As discussed in an earlier section, there is experimental evidence that platelets which have been exposed to the stimuli involved in thrombus formation can escape from the thrombus, return to the circulation, and survive normally. Although platelets exposed to thrombin will not readily aggregate on a second exposure to thrombin, they do aggregate upon exposure to collagen and may show increased sensitivity to ADP-induced aggregation (103). Furthermore, platelets that have been stimulated to release materials from their granules should be detectable in the circulation and the released material should also be detectable.

Citrated platelet-rich plasma prepared from the blood of patients during episodes of thrombosis shows increased sensitivity to ADP- and epinephrine-induced aggregation. However, when platelets are taken from these subjects several weeks later when the process has become quiescent, the increased sensitivity is no longer apparent (104).

There are many other studies showing apparent increased sensitivity of platelets to aggregating- and release-inducing agents in association with the clinical manifestations of vascular disease. However, none of these studies shows any sharp discrimination between individual subjects and the evidence strongly suggests that most of the altered platelet sensitivity may be a consequence of the underlying process rather than its cause.

Methods for detecting intravascular platelet aggregates are open to some debate as to whether the aggregates actually occur in the circulation or form during blood sampling (105,106). In subjects with transient attacks of cerebral ischemia, increased numbers of intravascular platelet aggregates were found using the Wu and Hoak method and these aggregates were not observed when the clinical manifestations disappeared (104). This subject has been reviewed recently (107,108). In most cases in which increased platelet sensitivity to aggregating agents has been detected, it could be abolished by aspirin administration. This indicates that the increased sensitivity is a consequence of increased activity of the arachidonate pathway, possibly as a result of the intravascular reactions (107).

Detection of altered platelets in the circulation is more difficult but perhaps more directly related to the question of whether intravascular thrombus formation is occurring. The "acquired storage pool disease" (80) described in some patients with intravascular immune reactions probably results from release of platelet storage granule contents from platelets that have been exposed to a release-inducing agent in the circulation.

When thrombosis is induced in rabbits by a cannula placed in the aorta, the proportion of light platelets in the circulation is increased (79). (Platelets of different densities can be separated by density gradient centrifugation through stractan or albumin.) The least dense platelets have a slight reduction in some of their granule contents, most likely because of exposure to a release-inducing agent. It is not yet known how useful this method will be for detecting altered platelets that may have taken part in thrombus formation. The method may be of use to examine the possible correlation of increased numbers of light platelets with shortened platelet survival. It has been shown that the light platelets from the stractan gradient are the older platelets and that these platelets have a diminished amount of surface sialic acid (109).

The other approach that has been used to detect intravascular thrombosis is to assay plasma for products released from platelets such as platelet factor 4 and β-thromboglobulin (76-78). Two problems with this approach are that the platelets may not be the only cells that release these materials, and the half-life of these materials in the circulation is short.

Finally, platelet survival can be altered by diet and smoking (99,110). An association has been shown in a number of studies between platelet survival and the clinical manifestations of arterial disease (111-113). However, the significance of shortened platelet survival is not entirely clear. Platelets that have taken part in thrombus formation are likely to have been exposed to ADP and thrombin, but these agents do not shorten platelet survival (63,103). However, removal of platelet membrane sialic acid does shorten platelet survival (114). Whether this can occur *in vivo* is unclear, although there are some viruses with neuraminidase activity which can remove membrane sialic acid and shorten platelet survival (115). The fact that endothelial damage shortens platelet survival in monkeys (23) but not in rabbits (20) raises the possibility of a species difference in the mechanisms responsible for shortened platelet survival. The difference between the results with balloon injury to a rabbit aorta and balloon injury to a monkey aorta could be the extent of thrombus formation that occurs following the injury. It appears that monkeys form a more extensive thrombus and this could be the reason shortened platelet survival has been observed in this species.

It is clearly important in these tests for the detection of altered platelet function to keep in mind the need to differentiate between results that are a manifestation of the intravascular ischemic episode, and results that may indicate a fundamental change in the platelets or blood coagulation which contribute to the development of thromboembolism. At the present time it appears likely that altered platelets are the result of the intravascular events rather than their cause.

DRUGS, PLATELET FUNCTION, THROMBOSIS, AND ATHEROSCLEROSIS

The effects of three drugs are currently being evaluated in clinical trials for the management of arterial thromboembolic disease. These drugs are aspirin, sulfinpyrazone, and dipyridamole.

Aspirin inhibits platelet cyclo-oxygenase and thereby prevents the formation of the prostaglandin endoperoxides (PGG_2 and PGH_2) and thromboxane A_2 (116). This effect of aspirin does not inhibit primary ADP-induced platelet aggregation, thrombin-induced aggregation, or the thrombin-induced release reaction (60). Furthermore, we have recently observed that aspirin blocks neither the adherence of platelets to collagen nor the release reaction of platelets adherent to collagen (117). It is therefore not surprising that aspirin is unable to inhibit the smooth muscle cell proliferation that occurs after the endothelium is removed with a balloon catheter (118). Finally, aspirin has not been found to have any effect on platelet survival (119).

Sulfinpyrazone is a weaker inhibitor than aspirin of platelet cyclo-oxygenase (120). It also does not inhibit platelet adhesion to collagen or the release reaction of the platelets that are adherent to collagen (117). Sulfinpyrazone does lengthen shortened platelet survival (121,122). The mode of action of sulfinpyrazone is not clear, but one possible mechanism is that it may diminish injury to the endothelium (123).

Dipyridamole increases platelet cyclic-AMP levels (124). It also inhibits platelet adherence to the subendothelium and collagen (117). Dipyridamole prolongs shortened platelet survival (119). In homocystinemia-induced endothelial injury in monkeys, dipyridamole reduces the extent of smooth muscle cell proliferation (125). This may be related to the ability of dipyridamole to diminish platelet adherence to damaged vessel walls.

Currently aspirin, sulfinpyrazone, and dipyridamole are being used in clinical trials to prevent death in individuals who have had a myocardial infarction or to prevent strokes and death in patients who have had transient attacks of cerebral ischemia. Aspirin was found to produce a significant reduction in the incidence of strokes and death in patients who had clinical evidence of transient attacks of cerebral ischemia (126). At this Workshop Dr. Barnett will describe the results of the Canadian trial showing that sulfinpyrazone has little or no effect, but that aspirin has a protective effect in some males. A number of studies of individuals with myocardial infarction have demonstrated that there is a tendency for those taking aspirin to show lower incidence of death. This subject is discussed in more detail by Dr. Genton at this Workshop. The only conclusive evidence that dipyridamole may have some effect comes from an early study of the use of this drug in preventing embolic phenomena in subjects with prosthetic heart valves who were also receiving oral anticoagulants (127). It seems likely that in these clinical conditions, these drugs may be beneficial for certain groups or subgroups of patients. The results of these trials may make it possible to identify subgroups who are likely to benefit from treatment with the drugs. The results may also help clarify the nature of the mechanisms involved and provide some opportunity to select drugs which may be more appropriate for affecting the underlying mechanisms.

REFERENCES

1. Wissler RW: Overview of problems of atherosclerosis. In CEREBROVASCULAR DISEASES, edited by Scheinberg P. New York, Raven Press, 1976, pp. 59-75.

2. Geer JC, Haust MD: Smooth muscle cells in atherosclerosis. In MONOGRAPHS ON ATHEROSCLEROSIS 2, edited by Pollak OJ, Simms HS, Kirk JE. New York, Karger, 1972.

3. Strong JB, McGill HC, Jr: The natural history of coronary atherosclerosis. AM J PATHOL 40:37-49, 1962.

4. Mustard JF, Packham MA: The role of blood and platelets in atherosclerosis and the complications of atherosclerosis. THROMB DIATH HAEMORRH 33:444-456, 1975.

5. Taylor CB, Hass GM, Ho K-J: The role of repair of arterial injury and degeneration in arteriosclerosis. In LE RÔLE DE LA PAROI ARTÉRIELLE DANS L'ATHÉROGÉNÈSES. Colloques Internationaux du Centre National de la Recherche Scientifique No. 169, 853-872, Paris, 1968.

6. Moore S: Thromboatherosclerosis in normolipemic rabbits. A result of continued endothelial damage. LAB INVEST 29:478-487, 1973.

7. Alonso DR, Starek PK, Minick CR: Studies on the pathogenesis of atheroarteriosclerosis induced in rabbit cardiac allografts by the synergy of graft rejection and hypercholesterolemia. AM J PATHOL 87:415-442, 1977.

8. Packham MA, Rowsell HC, Jørgensen L, Mustard JF: Localized protein accumulation in the wall of the aorta. EXP MOL PATHOL 7:214-232, 1967.

9. McGill HC, Geer JC, Holman RL: Sites of vascular vulnerability in dogs demonstrated by Evans blue. ARCH PATHOL 64:303-311, 1957.

10. Jørgensen L, Packham MA, Rowsell HC, Buchanan MR, Mustard JF: Focal aortic injury caused by cannulation: Increased plasma protein accumulation and thrombosis. ACTA PATHOL MICROBIOL SCAND [A] 82:637-647, 1974.

11. Baumgartner HR, Muggli R, Tschopp TB, Turitto VT: Platelet adhesion, release and aggregation in flowing blood: Effects of surface properties and platelet function. THROMB HAEMOSTAS 35:124-138, 1976.

12. Rutherford RB, Ross R: Platelet factors stimulate fibroblasts and smooth muscle cells quiescent in plasma serum to proliferate. J CELL BIOL 69:196-203, 1976.

13. Ihnatowycz IO, Cazenave J-P, Moore S, Mustard JF: Platelet-derived growth factor production during the platelet release reaction independent of the arachidonate pathway. THROMB HAEMOSTAS 38:229, 1977.

14. Stemerman MB, Ross R: Experimental arteriosclerosis. I. Fibrous plaque formation in primates, an electron microscope study. J EXP MED 136:769-789, 1972.

15. Ross R, Glomset JA: Atherosclerosis and the arterial smooth muscle cell. Proliferation of smooth muscle is a key event in the genesis of the lesions of atherosclerosis. SCIENCE 180: 1332-1339, 1973.

16. Moore S, Friedman RJ, Singal DP, Gauldie J, Blajchman MA, Roberts RS: Inhibition of injury-induced thromboatherosclerotic lesions by anti-platelet serum in rabbits. THROMB HAEMOSTAS 35:70-81, 1976.

17. Friedman RJ, Stemerman MB, Wenz B, Moore S, Gauldie J, Gent M, Tiell ML, Spaet TH: The effect of thrombocytopenia on experimental arteriosclerotic lesion formation in rabbits: I. Smooth muscle cell proliferation and re-endothelialization. J CLIN INVEST 60:1191-1201, 1977.

18. Ross R: Personal communication.

19. Baumgartner HR, Muggli R: Adhesion and aggregation: Morphological demonstration and quantitation *in vivo* and *in vitro*.

In PLATELETS IN BIOLOGY AND PATHOLOGY, edited by Gordon JL. Elsevier/North Holland Biomedical Press, 1976, pp. 23-60.

20. Groves HM, Kinlough-Rathbone RL, Richardson M, Mustard JF: Platelet survival and interaction with damaged rabbit aorta. BLOOD 50(Suppl 1):241, 1977.

21. Friedman RJ: Personal communication.

22. Stemerman MB: Thrombogenesis of the rabbit arterial plaque. AM J PATHOL 73:7-26, 1973.

23. Ross R, Harker L: Hyperlipidemia and atherosclerosis. Chronic hyperlipidemia initiates and maintains lesions by endothelial cell desquamation and lipid accumulation. SCIENCE 193:1094-1100, 1976.

24. Meuleman DG, Buchanan MR, Giles AR, Hirsh J: Normalization of platelet survival in an experimental model after platelet exposure to thrombin *in vitro* or to ADP *in vivo*. THROMB HAEMOSTAS 38:124, 1977.

25. Somer JB, Schwartz CJ: Focal ^{3}H-cholesterol uptake in the pig aorta. ATHEROSCLEROSIS 13:293-304, 1971.

26. Ross R, Glomset JA: The pathogenesis of atherosclerosis. N ENGL J MED 7:369-377, 1976.

27. Goldstein JL, Brown MS: Lipoprotein receptors, cholesterol metabolism and atherosclerosis. ARCH PATHOL 99:181-184, 1975.

28. Goldstein JL, Anderson RGW, Buja LM, Basu SK, Brown MS: Overloading human aortic smooth muscle cells with low density lipoprotein-cholesteryl esters reproduces features of atherosclerosis *in vitro*. J CLIN INVEST 59:1196-1202, 1977.

29. Iverius P-H: Possible role of glycosaminoglycans in the genesis of atherosclerosis. In ATHEROGENESIS: INITIATING FACTORS. Ciba Foundation Symposium No. 12 (New Series). Amsterdam and New York, Associated Scientific Publishers, 1973, pp. 185-196.

30. Minick CR, Alonso DR, Litrenta M, Silane MF, Stemerman MB: Regenerated endothelium and intimal proteoglycan accumulation. CIRCULATION 56:27, 1977.

31. Smith EB: The relationship between plasma and tissue lipids in human atherosclerosis. ADV LIPID RES 12:1-49, 1974.

32. Caplan BA, Gerrity RG, Schwartz CJ: Endothelial cell morphology in focal areas of *in vivo* Evans blue uptake in the young pig aorta. I. Quantitative light microscopic findings. EXP MOL PATHOL 21:102-117, 1974.

33. Gutstein WH, Farrell GA, Armellini C: Blood flow disturbance and endothelial cell injury in preatherosclerotic swine. LAB INVEST 29:134-149, 1973.

34. Jørgensen L, Packham MA, Rowsell HC, Mustard JF: Deposition of formed elements of blood on the intima and signs of intimal injury in the aorta of rabbit, pig and man. LAB INVEST 27: 341-350, 1972.

35. Wright HP: Mitosis patterns in aortic endothelium. ATHEROSCLEROSIS 15:93-100, 1972.

36. Caplan BA, Schwartz CJ: Increased endothelial cell turnover in areas of *in vivo* Evans blue uptake in the pig aorta. ATHEROSCLEROSIS 17:401-417, 1973.

37. Stary HC, McMillan GC: Kinetics of cellular proliferation in experimental atherosclerosis. Radioautography with grain counts in cholesterol-fed rabbits. ARCH PATHOL 89:173-183, 1970.

38. Fry DL: Response of the arterial wall to certain physical factors. In ATHEROGENESIS: INITIATING FACTORS Ciba Foundation Symposium 12 (New Series). Amsterdam and New York, Associated Scientific Publishers, 1973, pp. 93-125.

39. Nerem RM: Vibration-induced arterial shear stresses. LANCET 1:78, 1971.

40. Mustard JF, Moore S, Packham MA, Kinlough-Rathbone RL: Platelets, thrombosis and atherosclerosis. In PROCEEDINGS OF THE FIRST INTERNATIONAL ATHEROSCLEROSIS CONFERENCE. Prog Biochem Pharmacol. Basel, Karger (In Press).

41. Kniker WT, Cochrane CG: The localization of circulating immune complexes in experimental serum sickness. The role of vasoactive amines and hydrodynamic forces. J EXP MED 127:119-135, 1968.

42. Friedman RJ, Moore S, Singal DP: Repeated endothelial injury and induction of atherosclerosis in normolipemic rabbits by human serum. LAB INVEST 30:404-415, 1975.

43. Moore S, Ihnatowycz IO: Vessel injury and atherosclerosis. In THROMBOSIS: ANIMAL AND HUMAN MODELS, edited by Day HJ, Molony BA, Nishizawa EE, Rynbrandt RH. New York, Plenum Publishing Corp., 1978, pp. 145-163.

44. Minick CR, Stemerman MB, Insull W, Jr.: Effect of regenerated

endothelium on lipid accumulation in the arterial wall. PROC NATL ACAD SCI USA 74:1724-1728, 1977.

45. Bjorkerud S, Bondjers G: Repair responses and tissue lipid after experimental injury to the artery. ANN NY ACAD SCI 275:180-198, 1976.

46. Nam SC, Lee WM, Jarmolych J, Lee KT, Thomas WA: Rapid production of advanced atherosclerosis in swine by a combination of endothelial injury and cholesterol feeding. EXP MOL PATHOL 18:369-379, 1973.

47. Clowes AW, Ryan GB, Breslow JL, Karnovsky MJ: Absence of enhanced intimal thickening in the response of the carotid artery wall to endothelial injury in hypercholesterolemic rats. LAB INVEST 35:6-17, 1976.

48. Minick CR, Murphy GE: Experimental induction of atheroarteriosclerosis by the synergy of allergic injury to arteries and lipid-rich diet. AM J PATHOL 73:265-300, 1973.

49. Mustard JF: Function of blood platelets and their role in thrombosis. TRANS AM CLIN CLIMATOL ASSOC 87:104-127, 1976.

50. Leonard EF, Grabowski EF, Turitto VT: The role of convection and diffusion on platelet adhesion and aggregation. ANN NY ACAD SCI 201:329-342, 1972.

51. Holmsen H: Biochemistry of the platelet release reaction. In BIOCHEMISTRY AND PHARMACOLOGY OF PLATELETS, Ciba Foundation Symposium 35 (New Series). New York, Elsevier - Excerpta Medica - North Holland, 1975, pp. 175-205.

52. Baumgartner HR: Platelet interaction with collagen fibrils in flowing blood. I. Reaction of human platelets with α chymotrypsin-digested subendothelium. THROMB HAEMOSTAS 37:1-16, 1977.

53. Smith JB, Ingerman CM, Kocsis J, Silver MJ: Formation of an intermediate in prostaglandin biosynthesis and its association with the platelet release reaction. J CLIN INVEST 53:1468-1472, 1974.

54. Smith JB, Ingerman CM, Silver MJ: Effects of arachidonic acid and some of its metabolites on platelets. In PROSTAGLANDINS IN HEMATOLOGY, edited by Silver MJ, Smith JB, Kocsis JJ. New York, Spectrum Publications Inc., 1977, pp. 277-292.

55. Svensson J, Hamberg M, Samuelsson B: On the formation and effects of thromboxane A_2 in human platelets. ACTA PHYSIOL

SCAND 98:285-294, 1976.

56. Niewiarowski S, Stuart RK, Thomas DP: Activation of intravascular coagulation by collagen. PROC SOC EXP BIOL MED 123: 196-200, 1966.

57. Nemerson Y, Pitlick FA: The tissue factor pathway of blood coagulation. In PROGRESS IN HEMOSTASIS AND THROMBOSIS Vol. 1, edited by Spaet TH, New York, Grune and Stratton, Inc., 1972, pp. 1-37.

58. Walsh PN: The role of platelets in the contact phase of blood coagulation. BR J HAEMATOL 22:237-254, 1972.

59. Joist JH, Dolezel G, Lloyd JV, Kinlough-Rathbone RL, Mustard JF: Platelet factor-3 availability and the platelet release reaction. J LAB CLIN MED 84:474-482, 1974.

60. Kinlough-Rathbone RL, Packham MA, Reimers H-J, Cazenave J-P, Mustard JF: Mechanisms of platelet shape change, aggregation and release induced by collagen, thrombin or A23,187. J LAB CLIN MED 90:707-719, 1977.

61. Bills TK, Smith JB, Silver MJ: Selective release of arachidonic acid from the phospholipids of human platelets in response to thrombin. J CLIN INVEST 60:1-6, 1977.

62. Niewiarowski S, Regoeczi E, Stewart GJ, Senyi A, Mustard JF: Platelet interaction with polymerizing fibrin. J CLIN INVEST 51:685-700, 1972.

63. Mustard JF, Rowsell HC, Murphy EA: Platelet economy (platelet survival and turnover). BR J HAEMATOL 12:1-24, 1966.

64. Reimers H-J, Cazenave J-P, Senyi AF, Hirsh J, Kinlough-Rathbone RL, Packham MA, Mustard JF: *In vitro* and *in vivo* functions of thrombin-treated platelets. THROMB HAEMOSTAS 35:151-166, 1976.

65. Turner SR, Tainer JA, Lynn WS: Biogenesis of chemotactic molecules by the arachidonate lipoxygenase system of platelets. NATURE 257:680-681, 1975.

66. Weksler BB, Coupal CE: Platelet-dependent generation of chemotactic activity in serum. J EXP MED 137:1419-1430, 1973.

67. Nilsson IM, Pandolfi M: Fibrinolytic response of the vascular wall. THROMB DIATH HAEMORRH (Suppl) 40:231-242, 1970.

68. Kaplan AP, Meier HL, Mandle R, Jr.: The Hageman factor dependent pathways of coagulation, fibrinolysis, and kinin-

generation. SEMIN THROMB HEMOSTAS 3:1-26, 1976.

69. Yecies LD, Kaplan AP: The activation of plasminogen by the Hageman factor dependent plasminogen activator. FED PROC 35:731, 1976.

70. Stein PD, Sabbah HN: Measured turbulence and its effect on thrombus formation. CIRC RES 35:608-614, 1974.

71. Murphy EA, Rowsell HC, Downie HG, Robinson GA, Mustard JF: Encrustation and atherosclerosis: The analogy between early *in vivo* lesions and deposits which occur in extracorporeal circulations. CAN MED ASSOC J 87:259-274, 1962.

72. Goldsmith HL: The flow of model particles and blood cells and its relation to thrombogenesis. In PROGRESS IN HEMOSTASIS AND THROMBOSIS, Vol. 1, edited by Spaet TH. New York, Grune and Stratton, 1972, pp. 97-139.

73. Goldsmith HL: Bloow flow and thrombosis. THROMB DIATH HAEMORRH 32:35-48, 1974.

74. Fulton GP, Akers RP, Lutz BR: White thrombo-embolism and vascular fragility in hamster cheek pouch after anticoagulants. BLOOD 8:140-152, 1953.

75. Baumgartner HR: The role of blood flow in platelet adhesion, fibrin deposition, and formation of mural thrombi. MICROVASC RES 5:167-179, 1973.

76. Niewiarowski S, Lowery CT, Hawiger J, Millman M, Timmons S: Immunoassay of human platelet factor 4 (PF_4, antiheparin factor) by radial immunodiffusion. J LAB CLIN MED 87:720-733, 1976.

77. Kaplan KL, Drillings M, Nossel HL, Lesnik G: Radioimmunoassay of β-thromboglobulin (BTG) and platelet factor 4 (PF4). In THE SIGNIFICANCE OF PLATELET FUNCTION TESTS IN THE EVALUATION OF HEMOSTATIC AND THROMBOTIC TENDENCIES, WORKSHOP ON PLATELETS Philadelphia, 1976, edited by Day HJ, Zucker MB, Holmsen H. US Govt. Printing Office (In Press).

78. Ludlam CA, Cash JD: Studies on the liberation of β-thromboglobulin from human platelets *in vitro*. BR J HAEMATOL 33:239-247, 1976.

79. Cieslar P, Greenberg JP, Packham MA, Kinlough-Rathbone RL, Mustard JF: Separation of degranulated platelets from normal platelets. THROMB HAEMOSTAS 38:122, 1977.

80. Zahavi J, Marder VJ: Acquired "storage pool disease" of platelets associated with circulating anti-platelet antibodies. AM J MED 56:883-890, 1974.

81. Duguid JB: Thrombosis as a factor in the pathogenesis of aortic atherosclerosis. J PATH BACT 60:57-61, 1948.

82. Hand RA, Chandler AB: Atherosclerotic metamorphosis of autologous pulmonary thromboemboli in the rabbit. AM J PATHOL 40:469-486, 1962.

83. Woolf N, Bradley JWP, Crawford T, Carstairs KC: Experimental mural thrombi in the pig aorta. The early natural history. BR J EXP PATHOL 49:257-264, 1968.

84. Mitchell JRA, Schwartz CJ: The relationship between myocardial lesions and coronary artery disease. II. A selected group of patients with massive cardiac necrosis or scarring. BR HEART J 25:1-24, 1963.

85. Chandler AB, Chapman I, Erhardt LR, Roberts WC, Schwartz CJ, Sinapius D, Spain DM, Sherry S, Ness PM, Simon TL: Coronary thrombosis in myocardial infarction. Report of a workshop on the role of coronary thrombosis in the pathogenesis of acute myocardial infarction. AM J CARDIOL 34:823-833, 1974.

86. Erhardt LR, Lundman T, Mellstedt H: Incorporation of ^{125}I-labelled fibrinogen into coronary arterial thrombi in acute myocardial infarction in man. LANCET 1:387-390, 1973.

87. Cade JF, Hirsh J, Regoeczi E, Gent M, Buchanan MR, Hynes DM: Resolution of experimental pulmonary emboli with heparin and streptokinase in different dosage regimens. J CLIN INVEST 54:782-791, 1974.

88. Coleman RE, Harwig SSL, Harwig JF, Siegel BA, Welch MJ: Fibrinogen uptake by thrombi: Effect of thrombus age. J NUCL MED 16:370-373, 1975.

89. Moore S, Belbeck LW, Evans G: Myocardial lesions associated with partial, compared to complete, thrombotic occlusion of a coronary artery. CIRCULATION 54 (Suppl II):202, 1976.

90. Haerem JW: Myocardial lesions in sudden, unexpected coronary death. AM HEART J 90:562-568, 1975.

91. Haerem JW: Platelet aggregates in intramyocardial vessels of patients dying suddenly and unexpectedly of coronary artery disease. ATHEROSCLEROSIS 15:199-213, 1972.

92. Haerem JW: Mural platelet microthrombi and major acute lesions of main epicardial arteries in sudden coronary death. ATHEROSCLEROSIS 19:529-541, 1974.

93. Renaud S, Kinlough-Rathbone RL, Mustard JF: Relationship between platelet aggregation and the thrombotic tendency in rats fed hyperlipemic diets. LAB INVEST 22:339-343, 1970.

94. Hornstra G: Dietary fats and arterial thrombosis. HAEMOSTASIS 2:21-52, 1973-74.

95. Hornstra G, Chait A, Karvonen MJ, Lewis B, Turpeinen O, Vergroesen AJ: Influence of dietary fat on platelet function in men. LANCET 1:1155-1157, 1973.

96. Fleischman AI, Justice D, Bierenbaum ML, Stier A, Sullivan A: Beneficial effect of increased dietary linoleate upon *in vivo* platelet function in man. J NUTR 105:1286-1290, 1975.

97. Seyberth HW, Oelz O, Kennedy T, Sweetman BJ, Danon A, Frölich JC, Heimberg M, Oates JA: Increased arachidonate in lipids after administration to man: Effects on prostaglandin biosynthesis. CLIN PHARMACOL THER 18:521-529, 1975.

98. Kernoff PBA, Davies JA, McNicol GP, Willis AL, Stone KJ: The antithrombotic potential of dihomo-γ-linolenic acid. THROMB HAEMOSTAS 38:194, 1977.

99. Mustard JF, Murphy EA: Effect of different dietary fats on blood coagulation, platelet economy, and blood lipids. BR MED J 1:1651-1655, 1962.

100. Jonker JJ, Veen MR, Schopman W, den Ottolander GJG: Platelet survival time in angina pectoris and hyperlipoproteinemia. THROMB RES 4 (Suppl 1):65-67, 1974.

101. Kim WM, Merskey C, Deming QB, Adel HN, Wolinsky H, Clarkson TB, Lofland HB: Hyperlipidemia, hypercoagulability and accelerated thrombosis: Studies in congenitally hyperlipidemic rats and in rats and monkeys with induced hyperlipidemia. BLOOD 47:275-286, 1976.

102. Florentin RA, Nam SC, Lee KT, Thomas WA: Increased ^{3}H-thymidine incorporation into endothelial cells of swine fed cholesterol for 3 days. EXP MOL PATHOL 10:250-255, 1969.

103. Reimers HJ, Packham MA, Kinlough-Rathbone RL, Mustard JF: Effect of repeated treatment of rabbit platelets with low concentrations of thrombin on their function, metabolism and survival. BR J HAEMATOL 25:675-689, 1973.

104. Dougherty JH, Jr., Levy DE, Weksler BB: Platelet activation in acute cerebral ischaemia. LANCET 1:821-824, 1977.

105. Wu KK, Hoak JC: Spontaneous platelet aggregation in arterial insufficiency: Mechanisms and implications. THROMB HAEMOSTAS 35:702-711, 1976.

106. Hornstra G, ten Hoor F: The filtragometer: A new device for measuring platelet aggregation in venous blood of man. THROMB DIATH HAEMORRH 34:531-544, 1975.

107. Packham MA, Mustard JF: Methods for detection of hypersensitive platelets. Working Party VIth Cong. of Int. Soc. on Thromb. and Haemostas. Philadelphia, June 1977. THROMB HAEMOSTAS (In preparation).

108. Packham MA, Mustard JF: Platelet aggregation, relevance to thrombotic tendencies. In THROMBOSIS: ANIMAL AND HUMAN MODELS, edited by Day HJ, Molony BA, Nishizawa EE, Rynbrandt RH. New York, Plenum Publishing Corp., 1978, pp. 51-72.

109. Greenberg JP, Rand ML, Packham MA: Relation of platelet age to platelet sialic acid. FED PROC 36:453, 1977.

110. Mustard JF, Murphy EA: Effect of smoking on blood coagulation and platelet survival in man. BR MED J 1:846-849, 1963.

111. Mustard JF, Packham MA, Kinlough-Rathbone RL: Platelet survival. In THE SIGNIFICANCE OF PLATELET FUNCTION TESTS IN THE EVALUATION OF HEMOSTATIC AND THROMBOTIC TENDENCIES, WORKSHOP ON PLATELETS, Philadelphia, 1976, edited by Day HJ, Zucker MB, Holmsen H. US Govt. Printing Office (In Press).

112. Steele PP, Weily HS, Davies H, Genton E: Platelet function studies in coronary artery disease. CIRCULATION 48:1194-1200, 1973.

113. Harker LA, Slichter SJ: Arterial and venous thromboembolism: Kinetic characterization and evaluation of therapy. THROMB DIATH HAEMORRH 31:188-203, 1974.

114. Greenberg J, Packham MA, Cazenave J-P, Reimers H-J, Mustard JF: Effects on platelet function of removal of platelet sialic acid by neuraminidase. LAB INVEST 32:476-484, 1975.

115. Scott S, Reimers H-J, Chernesky MA, Greenberg JP, Kinlough-Rathbone RL, Packham MA, Mustard JF: The effect of viruses on platelet aggregation and platelet survival in rabbits. (Submitted for publication).

116. Roth GJ, Majerus PW: The mechanism of the effect of aspirin on human platelets. I. Acetylation of a particulate fraction protein. J CLIN INVEST 56:624-632, 1975.

117. Cazenave J-P, Packham MA, Kinlough-Rathbone RL, Mustard JF: Platelet adherence to the vessel wall and to collagen-coated surfaces. In THROMBOSIS: ANIMAL AND HUMAN MODELS, edited by Day HJ, Molony BA, Nishizawa EE, Rynbrandt RH. New York, Plenum Publishing Corp., 1978, pp. 31-49.

118. Baumgartner HR, Studer A: Platelet factors and the proliferation of vascular smooth muscle cells. Workshop on Thrombosis and Atherosclerosis IVth International Symposium on Atherosclerosis, Tokyo, 1976.

119. Harker LA, Slichter SJ: Platelet and fibrinogen consumption in man. N ENGL J MED 287:999-1005, 1972.

120. Ali M, Mcdonald JWD: Effects of sulfinpyrazone on platelet prostaglandin synthesis and platelet release of serotonin. J LAB CLIN MED 89:868-875, 1977.

121. Smythe HA, Ogryzlo MA, Murphy EA, Mustard JF: The effect of sulfinpyrazone (Anturan) on platelet economy and blood coagulation in man. CAN MED ASSOC J 92:818-821, 1965.

122. Steele P, Battock D, Genton E: Effects of clofibrate and sulfinpyrazone on platelet survival time in coronary artery disease. CIRCULATION 52:473-476, 1975.

123. Turpie AGG, Chernesky MA, Larke RPB, Moore S, Regoeczi E, Mustard JF: Thrombocytopenia and vasculitis induced in rabbits by Newcastle disease virus. Proc. III Congr. Int. Soc. Thromb. Haemostas., Washington, 1972, p. 344 (Abstract).

124. Mustard JF, Packham MA: Platelets, thrombosis and drugs. DRUGS 9:19-76, 1975.

125. Harker LA, Ross R, Slichter SJ, Scott CR: Homocystine-induced arteriosclerosis. The role of endothelial cell injury and platelet response in its genesis. J CLIN INVEST 58:731-741, 1976.

126. Fields WS, Lemak NA, Frankowski RF, Hardy RJ: Controlled trial of aspirin in cerebral ischaemia. STROKE 8:301-316, 1977.

127. Sullivan JM, Harken DE, Gorlin R: Pharmacologic control of thromboembolic complications of cardiac-valve replacement. N ENGL J MED 284:1391-1394, 1971.

PLATELET ADHERENCE TO THE VESSEL WALL AND TO COLLAGEN-COATED SURFACES*

Jean-Pierre Cazenave, M.D.,Ph.D., Marian A. Packham, Ph.D., Raelene L. Kinlough-Rathbone, M.D.,Ph.D., and J. Fraser Mustard, M.D.,Ph.D.

Department of Pathology, McMaster University, Hamilton, Ontario, Canada; Department of Biochemistry, University of Toronto, Ontario, Canada

ABSTRACT

A rotating probe system has been developed to quantitate the adherence of ^{51}Cr-labeled platelets to collagen-coated glass rods or to the subendothelium of the rabbit aorta. The platelets were suspended in a medium containing physiological concentrations of calcium and magnesium, albumin, and apyrase to prevent aggregation. Chelation of divalent cations in the medium by addition of sodium citrate, EDTA, or EGTA markedly diminished platelet adherence. These observations indicate that the interpretation of platelet adherence studies performed in the presence of these agents is questionable. Increasing albumin concentrations in the medium decreased the number of adherent platelets, whereas increasing the hematocrit increased platelet adherence. Thus the factors influencing platelet adherence were studied in the presence of 4% albumin and 40% hematocrit.

When the platelet surface was modified by treatment with thrombin, plasmin, trypsin, chymotrypsin, or ADP, platelet adherence to the surfaces was decreased. Removal of surface sialic acid by neuraminidase had no effect on adherence. Exposing the endothelial surface of an aorta to thrombin resulted in a marked increase in

*This work was supported by Medical Research Council of Canada Grants MT 1309 and MT 2629 and by Senior Research Fellowships of the Ontario Heart Foundation to J.-P. Cazenave and R. L. Kinlough-Rathbone.

platelet adherence to the thrombin-treated surface; this effect was prevented by adding heparin to the platelet suspension. Platelet adherence to collagen and to subendothelium was inhibited by several drugs that are used in man: dipyridamole, RA 433, methylprednisolone, and the antibiotics penicillin G and cephalothin. Under the experimental conditions used, ASA did not inhibit adherence to collagen, although indomethacin and a high concentration of sulfinpyrazone did. None of these three drugs inhibited release of granule contents from the adherent platelets. Therefore, it is unlikely that they would inhibit smooth muscle proliferation in response to the platelet growth factor released from platelets adherent to collagen in the subendothelium at a site of vessel wall injury.

INTRODUCTION

One of the first events in thrombus formation is adherence of platelets to an injury site on a blood vessel wall. Platelets adhere to collagen, to the basement membrane, and to the microfibrils around elastin, but only collagen has been shown to induce release of the granule contents of the adherent platelets (1). A number of investigators have developed methods to study platelet adherence to damaged vessel walls or to protein-coated surfaces (1-20). Most of these determinations have been made *in vitro* with collagen-coated surfaces (5,7,13,19,22-24), sepharose beads to which collagen has been covalently attached (25), or segments of vessels from which the endothelium has been removed (1-10). Most of the *in vivo* experiments in which platelet adherence to the subendothelium has been examined have been done by the morphometric technique of Baumgartner and his colleagues (3,5).

All of these investigations have been directed toward determining the factors, conditions, and drugs that affect platelet adherence to the subendothelium. The main advantage of the *in vivo* technique (3,5,26) is that the platelets are in their natural medium and it is not necessary to add anticoagulants to the blood. In the *in vitro* studies in which whole blood or platelet-rich plasma is used, chelating agents or other anticoagulants have to be used and these affect platelet adherence (5-7,27-29). Without anticoagulants, the products of coagulation increase the number of platelets associated with the surface (30,31).

One of the advantages of using suspensions of isolated platelets in an artificial medium to study adherence is that the composition of the medium can be varied to determine the effects of divalent cations, protein concentration, hematocrit,or other constituents. It is also possible to alter the platelets by enzymatic or chemical treatment and then resuspend them in a fresh medium for adherence determinations.

Morphometric techniques in which adherent platelets and platelet thrombi are examined microscopically are of necessity confined to a small surface area and are time-consuming. Techniques with radioisotopically labeled platelets (^{51}Cr is most often used) permit quantitation of platelet adherence over a large surface area, but it is not possible to distinguish between adherent single platelets and adherent thrombi. If the adherence of only single platelets is to be studied, platelet aggregation on the surface must be prevented. This can be done by removing released ADP with enzyme systems such as apyrase (19,32) or creatine phosphate-creatine phosphokinase (32-34).

ROTATING PROBE METHOD

We have developed a rotating probe system to quantitate platelet adherence to collagen or to the subendothelium of the rabbit aorta (6,7,34). In this system, collagen-coated glass rods or everted segments of rabbit aorta are mounted on vertical probes which are rotated in suspensions of washed platelets at 37°C for 10 min at 200 rpm. The platelets are prelabeled with ^{51}Cr so that the number of platelets that adhere can be determined. The suspending medium for the platelets is Tyrode's solution or Eagle's minimal essential medium, both of which contain physiological concentrations of calcium and magnesium. The suspending medium also contains albumin, apyrase, and washed red blood cells (7,34).

The endothelium is removed from rabbit aortas *in situ* by passage of a balloon catheter according to the method developed by Baumgartner (5,35). Glass rods are coated with collagen as described elsewhere (7,34).

After the surfaces on the probes have been rotated in the platelet suspension, they are rinsed at 37°C for 5 min at 200 rpm in a solution containing EDTA to ensure that if even a few small aggregates are present on the surface, they are removed.

The technique measures the adherence of individual platelets to subendothelial constituents, or to collagen, rather than formation of platelet thrombi on the surfaces. Most of the studies have been done with rabbit platelets and rabbit aortas, but similar results have been obtained with human platelets and collagen-coated surfaces.

EFFECT OF DIVALENT CATIONS ON PLATELET ADHERENCE

If chelating agents are added to the platelet suspending medium, platelet adherence is strongly inhibited. Sodium citrate, EDTA, and EGTA at concentrations that chelate all the divalent cations in the medium diminish human and rabbit platelet adherence to collagen to approximately 25% of the control value obtained in a medium containing physiologic concentrations of calcium and magnesium. Adherence to the damaged aorta is decreased to approximately 5% of the control value by these chelating agents. These observations complicate the interpretation of platelet adherence studies in which chelating agents have been added to blood or platelet-rich plasma to prevent coagulation. Baumgartner and his colleagues (1, 5,27-29) have also reported an inhibitory effect of EDTA and of high concentrations of citrate on platelet adherence to the subendothelium. We have found that under some conditions, citrate obscures the effect of aspirin on platelet adherence (6).

EFFECT OF ALBUMIN CONCENTRATION AND HEMATOCRIT ON PLATELET ADHERENCE

We have reported previously that increasing the albumin concentration in the platelet suspending medium decreases the number of adherent platelets and reduces the variance of the results (6,7). The addition of washed red blood cells to the medium increases the number of adherent platelets (7). This observation agrees with those of other investigators who showed that red cells increased diffusion of platelets to the surfaces in several types of flow systems (36-38). The effect of red cells in the Couette flow system used in the present studies has also been demonstrated by Brash *et al.* (24).

In our early experiments in which red blood cells were not included in the platelet suspending medium, we demonstrated that aspirin and other nonsteroidal anti-inflammatory drugs inhibited platelet adherence to the surfaces (6,39). When it became apparent that aspirin did not inhibit platelet adherence in a vessel segment perfused with a suspension of rabbit platelets and red blood cells (8), we investigated the effect of the hematocrit in the rotating probe system on inhibition of platelet adherence by aspirin (Table 1). ^{51}Cr-labeled platelets were suspended in Tyrode s lution containing albumin, apyrase, and 5 mM Hepes buffer. They were incubated for 10 min with ASA or modified Tyrode solution. Then red blood cells were added. The final platelet count was 300,000 per mm^3. The collagen-coated glass rods were rotated in the platelet suspension at 200 rpm for 10 min at 37°C. The rods were then rinsed at 200 rpm for 5 min at 37°C in modified Tyrode solution containing 10 mM EDTA.

When the hematocrit was increased to 40%, inhibition of platelet adherence by aspirin was no longer evident. This may indicate that the weak inhibiting effect of aspirin on platelet adherence is overcome when diffusion of platelets to the surface is increased by the presence of red blood cells.

TABLE 1. EFFECT OF ASA ON ADHERENCE OF ^{51}Cr-LABELED RABBIT PLATELETS TO A COLLAGEN-COATED ROD WHEN TESTED IN THE PRESENCE OF VARIOUS ALBUMIN AND RED BLOOD CELL CONCENTRATIONS

ASA (μM)	Albumin (%)	Hematocrit (%)	No. of Segments	Number of Platelets per mm^2 (mean ± SE)	P*
0	0.35	0	16	31,800±8,900	
100	"	0	16	8,200± 400	<0.02
0	"	10	16	100,200±4,400	
100	"	10	16	30,000±3,000	<0.001
0	"	20	16	126,400±4,400	
100	"	20	16	104,300±2,600	<0.001
0	"	40	16	127,800±2,000	
100	"	40	16	122,500±2,400	<0.2
0	4	0	16	5,400± 600	
250	"	0	16	6,400± 500	<0.3
0	"	10	16	25,600±1,300	
250	"	10	16	14,800±1,200	<0.001
0	"	20	16	63,700±2,500	
250	"	20	16	48,200±1,800	<0.001
0	"	40	16	65,300±1,900	
250	"	40	16	60,400±1,700	<0.1

*Compared with control in the unpaired two-tailed Student's t test.

EFFECT OF ENZYME TREATMENTS OF THE PLATELET SURFACE ON ADHERENCE

Attempts have been made to identify the platelet surface constituents involved in platelet adherence to collagen. It now seems unlikely that collagen:glucosyl transferase plays a role in platelet adherence to collagen (40-42), as originally proposed (43,44). However, more recently it has been suggested that collagen:glucosyl transferase may bind to collagen and function as a collagen receptor on the platelet surface (45,46).

Glycoprotein I which is exposed at the platelet surface (47) may be involved in adherence; Bernard-Soulier platelets, which lack this glycoprotein, show an impaired ability to adhere to the subendothelium of a damaged vessel wall (48,49).

We have examined the effects of a number of enzyme treatments of the platelet surface and of pretreatment with ADP (Table 2). Because these studies were done with suspensions of washed plate-

TABLE 2. EFFECT OF TREATMENTS OF PLATELET SURFACE ON PLATELET ADHERENCE

Treatments which reduce adherence	Treatment which has no effect
Thrombin	Removal of sialic acid
Plasmin	
Trypsin	
Chymotrypsin	
ADP	

lets, it was possible to treat the platelets in various ways during the isolation procedure and then resuspend them in the final suspending medium. Platelets can be treated with thrombin and recovered as individual platelets that have lost most of their granule contents (50). These "degranulated" platelets show a diminished ability to adhere to collagen-coated surfaces and to subendothelium. There are at least three possible reasons for thrombin's effect on adherence:

1) Thrombin may have a direct proteolytic effect on the platelet membrane (51,52). Recently it was reported that thrombin caused a loss of membrane glycoprotein V (53). It is conceivable that this membrane alteration may reduce the ability of platelets to adhere.

2) The effect of thrombin on the platelet surface is secondary to the release reaction (54), which may alter or may cause a structural rearrangement of platelet membrane proteins.

3) The effect of the ADP that is released by the thrombin pretreatment may be responsible for the diminished adherence. Pretreatment of platelets with ADP, which causes aggregation but no release of granule contents, followed by resuspension of the platelets in fresh medium containing apyrase so that they returned to their disc shape, resulted in diminished adherence to collagen. During ADP-induced aggregation platelets lose chrondroitin sulfate A from their surfaces (55). It may be that loss of this sulfated proteoglycan is responsible for the reduced adherence of the ADP-treated platelets to collagen.

We have also examined the effect of proteolytic enzymes other than thrombin on platelet adherence to collagen and to subendothelium

Treatment of platelets with trypsin, plasmin, or chymotrypsin (7, 34) diminished their ability to adhere to a collagen-coated surface or to the subendothelium, possibly because of proteolysis of platelet membrane glycoproteins. Platelet membrane glycoproteins were stained with periodic acid Schiff stain (PAS) and examined by sodium dodecyl sulfate (SDS) polyacrylamide gel electrophoresis. Trypsin removed glycoprotein I and II but had little effect on glycoprotein III at the concentration used (100 µg/ml). In contrast, chymotrypsin (10 U/ml) and plasmin (6 CU/ml) removed all three glycoproteins. It may be that loss of membrane glycoproteins was responsible for the diminished adherence observed when platelets had been pretreated with these proteolytic enzymes. Although plasmin and trypsin also caused the release of platelet ADP which could affect platelet adherence, chymotrypsin did not cause the release reaction, so its effect on adherence cannot be attributed to the released ADP.

It should be emphasized that plasmin is an enzyme that platelets are likely to encounter *in vivo*, particularly if they take part in reversible thrombus formation, and platelets that have been exposed to it may have a reduced ability to adhere to the subendothelium.

These results with various enzyme treatments do not prove that platelet membrane glycoproteins are involved in platelet adherence, although they may be. It should be noted, however, that removal of the terminal sialic acid from platelet membrane glycoproteins did not affect adherence (56). In contrast, ADP treatment which removes surface chondroitin sulfate A did diminish adherence. Thus there may be several components of the platelet membrane that govern adherence of platelets to collagen and to the subendothelium.

ADHERENCE OF PLATELETS TO ENDOTHELIUM EXPOSED TO THROMBIN

It is generally agreed that platelets do not adhere to normal endothelium (57,58). We have explored the possible effects of thrombin on platelet adhesion to the vessel wall by exposing the endothelial surface of everted segments of rabbit aorta to thrombin. Exposure of undamaged endothelium to thrombin, followed by rinsing and rotating in a platelet suspension, led to much increased platelet adherence to the thrombin-treated surface. Addition of heparin to the platelet suspension prevented this effect of thrombin on platelet adherence. These results agree with those of other investigators (30) who have suggested that exposure of the endothelium to thrombin can lead to thrombin binding and to alteration of the endothelium. Thus inhibition of thrombin formation at a site of vessel injury or inhibition of the activity of thrombin would be expected to have inhibitory effects, not only on the coagulation pathway but on any aspects of platelet adherence in which thrombin is involved, and possibly also on the thrombin-induced release of granule contents including the mitogenic factor (59,60).

EFFECTS OF DRUGS ON PLATELET ADHERENCE

We have examined the effect of a number of drugs used in humans that inhibit platelet adherence to a collagen-coated surface when the platelets are suspended in 4% albumin and 40% hematocrit (Table 3). The methods were the same as those described in the section on effect of albumin concentration and hematocrit. Dipyridamole and its pyrimido-pyrimidine analogue RA 433 were both inhibitory. These drugs inhibit the phosphodiesterase of platelets which normally breaks down cyclic AMP (61). As a consequence, the level of cyclic AMP in the platelets rises, and it seems possible that this may be

TABLE 3. INHIBITION OF PLATELET ADHERENCE TO A COLLAGEN-COATED SURFACE BY SEVERAL INHIBITORS OF PLATELET FUNCTION

Drug	Concentration	Adherence (% of Control)	P*
None		100	
Dipyridamole	100 μM	72	<0.001
RA 433	100 μM	46	<0.001
PGE_1	1 μM	41	<0.001
Methylprednisolone	10 mM	16	<0.001
Methylprednisolone	1 mM	79	<0.001
Penicillin G	13.6 mM	38	<0.001
Cephalothin	13.6 mM	32	<0.001

*Compared with control in the unpaired two-tailed Student's t test.

responsible at least in part for the inhibitory effect. Evidence for this is the effect of prostaglandin E_1 (PGE_1) on platelet adherence. It is a strong inhibitor of platelet adherence at very low concentration (7,62) and raises platelet cyclic AMP levels by stimulating adenylate cyclase on the platelet membrane (61). Prostaglandin E_1 is an inhibitor not only of platelet adherence but also of the platelet release reaction, platelet aggregation, and the initial shape change of platelets which occurs in response to most aggregating agents (61). It may be that its ability to prevent the platelets from changing shape is responsible for its inhibitory effect on adherence.

Another drug which inhibits platelet adherence is methylprednisolone (7,63) but the concentrations required are much higher than those that would be achieved upon administration of this drug.

Penicillin G and related antibiotics are strong inhibitors of platelet adherence to a collagen-coated surface and to the damaged aorta (7,64,65). These antibiotics inhibit most platelet reactions (65,66) and are thought to coat the surface of platelets as they do red cells and prevent platelets from interacting with the aggregating and release-inducing agents (64,65). Similar results were obtained when these drugs were used to inhibit platelet adherence to subendothelium.

These results show that measuring platelet adherence to collagen-coated surfaces can be used as a screening test in attempts to determine how effectively drugs inhibit platelet interaction with the vessel wall at sites of vessel injury and thereby how effective they may be as inhibitors of thrombosis.

It has recently been shown that aspirin and sulfinpyrazone do not inhibit platelet adherence *in vivo* to rabbit aortas injured with a balloon catheter; in contrast, dipyridamole reduced adherence to half of the control values (Groves HM, Kinlough-Rathbone RL, Richardson M, Mustard JF, unpublished observations).

EFFECT OF NONSTEROIDAL ANTI-INFLAMMATORY DRUGS ON PLATELET ADHERENCE TO COLLAGEN AND RELEASE OF GRANULE CONTENTS

Our purpose was to study whether these drugs inhibited the release of granule contents from platelets that adhered to collagen, particularly because of the effect of the mitogen on the vessel wall. In this experiment the platelets were doubly labeled with ^{14}C-serotonin and ^{51}Cr. ^{14}C-serotonin is taken up into the platelet amine storage granules and is released when the platelets interact with collagen or thrombin. ^{51}Cr labels the platelet cytoplasmic constituents and is not lost unless the platelets actually lyse (67). Platelet adherence as determined by ^{51}Cr was measured in the usual way (6,7), and the percent release from adherent platelets was calculated by comparing the ratio of ^{14}C-serotonin to ^{51}Cr in the platelets before the reaction with the ratio in the adherent platelets after the reaction.

In these experiments (Table 4) the platelet count was 300,000 per mm^3, albumin concentration 4%, and hematocrit 40%. Aspirin did not have any significant effect on adherence, although indomethacin and a high concentration of sulfinpyrazone did inhibit adherence. At these concentrations all the drugs inhibit the platelet cyclo-oxygenase (34,61). However, none of the drugs inhibited release from the adherent platelets. In fact, it was observed consistently that the extent of release from platelets adherent to collagen tended to be higher in the presence of these drugs. It is apparent that if these

TABLE 4. RELEASE OF ^{14}C-SEROTONIN FROM PLATELETS ADHERENT TO A COLLAGEN-COATED SURFACE

Drug	Concentration	Adherence (% of Control)	% Release*
None		100	36
ASA	100 μM	97	59
Indomethacin	100 μM	69	56
Sulfinpyrazone	1 mM	61	74

*Release of ^{14}C-serotonin from adherent platelets (expressed as percent of total platelet ^{14}C-serotonin content).

drugs do not inhibit the release of the mitogenic factor from platelets (60) which has been shown to be released in parallel with serotonin (60,68,69), then they could not be expected to have a significant effect on the smooth muscle cell proliferation that occurs following damage to the vessel wall. In agreement with this theory, Baumgartner and Studer (70) and also Clowes and Karnovsky (71) have shown that aspirin does not inhibit the smooth muscle cell proliferation that follows the removal of the endothelium; and in unpublished experiments done with Dr. S. Moore we have shown that sulfinpyrazone does not inhibit smooth muscle cell proliferation in response to injury to the endothelium.

These studies have established that it is possible to measure quantitatively the adherence of ^{51}Cr-labeled platelets to surfaces in the presence of physiological concentrations of divalent cations, albumin, and red blood cells. Platelet aggregation on the surfaces was prevented by the inclusion of apyrase in the medium and by rinsing the surfaces in a solution containing EDTA. Thus the technique measures platelet adherence in the absence of platelet aggregation and thrombus formation. With this technique, it was possible to study the effect of various enzymatic treatments of the platelet surface and the effect of drugs on platelet adherence. Because the results of platelet adherence to subendothelium are similar to those with collagen-coated surfaces, the latter technique is useful to screen the effects of agents or conditions that modify platelet adherence.

ACKNOWLEDGMENT

We are grateful for the excellent technical assistance of Mrs. D. Blondowska.

REFERENCES

1. Baumgartner HR, Muggli R, Tschopp TB, Turitto VT: Platelet adhesion, release and aggregation in flowing blood: Effects of surface properties and platelet function. THROMB HAEMOSTAS 35:124-138, 1976.

2. Baumgartner HR, Haudenschild C: Adhesion of platelets to subendothelium. ANN NY ACAD SCI 201:22-36, 1972.

3. Baumgartner HR: The role of blood flow in platelet adhesion, fibrin deposition, and formation of mural thrombi. MICROVASC RES 5:167-179, 1973.

4. Blaisdell RK, Stemerman MB, Chen MM, Spaet TH: A new *in vitro* method for measuring platelet deposition on the vessel surface. THROMB DIATH HAEMORRH (Suppl) 60:35-38, 1974.

5. Baumgartner HR, Muggli R: Adhesion and aggregation: Morphological demonstration and quantitation *in vivo* and *in vitro*. In PLATELETS IN BIOLOGY AND PATHOLOGY, edited by Gordon JL. Elsevier/North-Holland Biomedical Press, 1976, p. 23.

6. Cazenave J-P, Packham MA, Guccione MA, Mustard JF: Inhibition of platelet adherence to damaged surface of rabbit aorta. J LAB CLIN MED 86:551-563, 1975.

7. Cazenave J-P, Packham MA, Davies JA, Kinlough-Rathbone RL, Mustard JF: Studies on platelet adherence to collagen and subendothelium. In THE SIGNIFICANCE OF PLATELET FUNCTION TESTS IN THE EVALUATION OF HEMOSTATIC AND THROMBOTIC TENDENCIES, edited by Day HJ, Holmsen H, Zucker MB. U.S. Government Printing Office, 1977, p. 181.

8. Davies JA, Essien E, Kinlough-Rathbone RL, Cazenave J-P, Mustard JF: Inhibitory effect of sulfinpyrazone and acetylsalicyclic acid on platelet adhesion to damaged aorta. BLOOD 46:1003, 1975.

9. Dosne A-M, Drouet L, Dassin E: Usefulness of ^{51}chromium-

platelet labelling for the measurement of platelet deposition on subendothelium. MICROVASC RES 11:111-114, 1976.

10. Essien EM, Mustard JF: Inhibition of platelet adhesion to rabbit aorta by sulphinpyrazone and acetylsalicyclic acid. ATHEROSCLEROSIS 27:89-95, 1977.

11. Packham MA, Evans G, Glynn MF, Mustard JF: The effect of plasma proteins on the interaction of platelets with glass surfaces. J LAB CLIN MED 73:686-697, 1969.

12. Zucker MB, Vroman L: Platelet adhesion induced by fibrinogen adsorbed onto glass. PROC SOC EXP BIOL MED 131:318-320, 1969.

13. Lyman B, Rosenberg L, Karpatkin S: Biochemical and biophysical aspects of human platelet adhesion to collagen fibers. J CLIN INVEST 50:1854-1863, 1971.

14. Mason RG, Read MS, Brinkhous KM: Effect of fibrinogen concentration on platelet adhesion to glass. PROC SOC EXP BIOL MED 137:680-682, 1971.

15. Vroman L, Adams AL, Klings M: Interactions among human blood proteins at interfaces. FED PROC 30:1494-1502, 1971.

16. Salzman EW: Nonthrombogenic surfaces: Critical review. BLOOD 38:509-523, 1971.

17. George JN: Direct assessment of platelet adhesion to glass: A study of the forces of interaction and the effects of plasma and serum factors, platelet function, and modification of the glass surface. BLOOD 40:862-874, 1972.

18. Jenkins CSP, Packham MA, Guccione MA, Mustard JF: Modification of platelet adherence to protein-coated surfaces. J LAB CLIN MED 81:280-290, 1973.

19. Cazenave J-P, Packham MA, Mustard JF: Adherence of platelets to a collagen-coated surface: Development of a quantitative method. J LAB CLIN MED 82:978-990, 1973.

20. Mohammad SF, Hardison MD, Glenn CH, Morton BD, Bolan JC, Mason RG: Adhesion of human blood platelets to glass and polymer surfaces. I. Studies with platelets in plasma. HAEMOSTASIS 3:257-270, 1974.

21. Mohammad SF, Hardison MD, Chuang HYK, Mason RG: Adhesion of human blood platelets to glass and polymer surfaces. II. Demonstration of the presence of a natural platelet adhesion inhibitor in plasma and serum. HAEMOSTASIS 5:96-114, 1976.

22. Feuerstein IA, Brophy JM, Brash JL: Platelet transport and adhesion to reconstituted collagen and artificial surfaces. TRANS AM SOC ARTIF INTERN ORGANS 21:427-434, 1975.

23. Muggli R, Baumgartner HR: Collagen coated gelatine tubes for the investigation of platelet adhesion and subsequent platelet aggregation under controlled flow conditions. THROMB DIATH HAEMORRH 34:333, 1975.

24. Brash JL, Brophy JM, Feuerstein IA: Adhesion of platelets to artificial surfaces: Effect of red cells. J BIOMED MATER RES 10:429-443, 1976.

25. Brass LF, Faile D, Bensusan HB: Direct measurement of the platelet:collagen interaction by affinity chromatography on collagen/sepharose. J LAB CLIN MED 87:525-534, 1976.

26. Groves HM, Kinlough-Rathbone RL, Richardson M, Mustard JF: Platelet survival and interaction with damaged rabbit aorta. BLOOD 50(Suppl 1):241, 1977.

27. Baumgartner HR, Stemerman MB, Spaet TH: Adhesion of blood platelets to subendothelial surface: Distinct from adhesion to collagen. EXPERIENTIA 27:283-285, 1971.

28. Baumgartner HR: Effects of anticoagulation on the interaction of human platelets with subendothelium in flowing blood. SCHWEIZ MED WOCHENSCHR 106:1367-1368, 1976.

29. Baumgartner HR: Platelet interaction with collagen fibrils in flowing blood. I. Reaction of human platelets with chymotrypsin-digested subendothelium. THROMB HAEMOSTAS 37:1-16, 1977.

30. Awbrey BJ, Owen WG, Fry GL, Cheng FH, Hoak JC: Binding of human thrombin to human endothelial cells and platelets. BLOOD 46:1046, 1975.

31. Niewiarowski S, Regoeczi E, Stewart GJ, Senyi AF, Mustard JF: Platelet interaction with polymerizing fibrin. J CLIN INVEST 51:685-700, 1972.

32. Haslam RJ: Mechanisms of blood platelet aggregation. In PHYSIOLOGY OF HEMOSTASIS AND THROMBOSIS, edited by Johnson SA, Seegers WH. Springfield, IL, Charles C Thomas, 1967, p. 88.

33. Tschopp TB, Baumgartner HR: Enzymatic removal of ADP from plasma: Unaltered platelet adhesion but reduced aggregation on subendothelium and collagen fibrils. THROMB HAEMOSTAS 35:334-341, 1976.

34. Cazenave J-P: Platelet adherence to collagen containing surfaces. Thesis, Ph.D., McMaster University, Hamilton, 1977.

35. Baumgartner HR: Eine neue Methode zur Erzeugung von Thromben durch gezielte Überdehnung der Gefässwand. Z GESAMTE EXP MED 137:227-246, 1963.

36. Goldsmith HL: The flow of model particles and blood cells and its relation to thrombogenesis. PROG HEMOSTASIS THROMB 1:97-139, 1972.

37. Turitto VT, Baumgartner HR: Platelet interaction with subendothelium in a perfusion system: Physical role of red blood cells. MICROVASC RES 9:335-344, 1975.

38. Leonard EF, Grabowski EF, Turitto VT: The role of convection and diffusion on platelet adhesion and aggregation. ANN NY ACAD SCI 201:329-342, 1972.

39. Cazenave J-P, Packham MA, Guccione MA, Mustard JF: Inhibition of platelet adherence to a collagen-coated surface by nonsteroidal anti-inflammatory drugs, pyrimido-pyrimidine and tricyclic compounds, and lidocaine. J LAB CLIN MED 83:797-806, 1974.

40. Cazenave J-P, Guccione MA, Mustard JF, Packham MA: Lack of effect of UDP, UDPG and glucosamine on platelet reactions with collagen. THROMB DIATH HAEMORRH 31:521-524, 1974.

41. Menashi S, Harwood R, Grant ME: Native collagen is not a substrate for the collagenglucosyltransferase of platelets. NATURE 264:670-672, 1976.

42. Anttinen H, Tuderman L, Oikarinen A, Kivirikko KI: Intracellular enzymes of collagen biosynthesis in human platelets. BLOOD 50:29-37, 1977.

43. Jamieson GA, Urban CL, Barber AJ: Enzymatic basis for platelet:collagen adhesion as the primary step in haemostasis. NATURE 234:5-7, 1971.

44. Bosmann HB: Platelet adhesiveness and aggregation: The collagen:glycosyl, polypeptide:N-acetyl-galactosaminyl and glycoprotein:galactosyl transferases of human platelets. BIOCHEM BIOPHYS RES COMMUN 43:1118-1124, 1971.

45. Jamieson GA, Smith DF, Kosow DP: Possible role of collagen: glucosyltransferase in platelet adhesion. Mechanistic considerations. THROMB DIATH HAEMORRH 33:668-671, 1975.

46. Smith DF, Kosow DP, Wu C, Jamieson GA: Characterization of human platelet UDP glucose-collagen glucosyltransferase using a new rapid assay. BIOCHIM BIOPHYS ACTA 483:263-278, 1977.

47. Nurden AT, Caen JP: Role of surface glycoproteins in human platelet function. THROMB HAEMOSTAS 35:139-150, 1976.

48. Weiss HJ, Tschopp TB, Baumgartner HR, Sussman II, Johnson MM, Egan JJ: Decreased adhesion of giant (Bernard-Soulier) platelets to subendothelium. Further implications on the role of the von Willebrand factor in hemostasis. AM J MED 57:920-925, 1974.

49. Caen JP, Nurden AT, Jeanneau C, Michel H, Tobelem G, Lévy-Toledano S, Sultan Y, Valensi F, Bernard J: Bernard-Soulier syndrome: A new platelet glycoprotein abnormality. Its relationship with platelet adhesion to subendothelium and with the factor VIII von Willebrand protein. J LAB CLIN MED 87: 586-596, 1976.

50. Reimers H-J, Kinlough-Rathbone RL, Cazenave J-P, Senyi AF, Hirsh J, Packham MA, Mustard JF: *In vitro* and *in vivo* functions of thrombin-treated platelets. THROMB HAEMOSTAS 35:151-166, 1976.

51. Steiner M: Effect of thrombin on the platelet membrane. BIOCHIM BIOPHYS ACTA 323:653-658, 1973.

52. Phillips DR, Agin PP: Thrombin substrates and the proteolytic site of thrombin action on human-platelet plasma membranes. BIOCHIM BIOPHYS ACTA 352:218-227, 1974.

53. Phillips DR, Agin PP: Platelet plasma membrane glycoproteins. Identification of a proteolytic substrate for thrombin. BIOCHEM BIOPHYS RES COMMUN 75:940-947, 1977.

54. Hagen I, Solum NO, Olsen T: Membrane alterations in connection with the release reaction in human platelets as studied by the lactoperoxidase-iodination technique and by agglutination with bovine factor VIII-related protein. BIOCHIM BIOPHYS ACTA 468: 1-10, 1977.

55. Ward JV, Radojewski-Hutt AM, Packham MA, Haslam RJ, Mustard JF: Loss of sulfated proteoglycan from the surface of rabbit platelets during adenosine 5'-diphosphate-induced aggregation. LAB INVEST 35:337-342, 1976.

56. Greenberg J, Packham MA, Cazenave J-P, Reimers H-J, Mustard JF: Effects on platelet function of removal of platelet sialic acid by neuraminidase. LAB INVEST 32:476-484, 1975.

57. Jørgensen L: Mechanisms of thrombosis. PATHOBIOL ANNU 1:139-204, 1971.

58. Baumgartner HR: Platelet interaction with vascular structures. THROMB DIATH HAEMORRH (Suppl) 51:161-176, 1972.

59. Ross R, Glomset J, Kariya B, Harker L: A platelet-dependent serum factor that stimulates the proliferation of arterial smooth muscle cells *in vitro*. PROC NATL ACAD SCI USA 71:1207-1210, 1974.

60. Ihnatowycz IO, Cazenave J-P, Moore S, Mustard JF: Platelet-derived growth factor production during the platelet release reaction independent of the endoperoxide pathway. THROMB HAEMOSTAS 38:229, 1977.

61. Packham MA, Mustard JF: Clinical pharmacology of platelets. BLOOD 50:555-573, 1977.

62. Cazenave J-P, Packham MA, Guccione MA, Mustard JF: Inhibition of platelet adherence to a collagen-coated surface by agents that inhibit platelet shape change and clot retraction. J LAB CLIN MED 84:483-493, 1974.

63. Cazenave J-P, Davies JA, Senyi AF, Blajchman MA, Hirsh J, Mustard JF: Effects of methylprednisolone on platelet adhesion to damaged aorta, bleeding time and platelet survival. BLOOD 48:1009, 1976.

64. Cazenave J-P, Packham MA, Guccione MA, Mustard JF: Effects of penicillin G on platelet aggregation, release, and adherence to collagen. PROC SOC EXP BIOL MED 142:159-166, 1973.

65. Cazenave J-P, Guccione MA, Packham MA, Mustard JF: Effects of cephalothin and penicillin G on platelet function *in vitro*. BR J HAEMATOL 35:135-152, 1977.

66. Brown CH III, Bradshaw MW, Natelson EA, Alfrey CP, Williams TW: Defective platelet function following the administration of penicillin compounds. BLOOD 47:949-956, 1976.

67. Kinlough-Rathbone RL, Packham MA, Mustard JF: Comparison of methods of measuring loss of cytoplasmic constituents from platelets. THROMB RES 9:669-673, 1976.

68. Busch C, Wasteson A, Westermark B: Release of a cell growth promoting factor from human platelets. THROMB RES 8:493-500, 1976.

69. Kaplan KL: Proteins secreted by platelets. Significance in

detecting thrombosis. IN THROMBOSIS: ANIMAL AND HUMAN MODELS, edited by Day HJ, Molony BA, Nishizawa EE, Rynbrandt RH. New York, Plenum Publishing Corp., 1978, pp. 105-120.

70. Baumgartner HR, Studer A: Platelet factors and the proliferation of vascular smooth muscle cells. ATHEROSCLEROSIS IV. PROCEEDINGS OF THE IVth INTERNATIONAL SYMPOSIUM ON ATHEROSCLEROSIS, Tokyo, 1976. Berlin, Springer, 1977.

71. Clowes AW, Karnovsky MJ: Failure of certain antiplatelet drugs to effect myointimal thickening following arterial endothelial injury in the rat. LAB INVEST 36:452-464, 1977.

SUMMARY OF DISCUSSION BY PARTICIPANTS

Dr. Salzman wondered why in this study aspirin increased platelet adhesion to the damaged wall, because aspirin inhibits PGI_2 synthesis by the endothelial cell, and in the system used, where the vessel wall was damaged, no endothelial cells were present and therefore presumably no PGI_2 synthesis was going on anyway. Dr. Cazenave replied that although he has no direct evidence, possibly the smooth muscle cells are the source for PGI_2 synthesis. Dr. Salzman cited the work of MacIntyre, Pearson, and Gordon[1] which indicated that in culture, only endothelial cells produced PGI_2.

Dr. Mustard said that while endothelial cells do make PGI_2, there is no evidence that smooth muscle cells do not make it, and he cited some animal studies that suggest they do. If a hole is made with a needle in the jugular vein of a thrombocytopenic rabbit, the bleeding persists but it can be stopped by 1) replacing platelets in the rabbit, 2) treating the vessel wall with hydrocortisone or methylprednisolone, or 3) treating the vessel wall with aspirin or indomethacin. If, however, arachidonic acid is added to the hydrocortisone- or methylprednisolone-treated vessel wall, the long bleeding time is restored in thrombocytopenic animals. In contrast, adding arachidonic acid to the aspirin- or indomethacin-treated vessel wall does not have this effect.[2] He inferred from the data that PGI_2 is made by the vessel wall and that by blocking this in thrombocytopenic animals, the bleeding process can be stopped. Steroids block phospholipase A_2 and thereby prevent release of arachidonate while aspirin inhibits the conversion of the arachidonate to PGI_2.

---

[1]MacIntyre DE, Pearson JD, Gordon JL: Localization and stimulation of prostaglandin I_2 production in vascular cells. NATURE (In Press).
[2]Blajchman MA, Senyi AS, Hirsh J, Mustard JF: The effect of prostaglandin inhibitors on the bleeding time in thrombocytopenic rabbits. BLOOD 50 (Suppl 1):259, 1977.

Dr. Ross said that in culture smooth muscle cells do not produce PGI_2. The evidence for this is that when smooth muscle cells are added to platelets they cause aggregation, while endothelial cells inhibit aggregation. Furthermore, indomethacin inhibits the endothelial cell effect. Dr. Cazenave suggested that the aggregation induced by smooth muscle cells might be due to collagen, but Dr. Ross said there was no direct evidence for this.

Dr. H. J. Day reported data of Moncada *et al.*[3] who indicated that all layers of the vessel wall produce a smooth muscle cell relaxing substance, presumably PGI_2, but the amount of this material produced decreases (on a tissue weight basis) as one moves from the endothelial cells to the adventitia.

Dr. Salzman said that when PGH_2 is added to endothelial cells in culture, a material appears in the medium which inhibits platelet aggregation, and the production of this material can be blocked by indomethacin. Smooth muscle cells and fibroblasts in culture do not produce this material.

Dr. Spaet was concerned about the use of ^{51}Cr for measuring platelet adhesion because Steiner and Baldini's studies[4] suggested that ^{51}Cr may be released, and that the degree of irreversible labeling is extremely variable. Dr. Mustard said that if the labeling is done carefully under controlled conditions, the labeling is irreversible, at least for acute studies. His group has compared morphometric observations with ^{51}Cr labeling results and found them to be similar. Dr. Packham supported the irreversible binding by saying that if the ^{51}Cr-labeled platelets are washed, then the labeling of the platelets is irreversible. Also, in another study, they showed that ^{51}Cr from lysed platelets did not adhere to endothelial cells or the damaged wall.

Dr. C. Day asked about the effect of thromboxane A_1 on platelets and aorta, and also about heparin's effect on thrombin-treated aorta. Dr. Cazenave replied that unless the aorta has been pretreated with thrombin, heparin at a concentration of 50 U/ml does not inhibit the adherence of platelets to the subendothelium. When damaged aortic surface has been pretreated with thrombin, heparin interacts with the thrombin and prevents it from promoting platelet adherence. Dr. Smith said that what is known about thromboxanes is

[3]Moncada S, Herman AG, Higgs EA, Vane JR: Differential formation of prostacyclin (PGX or PGI_2) by layers of the arterial wall. An explanation for the anti-thrombotic properties of vascular endothelium. THROMB RES 11:323-344, 1977.

[4]Tsukada T, Steiner M, Baldini M: Mechanism and kinetics of chromate transport in human platelets. AM J PHYSIOL 221:1699-1705, 1971.

inferential, for they have not been isolated. The effect of thromboxane A_1 is not known. What is known is that PGH_1, which can be isolated, does not cause aggregation and is a vasoconstrictor. Also, when 8,11,14-eicosatrienoic acid is used as a substrate for platelets, it is not as good a substrate as arachidonic acid.

Dr. Salzman commented that all of Dr. Cazenave's studies have been done in the presence of albumin. He said that in all systems containing protein, the protein will coat the surface first before any formed elements of the blood could get there. He wondered whether Dr. Cazenave has done any studies in plasma or plasma fractions. Dr. Cazenave said he has looked at platelet adhesion to a collagen-coated surface in the presence of various plasma ractions as well as citrated plasma. Plasma reduced platelet adherence, but he did not know whether this was due to the protein concentration or to citrate. Fibrinogen, previously treated with diisopropyl fluorophosphate to remove traces of thrombin, decreased platelet adherence in the presence of albumin. Clq, a subcomponent of the first component of complement, which is a large molecule with structural similarities to collagen, was also a powerful inhibitor of platelet adherence to collagen-coated surfaces.[5]

Dr. Honohan asked if neuraminidase-treated platelets aggregate and do not adhere or vice versa. Dr. Cazenave replied that removal of sialic acid from platelets does not diminish their sensitivity to normal aggregating agents and perhaps even increases their sensitivity to ADP, collagen, and thrombin. Neuraminidase treatment does not alter the ability of the platelets to adhere to collagen or the subendothelium.[6]

---

[5]Cazenave J-P, Assimeh SN, Painter RH, Packham MA, Mustard JF: Clq inhibition of the interaction of collagen with human platelets. J IMMUNOL 116:162-163, 1976.

[6]Greenberg J, Packham MA, Cazenave J-P, Reimers H-J, Mustard JF: Effects on platelet function of removal of platelet sialic acid by neuraminidase. LAB INVEST 32:476-484, 1975.

PLATELET AGGREGATION: RELEVANCE TO THROMBOTIC TENDENCIES*

M. A. Packham, Ph.D., and J. F. Mustard, M.D., Ph.D.

Department of Biochemistry, University of Toronto, Toronto, Ontario, Canada; Department of Pathology, McMaster University, Hamilton, Ontario, Canada

ABSTRACT

Platelets change shape, aggregate, and release their granule contents in response to a number of agents that they may encounter *in vivo*. Some understanding has been gained concerning the mechanisms involved in these platelet reactions; released ADP, products formed from platelet arachidonic acid when platelet phospholipase A_2 is activated, and at least one other mechanism contribute to aggregation responses. Many investigators have reported that platelets are more responsive to aggregating agents *in vitro* or aggregate spontaneously in some conditions associated with cardiovascular disease. Tests that are thought to detect circulating platelet aggregates have also been developed. However, the increased sensitivity demonstrated by all these tests may be a result of vascular disease rather than its cause.

Platelet hypersensitivity has also been noted in association with some dietary lipids, hyperbetalipoproteinemia, smoking, and stress. In many cases, the abnormal platelet responsiveness seems to be attributable to increased activation of the arachidonate pathway, possibly through increased sensitivity of phospholipase A_2 in the platelet membrane. Evidence for this concept is that drugs such as aspirin which block the action of the cyclo-oxygenase of this pathway and thus prevent the formation of prostaglandin endoperoxides PGG_2 and PGH_2, and of thromboxane A_2, abolish the platelet hypersensitivity that can be demonstrated by tests of biphasic aggregation responses to ADP or epinephrine. There is a large

*Supported by grants MT2629 and MT1309 from the Medical Research Council of Canada.

overlap, however, in the sensitivity of platelets from normal and abnormal groups, and it seems unlikely that platelet aggregation tests will prove to be of great value in assessing patients with thrombosis or in predicting the likelihood of the occurrence of the complications of atheroclerosis.

Other methods of detecting thrombosis include platelet survival measurements; determination of platelet coagulant activities; detection of materials (such as platelet factor 4 and β-thromboglobulin) released from platelets that have taken part in thrombus formation; and detection of such platelets on the basis of the reduction in platelet density that results from their exposure to thrombin and participation in reversible thrombus formation.

INTRODUCTION

Platelets change shape, aggregate and release their granule contents in response to a number of agents that they may encounter *in vivo*. These include collagen in damaged vessel walls, thrombin, ADP, short-lived compounds formed from arachidonic acid, antigen-antibody complexes, serotonin, epinephrine, vasopressin, platelet isoantibodies, viruses, and bacteria (1,2). The formation of a mass of aggregated platelets at an injury site on a blood vessel wall is one of the early events in the development of a thrombus. Circulating thromboemboli may occur if these thrombi embolize or if platelets encounter aggregating agents in the circulation (3).

Platelet Hypersensitivity and Thrombosis

A number of recent studies seem to indicate that subjects whose platelets show an increased susceptibility to aggregating agents also have an increased susceptibility to thrombosis (2). The question arises whether subjects whose platelets show an increased sensitivity to aggregating agents have an increased susceptibility to thrombosis as a result of the platelet abnormality, or whether the platelet hypersensitivity results from thrombotic processes which may or may not be clinically detectable. If increased platelet sensitivity is related to thrombotic processes, and suitable tests for platelet "hypersensitivity" can be developed, it might be possible to identify individuals who are at risk, institute treatments that are thought to inhibit thrombosis, and assess the effects of these treatments by tests of platelet function. In attempts to detect hypersensitive platelets, most investigators have examined platelet aggregation, although the platelet release reaction, platelet adherence and platelet survival have also been studied. This presentation will be confined mainly to a consideration of the results of *in vitro* tests of platelet aggregation.

CAUSES OF PLATELET HYPERSENSITIVITY

Theoretically, platelet hypersensitivity could be the result of congenital abnormalities or of acquired conditions. Two congenital conditions in which platelet hypersensitivity has been detected are cyanotic congenital heart disease (4) and type IIa hyperbetalipoproteinemia (5). However, the platelet hypersensitivity in these conditions is undoubtedly secondary and is not the result of a congenital platelet abnormality. In cyanotic congenital heart disease, the increased platelet responses to aggregating agents may be due to the presence of a high proportion of young platelets in the circulation; young platelets are thought to be more reactive than old platelets (4,6). In type IIa hyperbetalipoproteinemia, the platelet abnormality seems to be attributable to changes in platelet lipids resulting from abnormal plasma lipids (7). No congenital platelet abnormalities which are responsible for platelet hypersensitivity have been described.

In many cases, increased platelet sensitivity to aggregation is an acquired disorder. Conditions that have been identified as responsible for this include diet, particularly dietary lipids (8); smoking (9,10); stress (11-13); the use of oral contraceptives (14-16); and a number of disease processes associated with the cardiovascular system (2,17); see Table 1.

TABLE 1. CONDITIONS IN WHICH HUMAN PLATELET HYPERSENSITIVITY HAS BEEN REPORTED

Condition	References
Cardiovascular disease	70-75
Angina	18,20,45,50,60,76
Myocardial infarction	49,50,60,77
Peripheral occlusive atherosclerosis	20,78
or arterial insufficiency	60,79
Cerebrovascular disease	52,80,81
-stroke	47,49,51,82
-transient cerebral ischemia	23,47,60,63,82-84
Thromboembolism	48,49,85
Venous thrombosis	62,86
Diabetes	21,53,54,87-90
Hyperbetalipoproteinemia	5,7
Paroxysmal nocturnal hemoglobinuria	91
Pregnancy (particularly hypertensive)	92
Migraine	93,94
Myotonic dystrophy	95
Gout	96

AGGREGATION TESTS OF PLATELET HYPERSENSITIVITY

Most tests for detection of hypersensitive platelets involve observations of platelet aggregation. Some investigators have characterized hypersensitive platelets as those which aggregate with lower concentrations of aggregating agents than are required to aggregate platelets from so-called "normal" control subjects. The minimum concentration of ADP or epinephrine that causes a biphasic aggregation response in human, citrated, platelet-rich plasma has been determined in many studies (5,18-20). Some investigators have detected "spontaneous" aggregation upon stirring citrated platelet-rich plasma without adding aggregating agents (21). Spontaneous aggregation is not usually observed in plasma from normal subjects and seems to occur as the pH rises during stirring. There are two main tests that detect platelet aggregates in blood that has just been removed from the circulation. It has not been determined whether the platelet aggregates are actually present in the circulation, presumably as a result of platelet hypersensitivity *in vivo*, or whether the aggregates form as the blood is drawn. In Hornstra's filtragometer (22), pressure changes are measured as whole blood or plasma is forced through a screen with micropores and platelet aggregates block the pores. In Wu and Hoak's platelet aggregate ratio method (23), blood is taken both into EDTA-formalin in which platelet aggregates are preserved and into EDTA in which the aggregates break up; the ratio of the number of single platelets in the two suspensions is determined.

MECHANISMS OF PLATELET AGGREGATION

Three main mechanisms that cause platelet aggregation have been identified. ADP aggregates platelets and, when it is released from the platelet granules during platelet interactions with agents such as collagen or thrombin, it contributes to the aggregation response (1). Within the last few years it has been recognized that many of the agents that cause the platelets to release their granule contents also activate phospholipase A_2 of the platelet membrane. This results in the initiation of the pathway in which arachidonate is freed from platelet membrane phospholipids and is converted to the prostaglandin endoperoxides PGG_2 and PGH_2, and to thromboxane A2 (24-28). These short-lived intermediates of this pathway are themselves potent aggregating agents. They cause aggregation in the absence of releasable ADP (29) and hence must be able to induce aggregation through a mechanism that is independent of ADP. Their formation can be blocked with non-steroidal anti-inflammatory drugs which inhibit the cyclo-oxygenase that acts on arachidonic acid (30). There also appears to be an aggregating mechanism (or mechanisms) independent of ADP or of compounds formed from arachidonate. In experiments in which released ADP has been rapidly removed with the creatine phosphate/ creatine phosphokinase system and the arachidonate pathway has been blocked with aspirin or indomethacin, some aggregating agents (particularly thrombin and the divalent cation ionophore A23,187) cause extensive aggregation and release of granule contents (1,31). The ionophore apparently acts by causing internal calcium shifts in the platelets. Several investigators have speculated that thrombin may induce similar changes in internal platelet calcium (31-33). These three mechanisms appear to act synergistically with each other (1,34). Obviously, if any one of these mechanisms is abnormally sensitive to activation, platelet responses to aggregating agents will be enhanced.

The second phase of aggregation induced by ADP or epinephrine in human, citrated, platelet-rich plasma is thought to be associated with activation of the arachidonate pathway because it can be blocked by the nonsteroidal anti-inflammatory drugs that inhibit the cyclo-oxygenase of this pathway. Studies of secondary aggregation in response to ADP or epinephrine appear to be measuring the susceptibility of platelets to activation of their phospholipase A_2. In many instances, platelet hypersensitivity seems to be attributable to an increased activation of this enzyme with a resulting increase in the production of the short-lived intermediates of the arachidonate pathway; aspirin and other nonsteroidal anti-inflammatory drugs abolish the hypersensitivity (18,23,35). It may be that platelets that have been exposed to the intravascular events associated with vascular disease and ischemia are hypersensitive to activation of the arachidonate pathway.

EFFECTS OF DIETARY FATS

As summarized in Table 2, when animals or humans are fed diets rich in polyunsaturated fatty acids such as linoleic, γ-linolenic or dihomo-γ-linolenic acid, the sensitivity of the platelets to aggregation is decreased (36-40). This has been shown both by Hornstra's filtragometer technique and by aggregation studies with ADP. In contrast, platelets from subjects who have ingested large amounts of arachidonic acid are more sensitive to aggregating agents than platelets from subjects on a more normal diet (41). As noted earlier, arachidonic acid is the precursor of the potent aggregating agents PGG_2, PGH_2, and thromboxane A_2, whereas dihomo-γ-linolenic acid is the precursor of prostaglandin E_1, which is a strong inhibitor of platelet aggregation. Whether or not the effects of these lipids can be attributed to changes in the proportions of the various prostaglandins formed from platelet phospholipids when phospholipase A_2 is activated remains to be determined (38).

TABLE 2. EFFECT OF CHANGES IN DIETARY FAT ON PLATELET SENSITIVITY TO AGGREGATION

Dietary fat	Effect on Aggregation Response	Method of Study	Species	References
Low fat	Depressed	Aggregation to collagen or thrombin	Man	40
Linoleic	Decreased	Filtragometer	Man	8,36,37
Linoleic	No effect	Filtragometer	Man	97
Dihomo-γ-linolenic	Decreased	Aggregation to collagen or epinephrine	Rat and rabbit	98
Dihomo-γ-linolenic	No effect	Aggregation to ADP, collagen or arachidonate	Rabbit	99
Dihomo-γ-linolenic	Decreased	Aggregation to ADP	Baboon and man	39
γ-linolenic	Decreased	Aggregation to ADP	Baboon	39
Cholesterol	Increased	Platelet aggregate ratio	Monkey	100
Cholesterol	Increased	Rotating cone-plate	Rabbit	13
Butter or stearic	Increased	Aggregation to thrombin	Rat	101
Butter or stearic	Decreased	Aggregation to ADP or collagen	Rat	101
Arachidonic	Increased	Aggregation to ADP	Man	41

A number of other effects of increased dietary linoleic acid have been reported. A 12-year study by Miettinen *et al.* (42) demonstrated that a diet containing a large amount of linoleic acid was associated with a significantly reduced mortality from coronary heart disease. Hornstra and Lussenburg (43) have demonstrated that dietary linoleic acid increases the time required for thrombus formation in aortic loops in rats. Dietary linoleic acid has also been reported to increase the linoleic/arachidonic ratio in platelet phospholipids (Hornstra G, personal communication). Inhibition of the cyclo-oxygenase enzyme that acts on arachidonic acid by linoleic acid (Hornstra G, personal communication) and by dihomo-γ-linolenic acid (38) has been demonstrated *in vitro*. These latter two effects could be responsible for decreased PGG_2, PGH_2, and thromboxane A_2 formation and increased PGE_1 formation. It is tempting to speculate that the decreased thrombotic tendency associated with diets rich in linoleic acid may be attributable to the effect of this fatty acid or its derivatives on the arachidonate pathway. If some forms of platelet hypersensitivity are attributable to dietary lipids, it may be possible to reduce platelet sensitivity by changing the type of dietary fat.

Changes in dietary fat may influence the biophysical properties of platelet membranes as well as the biochemical reactions in which the membrane phospholipids are involved. Shattil and his colleagues (19,44) have shown that platelet responses to aggregating agents can be increased by increasing platelet membrane fluidity. This can be done by increasing the cholesterol content of the membrane. Platelets from patients with type IIa hyperbetalipoproteinemia have an increased ratio of cholesterol to phospholipid in their membranes and also show an increased sensitivity to aggregation with ADP or epinephrine (5,7). It is possible that membrane fluidity (microviscosity) may be the biophysical basis for the changes in the susceptibility of the platelets to activation of phospholipase A_2.

HYPERSENSITIVE PLATELETS AND VASCULAR DISEASE

Hypersensitive platelets have been observed in a number of conditions associated with vascular disease. Some of the observations are summarized in Table 1. In most of the conditions listed, it has not been possible to determine whether the changes in platelet sensitivity are a consequence of the disease process or a contributing factor to it. Results that are pertinent to this question have been reported by Frishman *et al.* (18,45). These investigators determined the minimum concentration of ADP required to produce a biphasic aggregation response in citrated, platelet-rich plasma from patients with angina pectoris and normal control subjects. Platelets from patients with angina were more sensitive to ADP-induced aggregation. Both propranolol and aspirin reduced platelet hypersensitivity but only propranolol increased the exercise tolerance of the patients with angina. Aspirin did not correct the electrocardiographic manifestations of ischemia associated with angina during exercise. Obviously, aspirin only affected the platelets, and thus it is clear that the hypersensitive platelets were not responsible for the ischemia associated with angina. However, on the basis of these experiments, it is not possible to determine whether propranolol affected the ischemia associated with angina independently of its effects on the platelets, or whether the decreased sensitivity of platelets during treatment with propranolol resulted, at least in part, from reduction of the ischemia. *In vitro* studies have demonstrated that propranolol inhibits ADP-induced aggregation (46) and hence propranolol may affect platelet hypersensitivity in two ways.

As noted earlier, an unresolved problem in all of the studies that have shown increased platelet sensitivity in association with vascular disease is that the change in the platelet sensitivity may be a result of the conditions in which it has been observed rather than their cause. There are apparently no prospective studies of changes in platelet sensitivity. However, there have been some reports that as acute conditions resolve, platelet sensitivity returns toward more normal values (47-49).

Dougherty *et al.* (47) found that platelets taken from patients during the acute phase of transient cerebral ischemic attacks or strokes showed increased sensitivity to ADP and adrenalin. However when these patients were tested 10 days or later after the acute event, their platelets had reverted to normal sensitivity to ADP. Aspirin corrected the increased sensitivity to normal during the acute phase, indicating that the increased sensitivity detectable by *in vitro* aggregation tests may be attributable to activation of the arachidonate pathway in platelets. However, in these studies, the increase in the percentage of circulating platelet aggregates observed during the acute attack was not changed by aspirin, although the circulating platelet aggregate ratio returned to normal 10 days or later after the acute attack. Thus it may be that the circulating platelet aggregate test detected a different type of platelet hypersensitivity than the test of ADP-induced aggregation, although both types of hypersensitivity may have had a common cause associated with the intravascular events.

Other investigators have also reported that platelet hypersensitivity detectable during the acute phase of thrombosis, hypertension, angina pectoris, myocardial infarction, or pulmonary embolism was not apparent when the patients were tested days or weeks later (48,49). In contrast, chronic platelet hypersensitivity has been reported in some patients with ischemic heart disease and in some patients who have had myocardial infarcts or repeated cerebrovascular occlusions (50,51). Platelet hypersensitivity to ADP and spontaneous platelet aggregation may not be due to the same platelet abnormalities, and may differ in persistence. Vos *et al.* (52) found that of 21 patients with a variety of vascular disorders 20 still showed platelet hypersensitivity after 6 months whereas of 14 exhibiting spontaneous platelet aggregation initially, only seven showed this abnormality after 6 months.

Although it is probably too soon for definite conclusions, it appears that increased platelet sensitivity is associated with conditions in which there is ischemia, trauma, or changes in lipids. In many if not all of the conditions listed in Table 1, the manifestation as hypersensitive platelets is probably secondary to some other event. Colwell and his colleagues reported that platelets from diabetic subjects have a hyperactive arachidonate pathway compared with platelets from control subjects (53,54). These observations constitute one of the first examples of the use of a test for platelet hypersensitivity that deals with a specific, known mechanism.

PLATELET AGGREGATION TESTS IN THE PREDICTION OF THROMBOTIC TENDENCIES

In patients with transient ischemic attacks or myocardial infarction, the results of the same type of tests for platelet hypersensitivity with similar patients in different laboratories do not always agree (Workshop on "Methods for Detection of Hypersensitive Platelets", Philadelphia, June 1977). This could be due to unrecognized differences in measuring platelet hypersensitivity, the status of the patients at the time they were studied, the choice of control groups, or the number of patients required for statistically significant differences to become apparent.

The extent of the response to human platelets to aggregating agents varies widely in the absence of any of the factors known to affect platelet responses (55,56). Platelet sensitivity depends to some extent on age and sex (57). As mentioned previously, diet may affect platelet sensitivity and it seems likely that there are other factors as yet unrecognized that also influence aggregation responses. The wide variation among the responses of platelets from "normal" individuals makes it difficult to identify any one subject as "abnormal", although statistically significant differences between some groups of subjects and groups of control subjects can be demonstrated. Hence, despite numerous reports that increased platelet sensitivity to aggregating agents is often associated with vascular disease and its complications, tests for abnormalities of platelet aggregation seem unlikely to be of great value in assessing patients with thrombosis (2,58). It is also unlikely that platelet aggregation tests will prove helpful in predicting the likelihood of complications of atherosclerosis (heart attacks and strokes).

EXPOSURE TO THROMBIN AS A CAUSE OF PLATELET HYPERSENSITIVITY

The only direct evidence that platelets which have taken part in thrombus formation may be more sensitive to other aggregating agents comes from *in vitro* experiments in which platelets were exposed to thrombin and then recovered as individual, disc-shaped platelets. These platelets were hypersensitive to ADP-induced aggregation and did not deaggregate readily (59). It seems possible that platelets exposed to thrombin *in vivo* may participate in thrombus formation and then return to the circulation as hypersensitive platelets when the thrombi embolize and the thromboemboli break up. Such a process would be compatible with the evidence of increased numbers of circulating platelet aggregates in some conditions associated with vascular disease (8,23,35,47,60).

OTHER METHODS TO DETECT THROMBOSIS

If detection of hypersensitive platelets does not prove to be a satisfactory way of determining that thrombosis is occurring, what other methods might detect this process? Several approaches to this question are being investigated.

It has been known for some time that platelet survival tends to be shortened in patients with clinical manifestations of arterial disease (61). This correlation is much better than that between platelet hypersensitivity and vascular disease, but the determination of platelet survival is technically much more difficult. Furthermore, sulfinpyrazone and dipyridamole, which tend to prolong shortened platelet survival, have little effect on platelet aggregation at concentrations that can be achieved *in vivo* (61). The lack of correlation between platelet hypersensitivity and shortened platelet survival is somewhat unexpected because platelet turnover is increased in association with shortened platelet survival and hence a high proportion of young platelets would be present. Karpatkin (6) demonstrated that young platelets are more reactive than old platelets; thus one would predict that platelet hypersensitivity would be associated with shortened platelet survival. Possibly the discrepancy between predicted and actual observations resides in differences between the tests used by Karpatkin (6) and those now being employed to detect hypersensitive platelets.

Walsh and his colleagues (62,63) have demonstrated increased platelet coagulant activities in association with venous thrombosis following hip surgery, and in transient cerebral ischemia in patients with normal serum lipids. Platelets from the latter group did not show hypersensitivity to aggregation induced by ADP, epinephrine, or collagen. Thus, in this study, platelet coagulant activities showed a better correlation with vascular disease than did platelet aggregation tests.

It seems feasible to detect in plasma materials that have been released from platelets that have interacted with collagen, thrombin, or other intravascular agents that stimulate platelets to release their granule contents. Dr. Kaplan's presentation to this Workshop (pages 105 to 120) deals with this approach. The released materials on which interest is focused at the moment are platelet factor 4 and β-thromboglobulin (64-67).

We are developing a method to detect platelets that have been exposed to thrombin and induced to release their granule contents. These platelets are less dense than normal platelets and can be largely separated from normal platelets by centrifugation through a stractan density gradient (68). When platelets were "degranulated" by treatment with thrombin, labeled with ^{51}Cr, infused into rabbits, and allowed to circulate for 18 hours, it was possible to show that most of the platelets that had been exposed to thrombin were in the least dense layer of the stractan density gradient. Thus it is possible to isolate platelet populations that are enriched in these artificially degranulated platelets.

We also examined the question of whether platelets that have been degranulated *in vivo* by taking part in reversible thrombus formation can be isolated in the same way. When thrombosis was induced in rabbits with an indwelling aortic catheter over an 18-hour period, the proportion of platelets in the least dense layer of the stractan gradient was increased and their serotonin content was substantially reduced (Cieslar P, Kinlough-Rathbone, RL, Packham, MA, Mustard JF, unpublished observations). With this technique it may be feasible to detect platelets that have taken part in reversible thrombus formation. Perhaps the least dense platelets in the circulation at any time include those that have been partially degranulated. This would be in accord with our finding (69) that the least dense platelet population is enriched in old platelets, because old platelets would have had the most chances to encounter release-inducing agents in the circulation. If thromboemboli are forming and breaking up, an increased proportion of degranulated platelets should be detectable.

REFERENCES

1. Packham MA, Kinlough-Rathbone RL, Reimers H-J, Scott S, Mustard JF: Mechanisms of platelet aggregation independent of adenosine diphosphate. In PROSTAGLANDINS IN HEMATOLOGY, edited by Silver MJ, Smith JB, Kocsis JJ. New York, Spectrum Publications, Inc., 1977, pp. 247-276.

2. Packham MA, Kinlough-Rathbone RL, Mustard JF: Aggregation and agglutination. In PLATELET FUNCTION TESTING, edited by Day HJ, Holmsen H, Zucker MB. DHEW Publication No. 727, U.S. Govt. Printing Office, Washington, D.C. (In Press).

3. Mustard JF, Kinlough-Rathbone RL, Packham MA: Recent status

of research in the pathogenesis of thrombosis. THROMB DIATH HAEMORRH (Suppl. 59):157-188, 1974.

4. Goldschmidt B, Sørland SJ: The young platelet population in children with cyanotic congenital heart disease. THROMB HAEMOSTAS 35:342-349, 1976.

5. Carvalho ACA, Colman RW, Lees RS: Platelet function in hyperlipoproteinemia. N ENGL J MED 290:434-438, 1974.

6. Karpatkin S: Heterogeneity of human platelets. II. Functional evidence suggestive of young and old platelets. J CLIN INVEST 48:1083-1087, 1969.

7. Shattil SJ, Bennett JS, Colman RW, Cooper RA: Abnormalities of cholesterol-phospholipid composition in platelets and low-density lipoproteins of human hyperbetalipoproteinemia. J LAB CLIN MED 89:341-353, 1977.

8. Hornstra G: Dietary fats and arterial thrombosis. HAEMOSTASIS 2:21-52, 1973.

9. Hawkins RI: Smoking, platelets and thrombosis. NATURE 236: 450-452, 1972.

10. Levine PH: An acute effect of cigarette smoking on platelet function. A possible link between smoking and arterial thrombosis. CIRCULATION 48:619-623, 1973.

11. Haft JI, Fani K: Intravascular platelet aggregation in the heart induced by stress. CIRCULATION 47:353-358, 1973.

12. Fleischman AI, Bierenbaum ML, Stier A: Effect of stress due to anticipated minor surgery upon *in vivo* platelet aggregation in humans. J HUMAN STRESS 2:33-37, 1976.

13. Oversohl K, Bassenge E, Schmid-Schönbein H: Effect of hyperlipidemia and stress on platelet aggregation in rabbits. THROMB RES 7:481-492, 1975.

14. Zahavi J, Dreyfuss F, Kalef M, Soferman N: Adenosine diphosphate-induced platelet aggregation in healthy women with and without a combined and sequential contraceptive pill. AM J OBSTET GYNECOL 117:107-113, 1973.

15. Elkeles RS, Hampton JR, Mitchell JRA: Effect of oestrogens on human platelet behaviour. LANCET 2:315-318, 1968.

16. Mettler L, Selchow BM: Oral contraceptives and platelet function. THROMB DIATH HAEMORRH 28:213-220, 1972.

17. Stuart MJ: Inherited defects of platelet function. SEMIN HEMATOL 12:233-253, 1975.

18. Frishman WH, Christodoulou J, Weksler B, Smithen C, Killip T, Scheidt S: Aspirin therapy in angina pectoris: Effects on platelet aggregation, exercise tolerance, and electrocardiographic manifestations of ischemia. AM HEART J 92:3-10, 1976.

19. Shattil SJ, Anaya-Galindo R, Bennett J, Colman RW, Cooper RA: Platelet hypersensitivity induced by cholesterol incorporation. J CLIN INVEST 55:636-643, 1975.

20. Gormsen J, Nielsen JD, Andersen LA: ADP-induced platelet aggregation *in vitro* in patients with ischemic heart disease and peripheral thromboatherosclerosis. ACTA MED SCAND 201: 509-513, 1977.

21. Breddin K, Grun H, Krzywanek HJ, Schremmer WP: On the measurement of spontaneous platelet aggregation. The platelet aggregation test III. Methods and first clinical results. THROMB HAEMOSTAS 35:669-691, 1976.

22. Hornstra G, ten Hoor F: The filtragometer: A new device for measuring platelet aggregation in venous blood of man. THROMB DIATH HAEMORRH 34:531-544, 1975.

23. Wu KK, Hoak JC: Increased platelet aggregates in patients with transient ischemic attacks. STROKE 6:521-524, 1975.

24. Smith JB, Ingerman CM, Silver MJ: Effects of arachidonic acid and some of its metabolites on platelets. In PROSTAGLANDINS IN HEMATOLOGY, edited by Silver MJ, Smith JB, Kocsis JJ. New York, Spectrum Publications, Inc., 1977, pp. 277-292.

25. Samuelsson B: The role of prostaglandin endoperoxides and thromboxanes in human platelets. In PROSTAGLANDINS IN HEMATOLOGY, edited by Silver MJ, Smith JB, Kocsis JJ. New York, Spectrum Publications, Inc., 1977, pp. 1-10.

26. Willis AL, Vane FM, Kuhn DC, Scott CG, Petrin M: An endoperoxide aggregator (LASS), formed in platelets in response to thrombotic stimuli. Purification, identification and unique biological significance. PROSTAGLANDINS 8:453-507, 1974.

27. Svensson J, Hamberg M, Samuelsson B: On the formation and effects of thromboxane A_2 in human platelets. ACTA PHYSIOL SCAND 98:285-294, 1976.

28. Bills TK, Smith JB, Silver MJ: Selective release of arachi-

donic acid from the phospholipids of human platelets in response to thrombin. J CLIN INVEST 60:1-6, 1977.

29. Kinlough-Rathbone RL, Reimers HJ, Mustard JF, Packham MA: Sodium arachidonate can induce platelet shape change and aggregation which are independent of the release reaction. SCIENCE 192:1011-1012, 1976.

30. Rome LH, Lands WEM, Roth GJ, Majerus PW: Aspirin as a quantitative acetylating reagent for the fatty acid oxygenase that forms prostaglandins. PROSTAGLANDINS 11:23-30, 1976.

31. Kinlough-Rathbone RL, Packham MA, Reimers H-J, Cazenave J-P, Mustard JF: Mechanisms of platelet shape change, aggregation and release induced by collagen, thrombin or A23,187. J LAB CLIN MED 90:707-719, 1977.

32. Feinman RD, Detwiler TC: Absence of a requirement for extracellular calcium for secretion from platelets. THROMB RES 7:677-679, 1975.

33. Holmsen H: Classification and possible mechanisms of action of some drugs that inhibit platelet aggregation. SER HAEMATOL 8, 3:50-80, 1976.

34. Kinlough-Rathbone RL, Packham MA, Mustard JF: Synergism between platelet aggregating agents: The role of the arachidonate pathway. THROMB RES 11:567-580, 1977.

35. Hornstra G: The filtragometer in thrombosis research. (Submitted for Publication).

36. Hornstra G, Lewis B, Chait A, Turpeinen O, Karvonen MJ, Vergroesen AJ: Influence of dietary fat on platelet function in man. LANCET 1:1155-1157, 1973.

37. Fleischman AI, Justice D, Bierenbaum ML, Stier A, Sullivan A: Beneficial effect of increased dietary linoleate upon *in vivo* platelet function in man. J NUTR 105:1286-1290, 1975.

38. Willis AL, Stone KJ, Hart M, Gibson V, Marples P, Botfield E, Comai K, Kuhn DC: Dietary fatty acids, prostaglandin endoperoxides and the prevention of thrombosis. In PROSTAGLANDINS IN HEMATOLOGY, edited by Silver MJ, Smith JB, Kocsis JJ. New York, Spectrum Publications, Inc., 1977, pp. 371-410.

39. Sim AK, McCraw AP: The activity of γ-linolenate and dihomo-γ-linolenate methyl esters *in vitro* and *in vivo* on blood platelet function in non-human primates and in man. THROMB RES 10:385-397, 1977.

40. Iacono JM, Binder RA, Marshall NW, Schoene NW, Jencks JA, Mackin JF: Decreased susceptibility to thrombin and collagen platelet aggregation in man fed a low fat diet. HAEMOSTASIS 3:306-318, 1974.

41. Seyberth HW, Oelz O, Kennedy T, Sweetman BJ, Danon A, Frölich JC, Heimberg M, Oates JA: Increased arachidonate in lipids after administration to man: Effects on prostaglandin biosynthesis. CLIN PHARMACOL THER 18:521-529, 1975.

42. Miettinen M, Turpeinen O, Karvonen MJ, Elosuo R, Paavilainen E: Effect of cholesterol-lowering diet on mortality from coronary heart disease and other causes. A twelve-year clinical trial in men and women. LANCET 2:835-838, 1972.

43. Hornstra G, Lussenburg RN: Relationship between the type of dietary fatty acid and arterial thrombosis tendency in rats. ATHEROSCLEROSIS 22:499-516, 1975.

44. Shattil SJ, Cooper RA: Membrane microviscosity and human platelet function. BIOCHEMISTRY 15:4832-4837, 1976.

45. Frishman WH, Weksler B, Christodoulou JP, Smithen C, Killip T: Reversal of abnormal platelet aggregability and changes in exercise tolerance in patients with angina pectoris following oral propranolol. CIRCULATION 50:887-896, 1974.

46. Weksler BB, Gillick M, Pink J: Effect of propranolol on platelet function. BLOOD 49:185-196, 1977.

47. Dougherty JH, Jr, Levy DE, Weksler BB: Platelet activation in acute cerebral ischaemia. Serial measurements of platelet function in cerebrovascular disease. LANCET 1:821-824, 1977.

48. Yamazaki H, Sano T, Asano T, Hidaka H: Hyperaggregability of platelets in thromboembolic disorders. THROMB RES (Suppl. II) 8:217-225, 1976.

49. Larcan A, Stoltz J-F, Laprevote-Heully M-C, Lambert H: La pression de filtration du plasma riche en plaquettes (PRP) au cours de diverses agressions. AGRESSOLOGIE 17:379-388, 1976.

50. Zahavi J: Hyperaggregability of platelets in thromboembolic disorders. THROMB HAEMOSTAS 36:479-481, 1976.

51. Kalendovsky Z, Austin J, Steele P: Increased platelet aggregability in young patients with stroke. Diagnosis and therapy. ARCH NEUROL 32:13-20, 1975.

52. Vos J, Oosterhuis HJ, ten Cate JW: Increased platelet aggregability as a risk factor in the pathogenesis of ischemic

cerebrovascular disease. (Submitted for Publication).

53. Sagel J, Colwell JA, Crook L, Laimins M: Increased platelet aggregation in early diabetes mellitus. ANN INTERN MED 82: 733-738, 1975.

54. Colwell JA, Sagel J, Crook L, Chambers A, Laimins M: Correlation of platelet aggregation, plasma factor activity, and megathrombocytes in diabetic subjects with and without vascular disease. METABOLISM 26:279-285, 1977.

55. Harrison MJG, Emmons PR, Mitchell JRA: The variability of human platelet aggregation. J ATHEROSCLER RES 7:197-205, 1967.

56. O'Brien JR: Variability in the aggregation of human platelets by adrenaline. NATURE 202:1188-1190, 1964.

57. Johnson M, Ramey E, Ramwell PW: Sex and age differences in human platelet aggregation. NATURE 253:355-357, 1975.

58. McNichol GP, Mitchell JRA, Reuter H, van de Loo J, Born GVR: Platelets in thrombosis. Their clinical significance and the evaluation of potential drugs. THROMB DIATH HAEMORRH 31:379-394, 1974.

59. Reimers H-J, Kinlough-Rathbone RL, Cazenave J-P, Senyi AF, Hirsh J, Packham MA, Mustard JF: *In vitro* and *in vivo* functions of thrombin-treated platelets. THROMB HAEMOSTAS 35:151-166, 1976.

60. Wu KK, Hoak JC: Spontaneous platelet aggregation in arterial insufficiency: Mechanisms and implications. THROMB HAEMOSTAS 35:702-711, 1976.

61. Mustard JF, Packham MA, Kinlough-Rathbone RL: Platelet survival. In PLATELET FUNCTION TESTING, edited by Day JH, Holmsen H, Zucker MB. DHEW Publication No. 727, U.S. Govt. Printing Office. (In Press).

62. Walsh PN, Rogers PH, Marder VJ, Gagnatelli G, Escovitz ES, Sherry S: The relationship of platelet coagulant activities to venous thrombosis following hip surgery. BR J HAEMATOL 32:421-437, 1976.

63. Walsh PN, Pareti FI, Corbett JJ: Platelet coagulant activities and serum lipids in transient cerebral ischemia. N ENGL J MED 295:854-858, 1976.

64. Niewiarowski S, Lowery CT, Hawiger J, Millman M, Timmons S: Immunoassay of human platelet factor 4 (PF4, antiheparin factor)

by radial immunodiffusion. J LAB CLIN MED 87:720-733, 1976.

65. O'Brien JR, Etherington MD, Jamieson S, Lawford P, Lincoln SV, Alkjaersig NJ: Blood changes in atherosclerosis and long after myocardial infarction and venous thrombosis. THROMB DIATH HAEMORRH 34:483-497, 1975.

66. Kaplan KL, Drillings M, Nossel HL, Lesnik G: Radioimmunoassay of β-thromboglobulin (βTG) and platelet factor 4 (PF4). In PLATELET FUNCTION TESTING, edited by Day HJ, Holmsen H, Zucker MB. DHEW Publication No. 727, U.S. Govt. Printing Office, Washington D.C. (In Press).

67. Ludlam CA, Cash JD: Studies on the liberation of β-thromboglobulin from human platelets *in vitro*. BR J HAEMATOL 33:239-247, 1976.

68. Cieslar P, Greenberg JP, Packham MA, Kinlough-Rathbone RL, Mustard JF: Separation of degranulated platelets from normal platelets. THROMB HAEMOSTAS 38:122, 1977.

69. Greenberg JP, Rand ML, Packham MA: Relation of platelet age to platelet sialic acid. FED PROC 36:453, 1977.

70. Breddin K: Untersuchungen über die Agglutinationsbereitschaft der Thrombozyten bei Gefässkrankheiten. In GEFÄSSWAND UND BLUTPLASMA, edited by Emmrich R, Perlick E. II. Symp. Med. Klinik, Leipzig, 1963.

71. Breddin K: Die Thrombozytenfunktion bei hämorrhagischen Diathesen, Thrombosen und Gefässkrankheiten. THROMB DIATH HAEMORRH (Suppl) 27:1-200, 1968.

72. Zahavi J, Dreyfuss F: An abnormal pattern of adenosine diphosphate-induced platelet aggregation in acute myocardial infarction. THROMB DIATH HAEMORRH 21:76-88, 1969.

73. Steele PP, Weily HS, Davies H, Genton E: Platelet function studies in coronary artery disease. CIRCULATION 48:1194-1200, 1973.

74. Breddin K, Krzwanek HJ, Bald M, Kutschera J: Platelet aggregation control: Clinical potential - Is enhanced platelet aggregation a risk factor for thrombo-embolic complications in atherosclerosis? In PLATELET AGGREGATION AND DRUGS, edited by Caprino L, Rossi EC. New York, Academic Press, 1974, pp. 197-212.

75. Scrobohaci M-L, Cunescu V, Orha I: Recurrent thromboembolism with spontaneous platelet aggregation. THROMB HAEMOSTAS 36:

645-646, 1976.

76. Gjesdal K: Platelet function and plasma free fatty acids during acute myocardial infarction and severe angina pectoris. SCAND J HAEMATOL 17:205-212, 1976.

77. O'Brien JR, Heywood JB, Heady JA: The quantitation of platelet aggregation induced by four compounds: A study in relation to myocardial infarction. THROMB DIATH HAEMORRH 16:752-767, 1966.

78. Cotton RC, Bloor K, Archibald G: Inter-relationships between platelet response to adenosine diphosphate, blood coagulation and serum lipids in patients with peripheral occlusive atherosclerosis. ATHEROSCLEROSIS 16:337-348, 1972.

79. Vreeken J, van Aken WG: Spontaneous aggregation of blood platelets as a cause of idiopathic thrombosis and recurrent painful toes and fingers. LANCET 2:1394-1397, 1971.

80. Danta G: Second phase platelet aggregation induced by adenosine diphosphate in patients with cerebral vascular disease and in control subjects. THROMB DIATH HAEMORRH 23:159-169, 1970.

81. Kobayashi I, Fujita T, Yamazaki H: Platelet aggregability measured by screen filtration pressure method in cerebrovascular diseases. STROKE 7:406-409, 1976.

82. Couch JR, Hassanein RS: Platelet aggregation, stroke, and transient ischemic attack in middle-aged and elderly patients. NEUROLOGY 26:888-895, 1976.

83. Mundall J, Quintero P, von Kaulla KN, Harmon R, Austin J: Transient monocular blindness and increased platelet aggregability treated with aspirin. NEUROLOGY 22:280-285, 1972.

84. Andersen LA, Gormsen J: Platelet aggregation and fibrinolytic activity in transient cerebral ischemia. ACTA NEUROL SCAND 55:76-82, 1976.

85. Yamazaki H, Sano T, Shimamoto T, Mashimo N, Takahashi T, Shimamoto T: Platelet functions in thromboembolic disorders. THROMB DIATH HAEMORRH (Suppl 60):213-222, 1974.

86. Wu KK, Barnes RW, Hoak JC: Platelet hyperaggregability in idiopathic recurrent deep vein thrombosis. CIRCULATION 53:687-691, 1976.

87. Rathbone RL, Ardlie NG, Schwartz CJ: Platelet aggregation and

thrombus formation in diabetes mellitus: An *in vitro* study. PATHOLOGY 2:307-316, 1970.

88. Kwaan HC, Colwell JA, Cruz S, Suwanwela N, Dobbie JG: Increased platelet aggregation in diabetes mellitus. J LAB CLIN MED 80:236-246, 1972.

89. Bensoussan D, Levy-Toledano S, Passa P. Caen J, Canivet J: Platelet hyperaggregation and increased plasma level of von Willebrand factor in diabetics with retinopathy. DIABETOLOGIA 11:307-312, 1975.

90. Heath H, Bridgen WD, Canever JV, Pollock J, Hunter PR, Kelsey J, Bloom A: Platelet adhesiveness and aggregation in relation to diabetic retinopathy. DIABETOLOGIA 7:308-315, 1971.

91. Steinberg D, Carvalho AC, Chesney CM, Colman RW: Platelet hypersensitivity and intravascular coagulation in paroxysmal nocturnal hemoglobinuria. AM J MED 59:845-850, 1975.

92. van Kessel PH, Wallenburg HCS, van Vliet HHDM: Platelet aggregation in normal and hypertensive pregnancy. In ABSTRACTS OF THE 17TH DUTCH FEDERATIVE MEETING, Amsterdam, 1975, p. 17.

93. Kalendovsky Z, Austin JH: "Complicated Migraine" Its association with increased platelet aggregability and abnormal plasma coagulation factors. HEADACHE 15:18-35, 1975.

94. Deshmukh SV, Meyer JS, Mouche RJ: Platelet dysfunction in migraine: Effect of self-medication with aspirin. THROMB HAEMOSTAS 36:319-324, 1976.

95. Bousser MG, Conard J, Lecrubier C, Samama M: Increased sensitivity of platelets to adrenaline in human myotonic dystrophy. LANCET 2:307-309, 1975.

96. Newland HR, Chandler AB: Blood uric acid levels and ADP-induced platelet aggregation in the rat. FED PROC 27:321, 1968.

97. O'Brien JR, Etherington MD, Jamieson S, Vergroesen AJ, ten Hoor F: Effect of a diet of polyunsaturated fats on some platelet-function tests. LANCET 2:995-997, 1976.

98. Willis AL, Comai K, Kuhn DC, Paulsrud J: Dihomo-γ-linolenate suppresses platelet aggregation when administered *in vitro* or *in vivo*. PROSTAGLANDINS 8:509-519, 1974.

99. Oelz O, Seyberth HW, Knapp HR, Oates JA: Effects of oral administration of dihomo-γ-linolenic acid on prostaglandin biosynthesis and platelet aggregation in the rabbit. ADV

PROSTAGLANDIN THROMBOXANE RES 2:787-790, 1976.

100. Wu KK, Armstrong ML, Hoak JC, Megan MB: Platelet aggregates in hypercholesterolemic rhesus monkeys. THROMB RES 7:917-924, 1975.

101. Renaud S, Kinlough RL, Mustard JF: Relationship between platelet aggregation and the thrombotic tendency in rats fed hyperlipemic diets. LAB INVEST 22:339-343, 1970.

SUMMARY OF DISCUSSION BY PARTICIPANTS

Dr. Brinkhous asked if Dr. Packham had any evidence to back up her data on the change in density with the wear-and-tear of living, i.e., platelet aging in circulation. Dr. Packham replied that electron micrographs of the low density material had not been done but electron micrographs of thrombin degranulated platelets show smaller numbers of dense granules. When thrombin degranulated platelets are injected into animals and isolated, these platelets are found in the top layer. Furthermore, she said that Dr. Karpatkin has evidence that old platelets have lost cytoplasmic constituents.[1]

Dr. Smith commented that Dr. Franco Pareti in Milan has shown that there are two types of storage pool disease; one is acquired and the other is hereditary. The acquired storage pool deficient platelets resemble the thrombin degranulated platelets. He also said that Pareti can distinguish storage pool disease platelets by the use of the uptake blocker, imipramine. The storage pool disease platelets leak labeled serotonin faster in the presence of imipramine than in the absence of it. He asked why in Dr. Packham's study the least dense rabbit platelets showed low serotonin levels but normal levels of ATP. She responded that in their method, the data include cytoplasmic as well as granular ATP, and therefore it is more difficult to show differences from the whole platelet population; however, she felt that a statistically significant difference may be demonstrable with more experiments.

Dr. Nishizawa wondered if anyone could comment on the use of the filtragometer to detect hypersensitive platelets and whether it might be a useful adjunct to assay the circulating platelet aggregates which Dr. Hoak measures. Dr. Hoak said he had not used it, but commented that each group tends to use their own method and it is difficult for a laboratory to do all the different tests on many patients.

[1]Karpatkin S: Heterogeneity of platelet survival and platelet proteins within a total platelet population. BLOOD 50(Suppl 1):243, 1977.

Dr. H. J. Day commented on Dr. Gear's stop-flow aggregometry[2] which he used to show increased aggregation of platelets from diabetics. In normals 20% of the platelets are nonaggregated, but with diabetics only 1-2% do not aggregate. He was also able to show a difference with platelets from patients who had arterial thrombosis.

Dr. Mustard asked why anyone would want to know whether platelets are sensitive to aggregating agents or whether there are platelet aggregates around. Would the use of a filtrometer be just another instrument to keep laboratories occupied? Dr. Hoak said that there are patients who have had carotid endarterectomy and who continue to have evidence of platelet aggregates. Therefore, removing the obstructive lesion is not necessarily the answer, because they may still have surfaces to which platelets react, eventually resulting in embolus formation. In these cases it would be useful to know whether residual conditions exist where platelet aggregation is occurring. Dr. Mustard asked if the test showed an abnormality, and if you treated the abnormality, whether this would be a good thing. Dr. Hoak indicated that the use of anti-platelet agents was associated with improvement in both the clinical condition and test results, but more data are required to be certain of a cause and effect relationship.

Dr. Colwell has a population of diabetics who show no clinical evidence of vascular disease but do show evidence of hypersensitive platelets. This is a difficult situation to deal with, because no good mechanism is available to tell whether in recently acquired or in chemical diabetes, the patients do or do not have ischemia or thrombosis going on. He feels strongly that in very early diabetes, where no massive ischemia or thrombosis is going on, there is evidence of hypersensitive platelets. These observations might be relevant to the genesis of thrombosis, so we should not disregard the possibility that these abnormalities occur prior to ischemia and thrombosis in diabetics.

Dr. Genton was curious about Dr. Mustard's comments; the way he asked his questions seemed to imply that such tests would not be useful, and he wanted to know his line of reasoning. He thought that if there was a method which would identify a patient or a group of patients at a particular risk in terms of thromboembolic problems, and if a method was available to normalize that test which would correlate with benefit to the patient, it should be useful and clinically applicable. Dr. Mustard said that that was the response he was looking for. He said that if you could take a test in prospective studies and show that there was a relationship with a clinical manifestation, and if that test could show some

[2]Gear ARL: ANALYTICAL BIOCHEM 72:332-345, 1976.

correlation to change in the outcome, then it might be a useful exercise.

Dr. Salzman mentioned the work of Dr. Walsh and coworkers [reference 62 in Dr. Packham's paper] who have shown that the platelet coagulant test predicted deep vein thrombosis. They followed a group of patients through surgery and afterward, and showed that with this test they could predict a certain percentage of patients who developed DVT as indicated by the labeled fibrinogen test.

Dr. Spaet thought that there were really two phenomena being considered: one was the alteration of platelets as a consequence of trauma to the platelets and the other the increased turnover which results in a higher percentage of new platelets being delivered from the bone marrow. He thinks that the tests that are being used to assess one phenomenon may be applicable to the other. Full understanding will only come after these aspects can be separated.

ROLES OF BLOOD FLOW IN PLATELET ADHESION AND AGGREGATION*

Eric F. Grabowski, Ph.D.

Department of Laboratory Medicine, Mayo Clinic

Rochester, MN

ABSTRACT

The investigations described in this review concern platelet adhesion and aggregation as blood flow-dependent phenomena. The experimental approach utilizes a chamber in which are controlled both blood flow and, in aggregation studies, the rate at which ADP enters flowing blood by localized diffusion through a Cuprophan membrane. Videomicroscopy and densitometry of video recordings allow quantification of the *in situ* growth of surface-adherent platelet aggregates. Platelet adhesion is studied separately using phase contrast microscopy. As a result, with the present method one can distinguish adhesion from aggregation, utilize whole blood, simulate arterial (or extracorporeal) shear rate conditions, independently vary ADP entry rate, and quantify aggregate growth *in situ* continuously.

One finding with this experimental system is that human platelet adhesion to Cuprophan membrane (and to at least two other surfaces) exposed to flowing blood for 10 min to 3 hr is negligible in comparison to dog platelet adhesion to these same surfaces. The species difference is present in both citrated and heparinized blood and at surface shear rates comparable to those in mammalian arteries, i.e., 99 to 986 sec^{-1}. Tests for the thromboresistance of biomaterials and for platelet adhesion under controlled flow conditions must take into better account variations between humans and other species. More generally, initial rates of platelet ad-

*Supported by NIH Grants HL-17443, HL-17430, and the Minnesota Heart Association.

hesion to Cuprophan for eight species are either "diffusion-limited" (dog, rabbit) or "surface-reaction limited" (human and five other species). In either case there operates a macroscopic transport mechanism for platelets which involves blood flow.

With citrated dog blood and ADP in μmolal concentrations at the membrane-blood surface, another finding is that aggregate rate of growth prior to embolization passes through a maximum (between 394 and 635 sec^{-1}) with respect to surface shear rate. This result can be explained by competition between platelet convection and diminution of blood levels of ADP with increased flow and suggests the existence of flow regimens favoring or inhibiting aggregate growth. Furthermore, aggregate growth seems to depend upon degree of platelet adhesion prior to the onset of ADP entry and, consequently, species and the particular synthetic surface in question. Shear flow, but not the presence of erythrocytes, is essential to the aggregation process.

For shear rates up to 394 sec^{-1}, the above results suggest a role for platelets in thrombosis which increases as shear rate increases. Such a role is compatible with the greater importance of platelets in arterial thrombosis (shear rates above about 100 sec^{-1}) than in venous thrombosis (shear rates below about 100 sec^{-1}). Arterial thrombi, characteristically more whitish in color, are in large part composed of platelets and fibrin, while the more reddish venous thrombi are principally red blood cells entrapped in a fibrin mesh. As a result, anticoagulants are less effective in prevention of arterial than venous thrombosis; antiplatelet agents are being evaluated in the management of arterial thrombosis, particularly treatment of coronary artery disease and cerebrovascular disease (1,2).

INTRODUCTION

Platelets, 5'-adenosine diphosphate (ADP) released from platelets or other formed elements, and certain clotting proteins have been regarded for some time as important in the pathogenesis of arterial thrombosis and also perhaps in venous thrombosis. Now it is also recognized that these elements undergo convection by flow and diffusion and are therefore subject to the laws of momentum and mass transport.

The degree of platelet adhesion to synthetic surfaces exposed to flowing blood (3-6) and subendothelium (7-9) depends upon blood flow rate and exposure time. A layer of singly adherent platelets forms more rapidly at higher rates of flow.

The degree or rate of platelet aggregation shows divergent responses. The rate of platelet aggregation on synthetic surfaces exposed to flowing blood (10), subendothelium (8), or endothelium with ADP applied just outside a venule wall by iontophoresis (11) increases with increasing blood flow rate at low rates of flow. An example is Begent and Born's finding (11) that this applies at mean flow velocities of <400 μm/sec in a 40-49 μm diameter venule. In contrast, at higher rates of blood flow the aggregation rate decreases (8,10,11).

The rate of initial platelet adhesion on synthetic surfaces or subendothelium exposed to flowing blood is now thought to be proportional to the rate at which fresh platelets arrive at surface. This arrival rate in turn is proportional to blood flow rate via the microconvective ("mixing") motions of erythrocytes in a shear flow (5,12). The absence of red blood cells, as in platelet-rich plasma, diminishes the arrival rate and consequently the adhesion rate by a factor of approximately 100.

The platelet aggregation rate depends on flow and diffusion through at least three other mechanisms:

1) Shear flow, with or without red blood cells, allows platelets on faster-moving streamlines to catch up and interact with platelets on neighboring, slower-moving streamlines. This mechanism, which has been likened to gradient coagulation (13), predicts an aggregation rate proportional to shear rate, at least for "low" rates of flow. It operates in the aggregometer of Born (14) and O'Brien (15), in which, interestingly, the aggregation rate increases with increased stirring rate.

2) Fluid shear stress may promote aggregation by enhancing the release reaction due to thrombin (16) or other stimuli, or by enhancing release itself (17,18). On the other hand, shear stress may directly inhibit formation of platelet-platelet bonds or decrease platelet sensitivity to ADP by prior depletion of platelet adenine nucleotides (17,18).

3) Activation of platelets at a finite rate by ADP (or some other substance) which has diffused away from the surface and into the flowing blood (13,19-22). This ADP can be released by previously adherent or surface-aggregated platelets, or by injured endothelial or subendothelial cells.

Either mechanisms 2) or 3) or both may be limiting at higher rates of flow.

This review describes two investigations on some of the roles of blood flow in platelet adhesion and aggregation. The first, an investigation of species differences in platelet adhesion to foreign surfaces, provides examples of the special roles of platelet convection and red blood cell-augmented platelet transport in platelet adhesion. It is also relevant to the preclinical testing of biomaterials. The second focuses on the special roles played by platelet convection and ADP convective diffusion in platelet aggregation on a foreign surface.

PLATELET ADHESION STUDIES

Methods

Species. Heparinized or citrated blood was obtained from eight species: human, dog, rabbit, sheep, pig, calf, macaque, and baboon.

Blood Flow System. The *in vitro* system used (Figure 1) permitted control of surface shear rate, exposure time, temperature (37°C) and pH (range 7.4 to 7.5). A key component of the system is a Lucite chamber (Figures 2 and 3) prefilled with a divalent cation-free Tyrode's solution (pH 7.4) and mounted vertically to minimize effects of red blood cell sedimentation. The chamber is interposed between a withdrawal pump (Harvard Model 600-0, Harvard Apparatus Co., Inc, Millis MA) and polypropylene beaker containing blood. The blood in this beaker is magnetically stirred with a Teflon-coated bar and maintained at constant temperature with a water bath. A 60-cm length of 0.20-cm ID Silastic tubing (Dow Corning, Indianapolis IN) connected beaker to chamber.

An alternative flow system (23) utilizes a roller pump (Polystaltic, Buchler Insts., Fort Lee NJ) and also an additional 80-cm length of the Silastic tubing in order to return blood to the beaker. This system was used to extend the period of blood exposure in some experiments and also to study the effects of recirculation.

Surfaces. One of the chamber surfaces bounding the blood flow was comprised of a membrane made from one of four different biomaterials of clinical and research interest: Cuprophan PT-150, Avcothane 51, compressed Gore-Tex, or fluorinated ethylcellulose.

Blood Collection and Cell Counting. All blood samples were initially collected in a beaker containing a solution of heparin (mixed bovine and porcine mucosa; Connaught, Toronto, Canada) and isotonic saline (1 part solution to 6.6 parts blood).

The final heparin concentration was 4 U/ml. The blood sample remained unstirred in the beaker for 1 hour and then was used during the second hour (24). Human blood and dog blood were also collected in a beaker containing sodium citrate (1 part to 6.6 parts blood, pH 7.4-7.5, 9.8 mM final concentration in blood). These samples were used immediately.

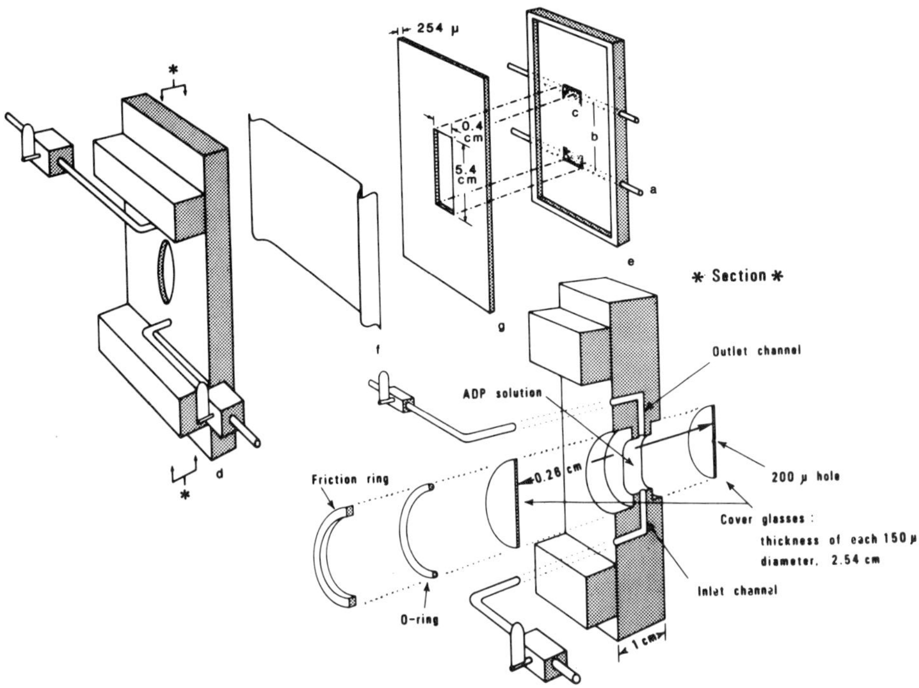

Figure 1. Blood flow chamber (Lucite): exploded view with inset showing details of passage for flow of ADP solution. Blood enters one of the two stainless steel lower ports (a), 0.20 cm inner diameter, and exits from the diagonally opposite upper one. Other ports, normally sealed, allow for cleaning. Headers (b), also 0.20 cm inner diameter, 0.10 ml volume each, are cylindrical and have carefully streamlined junctions (c) with the blood passage proper. When clamped together, the chamber lid (d) and base (e) are separated only by a Cuprophan membrane (f) and Silastic gasket-spacer (g).

Sodium pentobarbital (30 mg/kg, Diabutal, Diamond Laboratories Inc., Palo Alto CA) was administered i.v. prior to blood withdrawal from the jugular vein of dogs or the femoral vein of rabbits, while phencyclidine hydrochloride (1 mg/kg, Sernylan, Bio-Ceutic Lab., St. Joseph MO) was given i.v. before drawing blood from the antecubital or femoral vein of macaques and baboons. Control experiments with unanesthetized dogs and macaques indicated that the anesthetics did not affect the levels of platelet adhesion. Veins

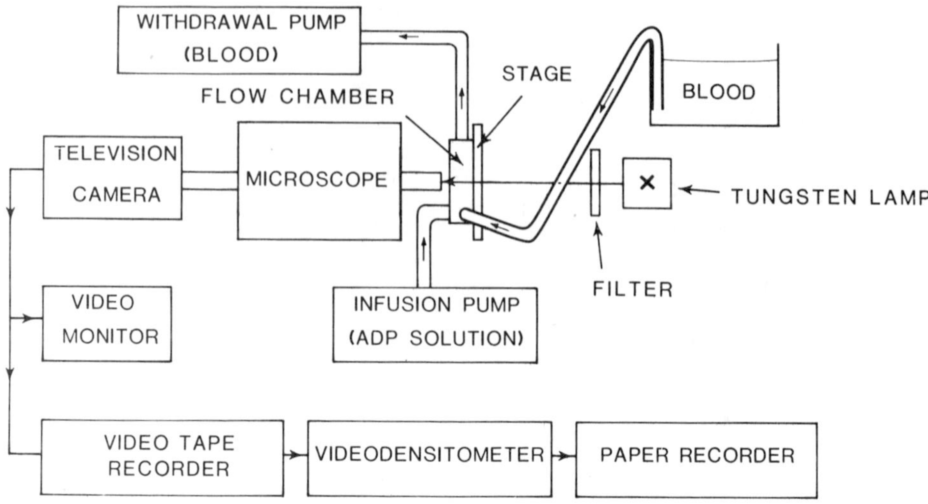

Figure 2. Block diagram showing the principal components of the present experimental system.

used for blood withdrawal for the other species were the antecubital (humans), jugular (calf and sheep), or antecubital or femoral (hogs). None of the animals or human subjects had received acetylsalicyclic acid or any other medication for at least 1 week before the blood samples were drawn.

In all species except sheep and calves, platelets were counted with a Coulter Counter Model B; blood samples were diluted by 13% with anticoagulant solution. In the case of sheep and calves, difficulty in sedimenting red blood cells and overlap between platelet and red blood cell volumes made it necessary to use manual counting (25) or the Technicon Auto Counter or Hemalog 8. Leukocytes were counted with a Coulter Counter Model A. Hematocrits were determined by the microhematocrit method.

Experiments. Membrane specimens were exposed to non-recirculated blood for 5 or 10 min at a surface shear rate (based on the bulk flow) of 986 sec^{-1}, or to recirculated blood for 30 or 180 min at the same shear rate. Additional 10-min experiments with human and dog blood were carried out at rates of 99, 197, and 394 sec^{-1}. After a 1-min chamber washout with prefill solution, membrane specimens were carefully removed from the chamber, fixed in 1% glutaraldehyde for 1 hr, stained with Wright's stain (except for Cuprophan), mounted between a microscope slide and cover slip, and examined at 625X by either phase contrast microscopy (Cuprophan) or light microscopy (other surfaces). Platelets were

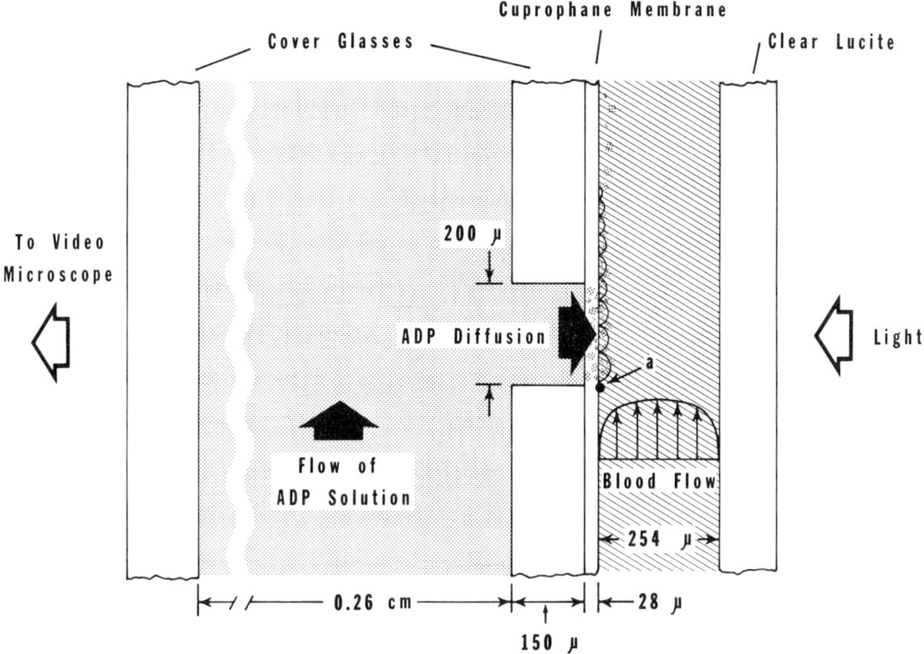

Figure 3. Chamber detail showing site of ADP entry by diffusion (membrane permeation). Surface irregularities represent adherent platelet aggregates, while dots in blood passage denote ADP molecules. Blunt blood velocity profile has been exaggerated for clarity. Wavelength of incident light is 800 ± 90 nm (mean ± half-width for half-maximum transmission). Not depicted is a light stop with a slit paralleling in size and orientation the blood passage (to avoid glare). ADP entry was not used in the platelet adhesion studies.

counted in several regions along the direction of flow. These regions were distributed over a distance that was small compared to the total length (5.4 cm) of the blood passage and were located midway between sides of the blood passage and midway between the chamber upstream and downstream ends.

In order to determine the sensitivity of the counting method (minimum detectable level of platelet adhesion) with Cuprophan, especially in the low count range, pre-wetted Cuprophan membranes were examined by phase microscopy for platelet-sized artifacts without exposure to flowing blood. The resulting count (mean ± SD) for 4 membranes was 31 ± 22/mm^2, so the sensitivity of the method with Cuprophan was taken to be ~100/mm^2. Sensitivity with the other biomaterials was judged to be at least as good. Therefore, levels of adhesion <100/mm^2 are simply reported as such rather than assigning a numerical value to them.

Scanning Electron Microscopy (SEM). Cuprophan and Avcothane membrane samples were examined by SEM (26).

Videomicroscopy. In situ observation and monitoring of the surface upon which the platelets adhered was possible by videomicroscopy (Figures 2 and 3), as described in the second part of this review. This capability was important in determining the presence or absence of surface-adherent platelet aggregates (as small as 25-50 microns in diameter) and flowing emboli in individual runs. Chamber design and streamlining ensured that such aggregates and emboli were not generated by chamber headers and/or inlet-outlet ports.

Results in Platelet Adhesion Studies

Table 1 summarizes heparinized blood platelet count, white cell count, hematocrit, and pH 1 hr after blood withdrawal for the 10-min studies. In addition, platelet counts are presented for blood collected into citrate (9.8 mM final concentration) and similarly diluted by 13% with the anticoagulant. The dog platelet counts were significantly lower in heparin than in citrate ($p < 0.01$ by the t test); similar differences observed with three other species were not statistically significant. The greatest species differences were in platelet counts, these counts ranging from 86,000 (dog) to 497,000/μl (hog). Significant, but lesser, variations are apparent in the other parameters.

Under phase microscopy, adherent dog (heparin and citrate) and rabbit (heparin) platelets generally appeared stellate on Cuprophan, due to pseudopod extension. Although usually single, platelets of both species occasionally appeared in chains of three or four in close proximity. Adherent platelets from the other six species were never positively identified, except for human platelets (heparin) at 30 min, which proved also to be stellate. With the other biomaterials, comparable observations were not possible because the membranes are relatively nontransparent and so their surfaces could not be studied well by light or phase contrast microscopy. Staining and light microscopy, however, generally revealed adherent platelets from all species, when present, to be single. SEM has confirmed the above impressions for dog (heparin and citrate) platelets (Figure 4) on Cuprophan, and for dog (heparin) platelets on Avcothane. Human (heparin and citrate) platelets have never been found on Cuprophan at 10 min by SEM (see below). Adherent *leukocytes* were almost never observed in 10-min Cuprophan runs.

Table 1. pH, Platelet and Leukocyte Counts, and Hematocrit [Mean ± SD, (N)*] of Blood Used for 10-min Experiments in Different Species§

Species	pH†	(Platelets/μl) x 10^{-3} Heparin	Citrate	Hematocrit(%)	Leukocytes/μl
Human	7.43±0.04(8)	170±59(8)	194±26(3)	40.3±2.1(8)	6,200±2,000(7)
Dog	7.45±0.02(5)	86±38(5)	270±70(4)	40.6±4.4(5)	14,600±3,000(5)
Rabbit	7.36±0.09(4)	453±101(3)	479±131(3)	32.0±2.5(4)	7,000±1,600(4)
Calf	7.47±0.02(9)	434±179(7)	359 (1)	30.4±3.5(10)	8,500±3,200(10)
Baboon	7.41±0.05(4)	246±137(3)	336±35(4)	38.9±4.8(4)	8,000±3,800(3)
Macaque	7.43±0.06(4)	322±160(4)		37.1±2.0(4)	6,200±2,300(4)
Hog	7.36±0.14(4)	497±180(4)		32.0±0.9(4)	21,700±4,800(4)
Sheep	7.47±0.05(4)	203 (1)		35.2±2.1(4)	8,200±2,500(4)

*N is the number of different human subjects or animals of a given species.

†pH values presented here are lower than those stated in a previous publication (23); the present values include a correction for a measurement artifact due to blood sample warming.

§In this and the succeeding table approximations to population standard deviations and standard errors are presented. These approximations were obtained by applying "small N" corrections to calculated sample standard deviations and standard errors.

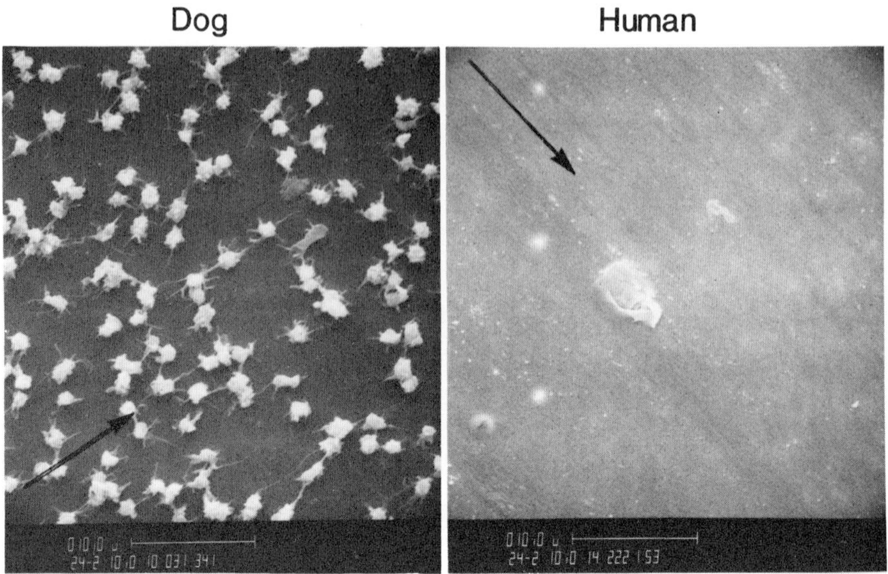

Figure 4: Scanning EM of Cuprophan exposed to citrated dog and human blood for 10 min at 986 sec^{-1}. Dog platelets but not human platelets are visible. Clarity of surface artifact of panel labeled "human" confirms that surface is in focus. Arrows indicate directions of the bulk flow.

Platelet Adhesion at 10 Minutes. Figures 4 and 5 show that in the 10-min runs on Cuprophan, adhesion of dog platelets was at least two to three orders of magnitude greater than that of human platelets. The difference increased as shear rate increased over the range of 99 to 986 sec^{-1}. Choice of anticoagulant had no significant effect on adhesion level.

Table 2 indicates that the species differed markedly in platelet adhesion on 10-min runs at a surface shear rate of 986 sec^{-1}; heparinized blood was used for these comparisons. Rabbit as well as dog platelet adhesion levels on Cuprophan were at least two to three orders of magnitude greater than those of human platelets or of platelets from any of the other five species. Dog platelet levels on Avcothane were comparable to those on Cuprophan or Gore-Tex, while human platelet adhesion to Avcothane, Cuprophan, or fluorinated ethylcellulose was virtually absent. In the two-sided Wilcoxon rank-sum test, these differences are all significant

Table 2. Platelets/mm^2 [Mean ± SE (N)*] After 10 Minutes of Blood Flow at a Surface Shear Rate of 986 sec^{-1}

Species	Cuprophan PT-150	Avcothane 51	Compressed Gore-Tex	Fluorinated Ethylcellulose
Human	<100 (4)	<100 (4)	6,000±3,200(8)	5,600±5,000(4)
Dog	27,400±4,600(5)	19,400±9,300(4)	16,200±8,300(8)	5,500±3,500(4)
Rabbit	78,400±6,400(4)	-	-	-
Calf	<100 (4)	-	13,500±9,800(5)	-
Baboon, macaque, hog, or sheep	<100 (4)†	-	-	-

*N is the number of different subjects or animals; heparinized blood was used for these comparisons.
†N = 4 for each of the four species grouped here.

($p = 0.05$). Further, a two-sided Student's t test shows the dog-rabbit difference on Cuprophan to be significant ($p < 0.005$).

Not only were there species differences, but platelets from the blood of a given species behaved differently on different biomaterials. Dog platelet adhesion to fluorinated ethylcellulose was significantly less than adhesion to Cuprophan or Avcothane ($p < 0.05$ by the t test). In contrast, human platelet adhesion to compressed Gore-Tex and fluorinated ethylcellulose far exceeded that to Cuprophan or Avcothane, while calf platelet adhesion to compressed Gore-Tex far exceeded that to Cuprophan ($p = 0.05$ by the Wilcoxon test in all three comparisons).

By videomicroscopy, surface-adherent platelet aggregates were not observed forming in any of these 10-min runs.

Adhesion Over 3-hr Period. Despite exposure times with recirculated blood of up to 3 hr, human platelet adhesion to Cuprophan remained negligible in comparison to that in the dog (23). Human platelet adhesion, in fact, exceeded 100/mm^2 only at 30 min and only for one subject, the value being 1300/mm^2. For the other three subjects adherent platelets were identified in isolated areas outside the counting region; such isolated areas were absent at 10 and 180 min. Dog platelet adhesion at 3 hr, however, was significantly less than adhesion at 30 min ($p < 0.05$ by the t test), suggesting removal (or detachment) of platelets (23).

Adherent *granulocytes* were observed on Cuprophan at 3 hr in three of six human subjects. Adhesion averaged 6.0/mm^2 (range 0 to 22/mm^2) for all six subjects. Unlike the case with platelets, even 1 leukocyte per microscopic field could be clearly identified. In 3-hr experiments with dog blood no adherent leukocytes were observed.

By videomicroscopy, isolated surface adherent platelet aggregates were transiently observed on Cuprophan in 3-hr runs with human, but not dog, blood. These aggregates, about 100 microns in diameter, appeared only after 15 to 20 min of blood flow and embolized completely after 1 to 2 hr of flow.

Discussion of Platelet Adhesion Studies

Species Differences. These studies showed surface-dependent differences between mammalian species with respect to platelet adhesion to foreign surfaces exposed to flowing blood. For example, on Cuprophan after 10 min at a surface shear rate of 986 sec^{-1}, adhesion of platelets from the human, calf, baboon, macaque, pig, or sheep was negligible compared to adhesion of dog or rabbit platelets. These differences 1) are present for surfaces of current clinical and research importance, 2) are present over the range of shear rates from 99 to 986 sec^{-1}, 3) are present in both citrated and heparinized blood, 4) persist at exposure times of up to 3 hr with recirculated blood, and 5) are unlikely only an artifact of the possible formation and embolization of surface-adherent platelet aggregates. The mechanism (or mechanisms) behind the species variations remains obscure, and could involve a plasma factor, the platelets, or both.

The *in situ*, continuous monitoring of the blood-biomaterial interfaces by means of video techniques was particularly valuable in evaluating surface-adherent aggregates and flowing emboli as complicating factors in the results. In particular, neither adherent aggregates nor flowing emboli (23) were detected in any of the 10-min runs. This suggests that embolization of surface adherent aggregates is unlikely to be a factor in the results shown in Table 2.

Species differences in some of the parameters in Table 1 might explain some differences in platelet adhesion. In particular, differences in hematocrit imply slight variations in whole blood viscosity. Yet none of these variations seems capable of accounting for differences in platelet adhesion of two to three orders of magnitude. If corrected upwards 13% for the effects of dilution with anticoagulant solution, the reported platelet and leukocyte counts and hematocrits are within known normal ranges for each species. An exception is the dog platelet counts, which initially are reduced in heparinized blood in comparison to citrated blood. The reduction appears to be due to in-bulk platelet aggregation, as is suggested by the early-time difference in frequency of flowing emboli for dog and human blood (23). The aggregation seems to be largely reversible, however, for the dog platelet count in heparin rises toward normal values by 3 hr (23).

Roles of Blood Flow. From the standpoint of macroscopic transport theory, platelet adhesion to a surface exposed to flowing blood may be considered a two-step process: 1) convection (delivery by flow) of fresh platelets to the surface, and 2) reaction, i.e., adhesion, of some or all of those platelets with the surface. In general, either or both steps may be rate-limiting.

If the rate of reaction is slow compared to convection, one should expect relatively low levels of platelet adhesion which are insensitive to changes in shear rate or flow rate. Such is the case for human platelet adhesion to Cuprophan, as shown in Figure 5. The reaction step appears also to be rate-limiting in the case of adhesion of calf, baboon, macaque, pig, or sheep platelets to Cuprophan.

On the other hand, if the rate of reaction is fast compared

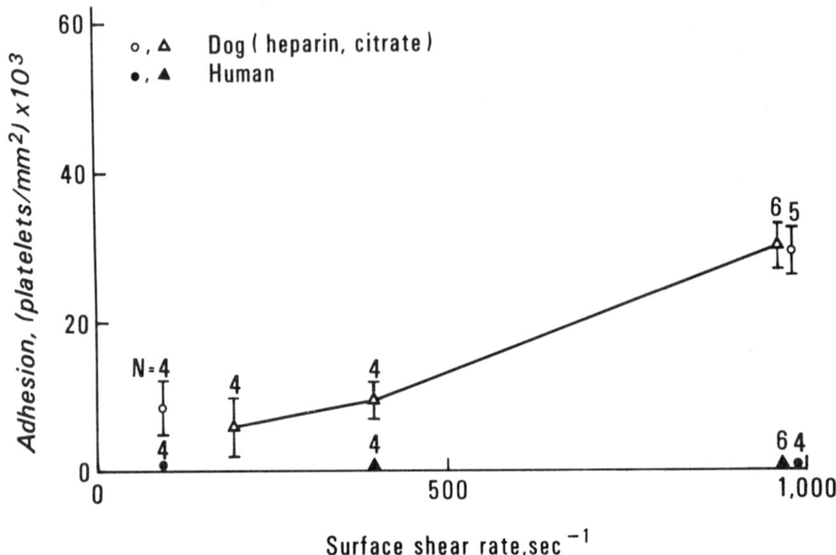

Figure 5. Human platelet and dog platelet adhesion to Cuprophan as a function of surface shear rate. Bars denote approximations to population standard errors.

to convection, one should anticipate relatively high levels of platelet adhesion which increase with increasing shear rates. Adhesion is then said to be"diffusion limited". Dog platelet adhesion fits this category, as also shown in Figure 5; so does rabbit platelet adhesion.

In brief, levels of human and animal platelet adhesion fall into one of two groups, and the groups represent extreme cases of a macroscopic transport mechanism which always involves blood flow.

A special effect of red blood cells which contributes to the convection or delivery step above is an augmentation of the effective diffusion coefficient for platelets. In platelet-rich plasma (PRP) only thermal fluctuations can impart diffusive motion to platelets, and one can calculate from the Stokes-Einstein equation a Brownian motion diffusivity of only about 1.6×10^{-9} cm^2/sec In the presence of erythrocytes and shear flow, however, the red cells appear to behave as "micro stirrers", tumbling as they do in response to a local fluid gradient in velocity (Figure 6). If one could neglect red cell-red cell interactions, the red cells would have approximately the same time-averaged vorticity, or

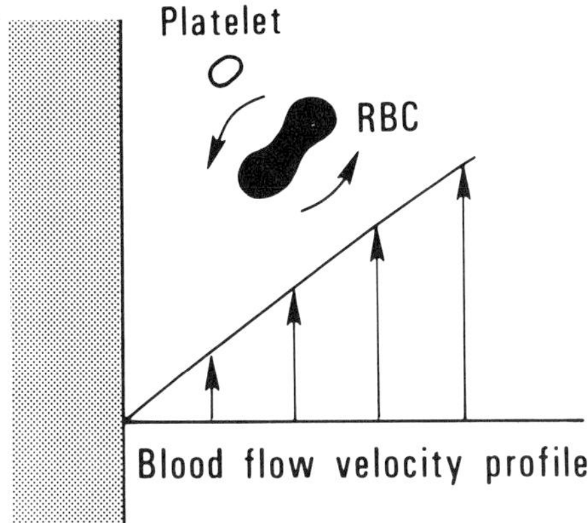

Figure 6. Red blood cell depicted as a "micro stirrer" of platelets. Erythrocyte turns, or tumbles, in response to a gradient in bulk flow velocity across the cell's breadth.

turning motion, as the local flow. But of course such interactions are important. The tumbling results in fluctuations in platelet position beyond those due to thermal motions.

Experiments and calculations suggest, in fact, that the effective diffusivity is actually of the order 10^{-7} cm^2/sec and increases with increasing shear rate (5,12). Moreover, initial rates of platelet adhesion achieved with whole blood are some two orders of magnitude greater than initial rates obtained using PRP and identical shear rates (9,12).

PLATELET AGGREGATION STUDIES

Methods

Blood Flow System. The flow system used was that described in the platelet adhesion studies. Citrated dog blood was used primarily.

ADP Entry. ADP (adenosine 5'-diphosphate from equine muscle, disodium salt, Sigma) was dissolved in divalent cation-free Tyrode's solution and stored in small aliquots at -20°C until immediately before use. ADP solution was pumped continuously (0.299 ml/min) through the chamber without contacting the blood directly (Figures 2 and 3), the ADP entering the blood by passive diffusion across a local region of Cuprophan membrane. This local region was an ultrasonically drilled, 200-μm diameter hole in a glass cover slip. The orifice itself was physically isolated from the flowing blood by the membrane, held against the cover slip by a blood-ADP solution hydrostatic pressure difference of 26 mmHg. This pressure difference also offset the osmotic pressure of blood proteins (27) which otherwise would have drawn water across the membrane from the ADP solution and even carried some ADP (and hydrated sodium and chloride ions) by solvent drag.

In order to assess the time course of ADP entry and to measure actual entry rates, a special procedure (28,29) was devised using tritiated ADP (50 μCi/ml in isotonic saline, New England Nuclear), to which was added sufficient non-labeled ADP to bring its final concentration to 50 mmolal. This allowed calculation of ADP entry rates from levels of ^{3}H-ADP appearing in the chamber outflow.

Video-optical System. Aggregate growth was visualized and quantified by means of videomicroscopy and dual window densitometry of video recordings. The videomicroscope consisted of a television camera (Model 2810-200, Cohu Electronics) with a broadcast-quality sync generator and a silicon diode tube (Model 4532, RCA) optically coupled to a microscope (Leitz Orthoplan). With the videomicroscope objective (6X) focused at the blood membrane interface near the site for ADP entry, adherent and growing platelet aggregates were observed with transmitted light (tungsten source; infrared transmitting visible absorbing filter No. 7-69, Dow Corning).

Wavelength of the incident light was 800 ± 90 nm (mean ± halfwidth for half-maximum transmission; peak transmission 82%). The choice of range of wavelength was based upon two considerations. First, by avoiding the absorption peaks for hemoglobin at 541 and 577 nm and the Soret band at still lower wavelength, one can avoid a range of wavelength over which the optical density of blood or packed platelets changes markedly with wavelength. This is advantageous for the mathematical formulation referred to below. Second, the mean wavelength is near an isobestic point (805 nm) of the hemoglobin and oxyhemoglobin absorption spectra, a wavelength at which light absorption by the two pigments is equal. For this particular isobestic point, at which the spectra cross at a relatively small angle, degree of transmitted light should be relatively independent of degree of oxygen saturation of the blood even for a modest (100 to 200 nm) range of wavelength about this point. Insofar as the incident light is in the near infrared range, use of the silicone diode tube provided special sensitivity. Moreover, the tube signal output is virtually linear with respect to illumination incident on the tube face over a dynamic range of 50.

As the aggregates locally displaced whole blood, the local blood film thickness and optical density were reduced, as is suggested in Figure 3. Increases in local light transmission were recorded continuously onto video tape (Ampex Model VR 1100 video recorder) for 5 to 10 min for subsequent analysis with a dual window videodensitometer (28,29).

Quantitative analysis was based on applicability of the Lambert-Beer Law, which expresses the relationship at a specific wavelength of light between optical density and the concentration and thickness of a solution. Details of this quantitative analysis appear elsewhere (28,29). Briefly the mean thickness of a local deposit of aggregates can be related to the difference between the intensity signals (voltages) produced by the two densitometer windows, one of which corrected for background transmission. The absorptivities (optical densities per unit path length) of both whole blood (hematocrit 35 to 45%) and packed platelets are required for this procedure and are determined separately over the range of wavelength from 700 to 900 nm. Calibration is achieved using gasket-spacers of known thicknesses.

A representative paper recording from the dual window densitometer appears in Figure 7, in which mean aggregate thickness is depicted as a function of time following the onset of ADP entry. One measureable parameter (shown) is the maximum growth rate. Note the embolization about 5 min into the experiment.

ADP entry rate $= 3.3 \times 10^3 \ \frac{\text{pmols}}{\text{cm}^2 \cdot \text{sec}}$

Surface shear rate $= 986 \ \text{sec}^{-1}$

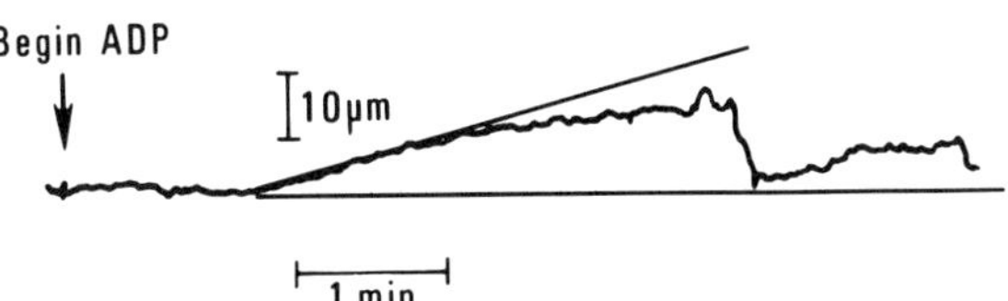

Figure 7. Paper recording of calibrated output from videodensitometer: mean aggregate thickness as a function of time.

Platelet Adhesion Before ADP Entry. Preliminary experiments with the present experimental system indicated that, at an ADP entry rate of 3.3 pmols/cm^2-sec and a shear rate of 986 sec^{-1}, 5 to 10 min of infusion of the ADP solution were required before visible aggregation occurred. On the other hand, when ADP entry was delayed for 10 min, visible aggregation began within 2 min after the infusion began. The latter time is similar to that required for washout of a pre-fill solution in the ADP solution passage (28,29). Such a phenomenon is compatible with the hypothesis that platelet aggregation on a foreign surface depends upon - perhaps requires - a certain degree of prior platelet adhesion and/or prior adsorption of one or more plasma proteins. Certainly platelet adhesion has been observed to precede as well as occur simultaneously with platelet aggregation on other synthetic surfaces see, for instance (3).

Experiments. In order to standardize the degree of prior platelet adhesion (or prior protein adsorption), in the principal experiments of this work the onset of ADP infusion was delayed for 10 min and only a shear rate of 986 sec^{-1} was used during that delay. Adjustment to the desired shear rate for the "aggregation phase" of a run was made at the time of onset of infusion.

ADP entry rate and shear rate were varied independently. One set of experiments was directed at characterizing aggregate growth rates as a function of reservoir ADP concentration (or entry rate) at one particular shear rate. The blood of each of three to four animals was studied on one to four occasions at each of four ADP concentrations (0.05, 0.50, 5.0 and 50 mmolal), or alternatively, four ADP entry rates (3.3 x 10^{-3}, 3.3 x 10^{-2}, 3.3 x 10^{-1} and 3.3 pmols/cm^2-sec). The main set of experiments aimed to characterize aggregate growth rates as a function of shear rate at each of two reservoir ADP concentrations (0.05 and 50 mmolal). Again, the blood of each animal was studied on one to four occasions for each experimental condition. In a few control runs, ADP entry was never begun, and we noted the extent of aggregation for periods of up to 60 min.

In order to explore the role of red blood cells in platelet aggregation, we used platelet-rich plasma (PRP) in four experiments in different dogs; the shear rate was 986 sec^{-1} and ADP entry rate, 3.3 pmols/cm^2-sec. PRP was obtained by centrifuging whole blood at 300 *g* for 10 min. In two of these experiments, PRP was used following 10 min of prior flow with whole blood. Start of the ADP pump coincided with the onset of the flow of PRP. In the other two experiments, only PRP was utilized. Onset of ADP entry followed 10 min of prior flow with PRP. In all four experiments, imaging was made possible by displacing the PRP with platelet-poor whole blood beginning 5 min after the ADP pump was started. Platelet-poor whole blood was prepared by centrifuging PRP at 200 *g* for 15 min, drawing off platelet-poor plasma (PPP), and then suspending the packed red blood cells in the PPP.

Throughout these quantitative studies, qualitative videomicroscopic observations were made on the nature of the surface-adherent platelet aggregates generated.

Results

Videomicroscopy. In general, a visible comet-shaped pattern of distinct platelet aggregates began to develop at and downstream from the ADP entry site within 1.5 to 5 min after the ADP infusion began. Repeated growth, embolization, and regrowth of the aggregates occurred, although the cycle required up to several minutes. Figure 8 shows aggregate growth before significant embolization of individual aggregates had occurred. When a solution of divalent cation-free Tyrode's solution was used to displace the ADP solution,

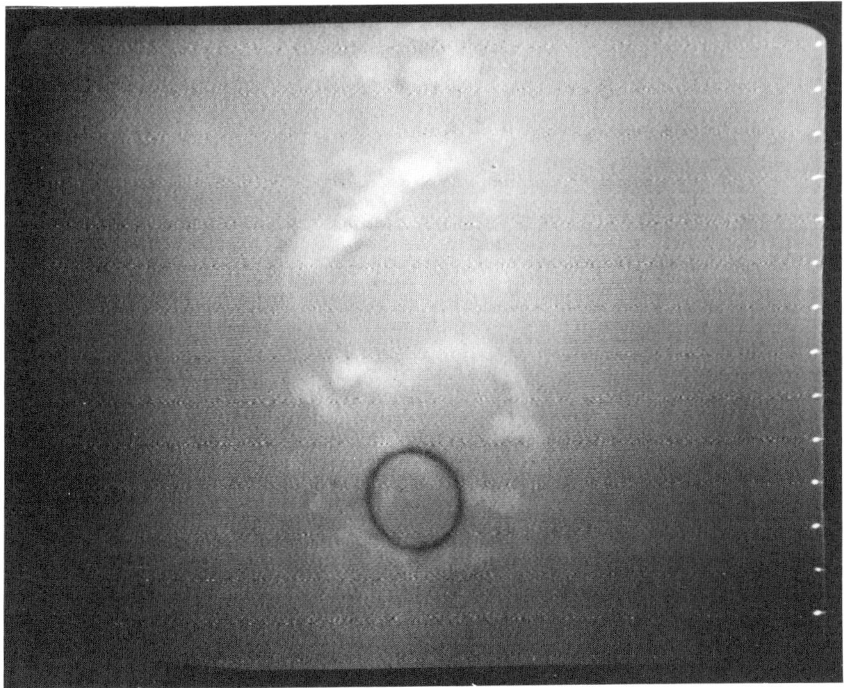

Figure 8. Aggregate growth pattern with infusion of 50 mmolal ADP solution and blood surface shear rate of 394 sec^{-1}; 4 minutes 36 seconds following onset of infusion. Blood flow is from bottom to top.

fresh aggregation ceased within a few minutes, while pre-existing aggregates embolized. Hence the surface adherence of aggregates, but not necessarily platelet cohesion, was reversible.

Rate of embolization and regrowth, although not quantified in this work, increased with increasing shear rate. Also, with increasing shear rate, there was an increasing tendency for adherent aggregates to "slide" slowly downstream and coalesce with other aggregates. The end result was fewer, but larger, platelet masses. With systematically heparinized dog blood (30) adherent aggregates tended to "peel off" the surface rather than slide. Initial rates of aggregate growth, however, were comparable.

The studies with PRP revealed that no aggregation occurred when PRP was used alone. However, aggregation with PRP readily took place after Cuprophan had been exposed to 10 min flow with whole blood.

Videodensitometry. Aggregate growth rates increased with increasing ADP entry rate, the values seeming to follow an "S"-shape curve (31). Figure 9 reveals that this same quantity had a complex dependence on shear rate and ADP entry rate. At the higher

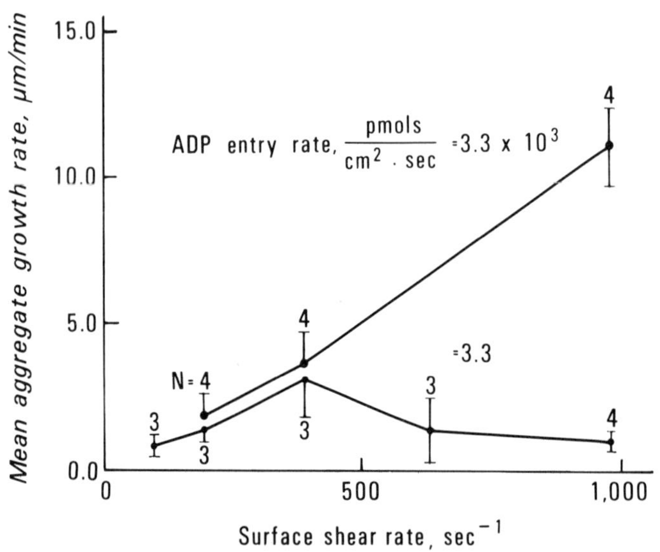

Figure 9. Mean aggregate growth rate as function of surface shear rate for two ADP entry rates. N = number of different animals. Bars again denote approximations to population standard errors. Sensitivity of method is about 1 micron per minute.

ADP entry rate, growth rate increased with increasing shear rate over the entire range of shear rates. At the lower ADP entry rate, on the other hand, this quantity passed through a maximum at a shear rate between 394 and 635 sec^{-1}. The maximum mean observed growth rate ($\pm$ SD) in three animals was 3.1 $\pm$ 1.9 µm/min and occurred at 394 sec^{-1}.

We did not try to normalize growth rates with respect to bulk platelet count because platelet aggregate growth rates should not depend on the platelet count but rather depend on the thrombocrit: the product of circulating platelet count and mean platelet volume. Although thrombocrits were not measured in this study, there is some evidence that the thrombocrit among different human subjects (32) and among species (33) may be constant despite variations in platelet count.

In the runs in which ADP entry was never begun, no visible aggregation occurred in the vicinity of the hole for up to 60 min and the densitometer output remained flat. Platelet counts taken at random times for blood samples from the chamber outflow did not differ significantly from those for beaker samples.

Discussion of Platelet Aggregation Studies

ADP Entry. The method used for ADP entry in these experiments has several advantages. First, the ADP entry rate is independent of blood flow rate, because the limiting resistance results from the membrane barrier itself and the "unstirred" layer within the orifice. Resistances associated with the flows of blood and ADP solution outside the orifice are neglible by comparison (28, 29). Second, entry rate is determined by and proportional to the inflow ADP concentration (0.05, 0.50, 5.0, or 50 mmolal). Third, the blood flow remains undisturbed, which would not be the case were ADP solution infused. Fourth, only a very narrow, boundary layer region of the blood film is affected by ADP. This feature leads to the formation of membrane-adherent platelet aggregates which grow and eventually embolize, yet leaves the platelets in the bulk of the blood unaffected.

The nature of this boundary layer and the relationship of ADP entry rate to the concentration distribution of ADP in blood are suggested in Figure 10, which is an enlargement of the neighborhood of the point "a" in Figure 3. Figure 10 depicts conceptually the boundary layer, where the local boundary layer thickness δ may be defined as the local distance from the membrane of a contour of constant concentration (1% of some surface reference). Both the ADP concentration and flow velocity depend on distance from the membrane and surface shear rate (dotted vs. solid arrows); ADP concentration additionally depends upon location along the membrane.

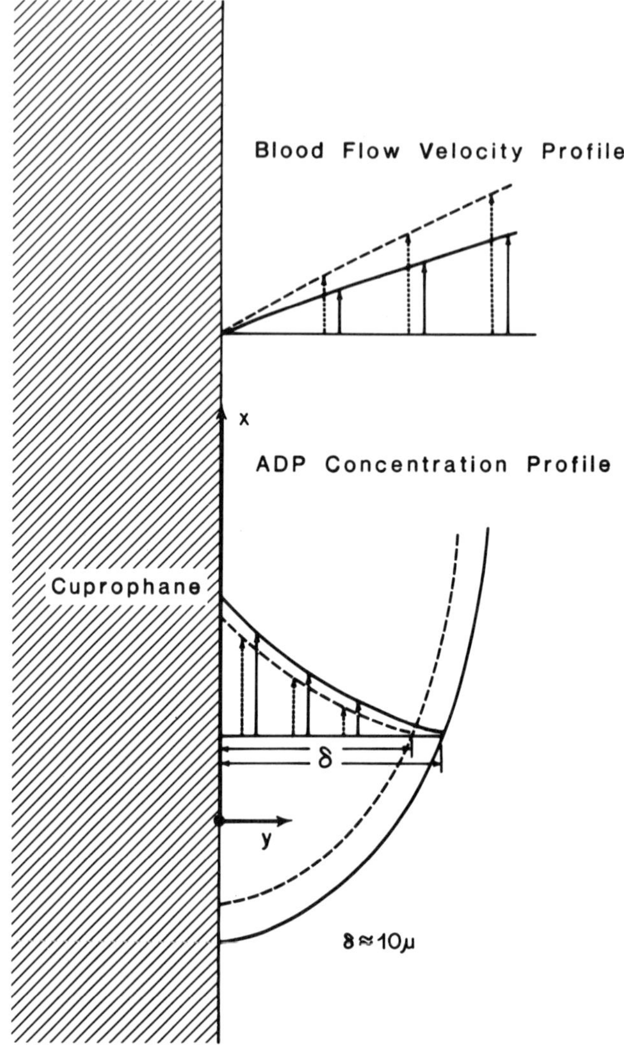

Figure 10. Enlargement of the neighborhood of point "a" of Figure 3, showing blood flow velocity and ADP concentration profiles for a lower (solid curves) and higher (dotted curves) surface shear rate.

Near the upstream end of the ADP entry site the thickness δ can be estimated to be of the order of ten microns or less (28,29). In principle one can determine the ADP concentration distribution upon numerical solution of an appropriate mathematical boundary value problem (20).

The ^{3}H-ADP studies indicated that some minutes are required for the ADP entry rate to attain a steady state; the 90% response time is 3 min. However, the dominant resistance to ADP transport is always the membrane itself (plus an "unstirred" fluid layer within the hole in the cover slip), provided that the shear rate in the blood passage is high enough. As a result, the ADP entry rate remains always essentially independent of blood shear rate in the range of the shear rates used.

The tracer studies also permitted calculation (28,29) of an effective permeability (cm/sec) of ADP to the membrane and unstirred layer. Deposition of plasma proteins on the membrane decreases the membrane's permeability to sucrose (molecular weight 342) by only 5% (33), so such deposition is unlikely to significantly reduce the permeability to ADP (MW 427). Therefore, we can estimate steady-state entry rates of ADP as the product of the permeability value for the membrane plus unstirred layer and the various inflow ADP concentrations. No correction for solvent drag is necessary (28,29).

Qualitative Observations. The observation of frequent and repetitive embolization and regrowth emphasizes the transient nature of surface-adherent aggregation and the need for its continuous *in situ* study. Thus, Baumgartner's conclusion (7) that mural thrombus formation is a transient phenomenon is certainly well founded. Therefore, evaluations of aggregate growth on subendothelium or synthetic surfaces exposed to flowing blood must take careful account of the dynamic, unstable nature of this growth.

It is not clear whether human platelets aggregate differently from dog platelets in the chamber. Preliminary observations suggest only that the number of individual aggregates comprising the comet-like pattern is far less with human blood, but this could be secondary to the negligible degree to which human platelets adhere to Cuprophan.

The presence of aggregation in PRP following prior exposure of Cuprophan to whole blood, but not prior exposure only to PRP itself implies that a pre-existing layer of adherent platelets may be required for aggregation. Clearly, red blood cells are not necessary for the aggregation process itself, provided only that a sufficient velocity gradient exists near the surface for platelets on faster moving streamlines to catch up with platelets on neighboring but slower moving streamlines.

Roles of Blood Flow. The strong positive dependence of aggregate growth rate on flow rate for the higher ADP entry rate (3.3×10^3 pmols/cm^2-sec) suggests growth limited by the rate of arrival by flow of fresh platelets, not finite platelet-ADP interaction times. The "reference ADP concentration", which occurs at the membrane-blood interface near the upstream end of the ADP entry region, is 1.5 mmolal at a shear rate of 394 sec^{-1}. This concentration is well above the threshold value for primary ADP-induced aggregation (35). It is particularly interesting, however, that the growth rate increases with increasing shear rate despite the simultaneous decrease in interface ADP concentration which must result from higher rates of flow and ADP dilution. Constancy of entry rate does not imply constancy of blood ADP levels, as is shown conceptually in Figure 10.

In contrast, at the lower rate of ADP entry (3.3 $pmols/cm^2$-sec) this flow dependence is markedly altered: the growth rate increases with increasing shear rate up to a shear rate of at least 394 sec^{-1}, but then decreases with increasing shear rate above that value.

One (or more) of three factors apparently becomes limiting at the higher shear rates: 1) levels of ADP, 2) finite platelet-ADP interaction times, and 3) shear stress in that such stress may oppose forces of platelet cohesion. Embolization is not involved, because the growth rates apply prior to any significant embolization.

The reference ADP concentration at 394 sec^{-1} is 1.5 μmolal, which is near threshold for primary ADP-induced aggregation. This suggests the hypothesis that a below-threshold level of ADP is the true limiting factor at higher shear rates. Such a hypothesis requires an ADP-platelet reaction time shorter than 200 msec (31) and the absence of major shear stress effects below a shear rate of about 1000 sec^{-1}.

Effects of shear stress are poorly understood. Brown *et al.* (17,18) have demonstrated shear stress levels (50 to 100 $dynes/cm^2$) in PRP above which platelets in bulk after several minutes show evidence of damage (release of acid phosphatase), liberation of ATP, ADP, and serotonin, and subsequent aggregation. Goldsmith (16) has reported that time- and space-averaged in-bulk shear stresses of 16.5 $dynes/cm^2$ in PRP subjected to oscillatory flow may, after several minutes, promote aggregation by enhancing the release reaction due to thrombin. Yet the importance of shear stress for platelet aggregation upon a surface exposed to whole blood at the shear stress levels of this work (5 to 50 $dynes/cm^2$) remains unclear.

SUMMARY OF ROLES OF BLOOD FLOW

Role of Blood Flow	Effect on: Platelet Adhesion	Effect on: Platelet Aggregation
Convection of platelets	↑	↑
Augmentation of platelet transport by red blood cell tumbling	↑	Qualitative not quantitative
Reduction of local levels of ADP and other aggregating substances	?	↓
Generation of shear stress	↓?	↓

ACKNOWLEDGEMENTS

I wish to express my warmest appreciation to Dr. Paul Didisheim for encouragement and helpful advice during the course of this work, to Kathleen K. Herther, James T. Franta, and John Q. Stropp for assistance with the experiments, to Dr. Jon C. Lewis and Joyce H. Borowick for the scanning electron micrographs, and to Rachael Baudoin for typing the manuscript.

REFERENCES

1. Didisheim P, Fuster V: Actions and clinical status in the management of platelet-suppressive agents. SEMIN HEMATOL, 1978. (In Press).

2. Genton E, Hirsh J, Gent M, Harker LA: Platelet-inhibiting drugs in thrombotic disease (in three parts). N ENGL J MED 293:1174-1178, 1236-1240, 1296-1300, 1975.

3. Petschek H, Adamis D, Kantrowitz AR: Stagnation flow thrombus formation. TRANS AM SOC ARTIF INTERN ORGANS 14:256-260, 1978.

4. Friedman LI, Leonard EF: Platelet adhesion to artificial surfaces: consequences of flow, exposure time, blood condition, and surface nature. FED PROC 30:1641-1646, 1971.

5. Grabowski EF, Friedman LI, Leonard EF: Effects of shear rate

on the diffusion and adhesion of blood platelets to a foreign surface. IND ENG CHEM FUNDAM 11:224-232, 1972.

6. Turitto VT, Leonard EF: Platelet adhesion to a spinning surface. TRANS AM SOC ARTIF INTERN ORGANS 18:348-354, 1972.

7. Baumgartner HR: The role of blood flow in platelet adhesion, fibrin deposition and formation of mural thrombi. MICROVASC RES 5:167-179, 1973.

8. Baumgartner HF: The subendothelial surface and thrombosis. THROMB DIATH HAEMORRH (Suppl) 59:91-105, 1974.

9. Turitto VT, Baumgartner HR: Platelet deposition on subendothelium exposed to flowing blood: Mathematical analysis of physical parameters. MICROVASC RES 9:335-344, 1975.

10. Poliwoda H, Hagemann G, Jacobi E: Velocity dependent interaction between platelets and different surfaces. In THEORETICAL AND CLINICAL HEMORHEOLOGY. Edited by Hartert HH, Copley AL, New York, Springer-Verlag, 1971, pp, 227-232.

11. Begent N, Born GVR: Growth rate *in vivo* of platelet thrombi, produced by iontophoresis of ADP, as a function of mean flow velocity. NATURE 227:926-930, 1970.

12. Turitto VT, Benis AM, Leonard EF: Platelet diffusion in flowing blood. IND ENG CHEM FUNDAM 11:216-223, 1972.

13. Richardson PD: Effect of blood flow velocity on growth rate of platelet thrombi. NATURE 245:103-104, 1973.

14. Born GVR: Quantitative investigations into the aggregation of blood platelets. J PHYSIOL 162:67P-68P, 1962.

15. O'Brien JR: Platelet aggregation. Part II. Some results from a new method of study. J CLIN PATHOL 15:446-455, 1962.

16. Goldsmith HL, Marlow JC, Yu SK: The effect of oscillatory flow on the release reaction and aggregation of human platelets. MICROVASC RES 11:335-359, 1976.

17. Brown CH, Lemuth RF, Hellums JD, Leverett JD, Alfrey CP: Response of human platelets to shear stress. TRANS AM SOC ARTIF INTERN ORGANS 21:35-38, 1975.

18. Brown CH, Leverett LB, Lewis CW, Alfrey CP, Hellums JD: Morphological, biochemical, and functional changes in human platelets subjected to shear stress. J LAB CLIN MED 86:462-471, 1975.

19. Monsler M, Morton W, Weiss R: The fluid mechanics of thrombus formation. In AMERICAN INSTITUTE OF AERONAUTICS AND ASTRONAUTICS 3rd FLUID AND PLASMA DYNAMICS CONFERENCE, Los Angeles, Calif. AIAA Paper No. 70-787, New York, 1970.

20. Grabowski EF: Momentum and mass transport in blood with application to thrombus formation. Doctoral Thesis, Columbia University, New York, 1972.

21. Arfors KE, Cockburn JS, Gross JF: Measurement of growth rate of laser-induced intravascular platelet aggregation and the influence of blood flow velocity. MICROVASC RES 11:79-87, 1976.

22. Ruckenstein E, Marmur A, Gill WN: Growth kinetics of platelet thrombi. J THEOR BIOL 66:147-168, 1977.

23. Grabowski EF, Didisheim P, Lewis JC, Franta JT, Stropp JQ: Platelet adhesion to foreign surfaces under controlled conditions of whole blood flow: Human vs rabbit, dog, calf, sheep, pig, macaque and baboon. TRANS AM SOC ARTIF INTERN ORGANS 23:141-149, 1977.

24. Grabowski EF, Herther KK, Didisheim P: Human versus dog platelet adhesion to Cuprophan under controlled conditions of whole blood flow. J LAB CLIN MED 88:368-374, 1976.

25. Brecher G, Cronkite EP: Morphology and enumeration of human blood platelets. J APPL PHYSIOL 3:365-377, 1950.

26. Lewis JC, Didisheim P, Grabowski EF, Zollman PE: Platelet adhesion to native and collagen coupled Cuprophan: A multispecies comparative SEM study. 35th Ann. Proc. Electron Microscopy Soc. Amer., pp. 648-649, 1977. (Abstract).

27. Landis EM, Pappenheimer JR: Exchange of substances through the capillary walls. In HANDBOOK OF PHYSIOLOGY, Amer. Physiol. Soc. Edited by Magoun HW, Washington, D.C., 1963, Williams and Wilkins, pp. 961-1034, Sect. 1, vol. II.

28. Grabowski EF: Platelet aggregation in flowing blood *in vitro*. I. Production by controlled ADP convective diffusion and quantification by videodensitometry. MICROVASC RES (In Press).

29. Grabowski EF, Herther KK, Didisheim P: Videomicroscopy and videodensitometry of platelet aggregation under controlled conditions of blood flow and ADP convective diffusion. In MICROCIRCULATION, edited by Grayson J, Zingg W, Plenum Press, vol. 1, 1976, pp. 197-199.

30. Grabowski EF, Herther KK, Didisheim P: Platelet aggregation quantified in an *ex vivo* chamber by means of videodensitometry. THROMB DIATH HAEMORRH (Suppl) 60:127-134, 1974.

31. Grabowski EF, Franta JT, Didisheim P: Platelet aggregation in flowing blood *in vitro*. II. Dependence of aggregate growth rate on ADP concentration and shear rate. MICROVASC RES (In Press).

32. Harker LA: Platelet production. N ENGL J MED 282:492-494, 1970.

33. Von Behrens WE: Evidence of phylogenetic canalisation of the circulating platelet mass in man. THROMB DIATH HAEMORRH 27: 159-172, 1972.

34. Colton CK, Smith KA, Merrill EW, Farrell PC: Permeability studies with cellulosic membranes. J BIOMED MATER RES 5:459-488, 1971.

35. Macmillan DC: Secondary clumping effect in human citrated platelet-rich plasma produced by adenosine diphosphate and adrenaline. NATURE 211:140-144, 1966.

SUMMARY OF DISCUSSION BY PARTICIPANTS

Dr. Spaet was concerned about the use of anticoagulants in this study because he thought that a similar conclusion about species differences might be drawn from platelet reactivity due at least in part to an artifact of anticoagulant addition. Dr. Grabowski replied that they were aware of this, and have begun to experiment with native whole blood, but this system does not lend itself to native blood. However, they have compared citrated and heparinized blood, and they found the same species differences with both preparations in terms of flow dependence on platelet adherence. The heparin concentration was 4U/ml and the citrate was 9.8 mM. Table 1 (in the paper) shows that heparin has a large effect on the initial bulk platelet concentration in dog blood. There is a general reduction of bulk concentration of platelets in the heparinized system, but the reduction is much greater in dogs than in humans. Dr. Didisheim remarked that these comparisons between platelet adhesion in heparinized and citrated blood would seem to rule out the role of ionized calcium concentration in the species difference. In the absence of anticoagulant, these experiments could only be done for a couple of minutes and would therefore not be satisfactory.[1]

Dr. Spaet also wondered about this flow system as compared to real life, because in blood flow through a blood vessel, there is a component of flow which is at a right angle to the main flow. In a flow chamber of this kind or in Dr. Baumgartner's model, in which the vessels are impermeable, the right angle component cannot be ascertained. According to Dr. Grabowski, Drs. Forstrom, Voss, and Blackshear (J FLUIDS ENGINEERING 96:168-172, 1974) have looked at this question as part of a study of particle deposition onto filtering surfaces. Such deposition, they state, is expected to occur when the drag force of filtration overcomes the fluid mechanic wall repulsive force. Since the latter force increases with surface shear rate, for a given filtration velocity there will exist a threshold shear rate below which deposition occurs (~50 sec^{-1} for platelets near arterial walls). Dr. Grabowski concludes from their work that for normal arterial walls, the right angle velocity component seems to be unimportant to platelet transport to the vessel intima for the range of surface shear rates (100-1000 sec^{-1}) he has investigated.

Dr. Spaet remarked that the closer the platelets get to the vessel wall where there is zero motion, the more important this component becomes because of the ability to suck the platelets in. Dr. Grabowski calculated that at a shear rate of 1000 sec^{-1}, the flow velocity at 1 micron from the surface (assuming this to be about the radius of a platelet) is of the order of a mm/sec (10^{-4} x 1000). Dr. Forstrom's estimate of the right angle velocity component, based on the experiments of Wilens (SCIENCE 114:389-393, 1951), is ~3 x 10^{-5} mm/sec. So the right angle velocity effect for the present shear rates is comparable to the bulk blood flow velocity only over distances from the surface which are small compared to the platelet itself. Although he does not dispute the possible

[1]Note added in proof:

Dr. Didisheim adds that recently it has been possible to study platelet adhesion by the method described by Dr. Grabowski, but in the absence of added anticoagulant. Using meticulous venipuncture technique (jugular vein in dogs, antecubital vein in humans) and a 16-gauge thin-wall needle attached to 60 cm of 2-mm (i.d.) Silastic tubing, satisfactory blood flow was maintained for 10 min at a surface shear rate of 986 sec^{-1} through the flow chamber. Under these conditions, the species difference in platelet adhesion persisted. The mean value for platelets per mm^2 Cuprophan membrane was 14,000 in four normal dogs in contrast to 0 in three normal human subjects.

importance of the effect in terms of platelet responses subsequent to platelet transport to the surface, Dr. Grabowski felt that the effect is not normally important within the context of the Forstrom analysis for the present shear rates.[2]

Dr. Mustard asked if Dr. Grabowski's data on species differences based mainly on Cuprophan membrane might not be due to the adsorption of different proportions of various proteins from the plasma of different species. Dr. Grabowski has not looked at different protein fractions in the various species, but prior exposure to the membrane of platelet-poor plasma (PPP) of a given dog increased that dog s platelet adherence without affecting observed differences in adhesion between dogs (intraspecies differences). Differences between species were observed with Avcothane and compressed Gore-Tex. Such observations support the idea of a plasma protein role but not one unique to Cuprophan.

Dr. Mustard wondered if Dr. Grabowski had done any work with collagen-coated surfaces and found species differences, because with Dr. Cazenave's method, no major differences in platelet adhesion could be demonstrated among species. Dr. Grabowski said that two colleagues, Drs. K. Mann and P. Didisheim, had used collagen-coupled Cuprophan in Dr. Grabowski's test system. Human, baboon, and sheep platelets all adhere to this surface in significant numbers; but the lack of species differences in numbers does not mean that the mechanism of adhesion is the same. In fact, the evidence is to the contrary. Dr. Lewis, another colleague, found that on collagen-coupled Cuprophan, dog and human platelets look different morphologically. Human platelets show evidence of cytoplasmic spread with a more filmy, lacy appearance. Dr. Mustard was not convinced that morphological differences gave key information, be-

[2]Note added in proof:

Dr. Grabowski adds that the Forstrom work assumes that the entire endothelial surface is uniformly available for filtration. If, however, filtration is confined to the interendothelial clefts, local right angle velocities would be higher approximately as the ratio of total endothelial surface area to cleft area. Given a sufficiently high ratio, Dr. Spaet's point might still be valid. In addition, Dr. Fernando Vargas (Department of Physiology, University of Minnesota, personal communication) is preparing to publish experimental results largely supporting Wilens' data. Vargas' estimate of the filtration coefficient for rabbit thoracic and abdominal aorta leads, for a 100-mmHg driving pressure, to a right angle velocity component comparable to Forstrom's. Equally important, total denudation of endothelium of his artery preparations by a "ballooning" technique increases the estimate of filtration coefficient only by a factor of 2.

cause many interpretations can be made of these pictures. He was more concerned about the point Dr. Salzman has made concerning the effects of adsorbed proteins on artificial surfaces. There is a high probability of protein adsorption and this could be an important factor in creating the species differences. Dr. Grabowski agreed that this indeed might be the case, as well as differences in platelets. He intended the term "platelet adhesion" in his paper to describe a phenomenon, not to identify platelets as necessarily being responsible for the observed species differences.

Dr. Salzman asked if on the basis of his study with dog and human platelets on Cuprophan, Gore-Tex, or fluorinated ethylcellulose, the species differences in platelet reactivity is surface related, i.e., on one type of surface more dog platelets stick and on another surface, fewer stick. Dr. Grabowski said yes. Dr. Salzman also asked if studies were done with other species. Dr. Grabowski said that he had looked at calf platelets on Gore-Tex and found a difference from human platelets, although on Cuprophan they were similar. Most of the studies have been done with human vs. dog platelets. He said that his system can double as an embolometer, i.e., it can measure numbers of flowing emboli using the videodensitometer. Using this as an endpoint, he sees further species differences between calf, human, and dog platelets.

PROTEINS SECRETED BY PLATELETS: SIGNIFICANCE IN DETECTING THROMBOSIS*

Karen L. Kaplan, M.D.,Ph.D.

Department of Medicine, Columbia University, College of Physicians and Surgeons, New York, NY

ABSTRACT

Because platelet survival measurements are time-consuming and may not completely reflect platelet involvement in hemostasis and thrombosis, other tests have been sought. Measurement of two proteins released by platelets, platelet factor 4 (PF4) and β-thromboglobulin (βTG), may provide simpler, more direct means of quantitating platelet involvement. The radioimmunoassays for these proteins reviewed in this paper are sensitive and specific. Although there are technical problems still to be resolved in their clinical application, clinical studies to date suggest that such assays will be useful in studying the pathogenesis and course of thromboembolic disorders. PF4 and βTG levels apparently do reflect *in vivo* platelet release. Because release of PF4 and βTG parallels release of platelet-derived growth factor, plasma PF4 and βTG levels should also reflect release of that protein. The PF4 and βTG assays along with an assay for fibrinopeptide A in clinical samples should help elucidate the relative importance of platelet release and fibrin formation in thromboembolic disorders.

*This work was supported by research grants from the National Institutes of Health (Program Project grants HL-15486 and HL-21006).

INTRODUCTION

When platelets are exposed to a vascular subendothelial surface *in vitro* they make contact, spread, degranulate, and aggregate to form platelet thrombi (1). There is evidence that a similar sequence of events occurs when endothelial loss is induced experimentally *in vivo*, e.g., by balloon catheterization (2), and it is very likely that platelet adhesion, release, and aggregation occur during platelet participation in normal hemostasis and pathologic thrombosis. Until recently the only method available for quantitating this platelet activation *in vivo* was measurement of the survival of radiolabeled platelets, and several studies have demonstrated shortened platelet survival in various thrombotic disorders (3-7). In humans degranulated platelets may, however, continue to circulate (8), and in animal systems disaggregated thrombin-degranulated platelets survive normally and partially correct the bleeding time when infused into a thrombocytopenic animal (9,10). Thus, platelet survival measurements may not completely reflect platelet involvement in hemostasis and thrombosis. Additionally, platelet survival studies are time-consuming and may be difficult to perform on large numbers of individuals or sequentially on patients at different stages of illness or therapy.

Measurement of a product of the platelet release reaction might provide a simpler, more direct means of quantitating *in vivo* platelet release (11). Materials released from the dense granules (ADP, ATP, serotonin, and calcium) are not practical for plasma measurements; however, over the last several years it has been recognized that proteins are released as well. The released proteins include platelet factor 4, which is a heparin-neutralizing protein (12-14); β-thromboglobulin (15,16), a factor which increases vascular permeability (17,18); a chemotactic factor (19); a bactericidal factor (20); fibrinogen (21); a protein which is mitogenic for smooth muscle cells, fibroblasts, and glial cells in tissue culture (22-25); and several acid hydrolases (26). At least two of these proteins, platelet factor 4 and β-thromboglobulin, appear to be platelet-specific. They have been isolated in several laboratories and immunoassays for them have been developed. A radioimmunoassay has also been developed for the mitogenic factor (27). The remainder of this report will review the isolation, characterization, and assay of platelet factor 4 and β-thromboglobulin and the potential use of such assays for detection of platelet involvement in thrombosis.

INITIAL DESCRIPTION, PURIFICATION, CHARACTERIZATION AND ASSAY

Platelet Factor 4 (PF4)

Several workers in the 1940's noted that thrombocytopenia was associated with increased sensitivity to heparin, suggesting that platelets contain a heparin-neutralizing material (28-30). A fraction responsible for the antiheparin activity was separated from platelets by VanCreveld and Paulssen (12,13) and termed platelet factor 4 by Deutsch (14). In the last few years workers in a number of laboratories have purified the protein responsible for most of the heparin-neutralizing activity of platelets, and it is suggested that the term PF4 be used for this protein rather than for heparin-neutralizing activity. Käser-Glanzmann *et al.* (31) purified PF4 from the supernatant of thrombin-treated washed platelets by chromatography on Sephadex G-200 and then Biogel A5M at 0.15M NaCl followed by chromatography on Sephadex G-75 at 0.75M NaCl. Moore and Pepper, also working with the supernatant of thrombin-treated washed platelets, used chromatography on Biogel A15M at 0.15M NaCl followed by chromatography on the same gel at 0.75M NaCl (32). Levine and Wohl (33) used heparin-EACA-agarose affinity chromatography to purify PF4 from the supernatant of outdated platelets, and Handin and Cohen (34) used heparin-agarose chromatography to purify PF4 from the supernatant of thrombin-treated washed platelets. Kaplan *et al.* have used either Biogel A15M chromatography or heparin-agarose chromatography (35). Deuel *et al.* used heparin-EACA-agarose chromatography (36) and Morgan *et al.* used heparin-agarose chromatography (37). Hermodsen *et al.* used chromatography on SP-Sephadex to purify PF4 (38). Nath *et al.* reported purification of PF4 by zinc precipitation and DEAE-cellulose chromatography (39); these workers now refer to this material as "low affinity PF4" because of its relatively weak heparin-binding capacity (40), and they state that "low affinity PF4" is responsible for 30% of the heparin-neutralizing activity of platelets, with PF4 accounting for the remainder.

PF4 is released from platelets bound to a proteoglycan carrier (31,32,41,42), and the PF4-carrier complex appears to have a molecular weight (MW) of about 350,000 by ultracentrifugal analysis (31,32, 41,42). PF4 can be dissociated from the carrier by high ionic strength (31,32,41,42). The carrier molecule is composed of four chondroitin sulfate chains of 12,000 MW and a polypeptide backbone of 11,000 MW, giving a total MW for the carrier of 59,000 (42). Each chondroitin sulfate chain binds one molecule of PF4 of about 29,000 MW as determined ultracentrifugally (31,32), and the complex occurs as a dimer giving rise to a material of 350,000 MW. The PF4 molecule appears to be composed of four identical subunits of 7,700 MW by amino acid sequence (36,38,43); thus, its actual MW is 31,000.

Several different subunit molecular weights have been reported based on sodium dodecyl sulfate polyacrylamide gel electrophoresis: 11,000 (33), 9,600 (34), and 5,500 (Kaplan, unpublished). This variation may be due to the difficulty of estimating molecular weights in this range by this technique (44) or it may reflect anomalous behavior of the PF4 molecule. The molecule has an interesting amino acid sequence with a concentration of acidic residues in the N-terminal end and a concentration of basic and hydrophobic residues at the C-terminal end (36,38,43). Evidence has been presented that lysine residues are responsible for the binding of PF4 to heparin (34) and it has been suggested that the C-terminal end with its high content of lysine is the heparin-binding site (36).

Workers in several laboratories have developed specific immunoassays for PF4. Gjesdahl has reported an electroimmunoassay for PF4 which requires concentration of both antiserum and plasma in order to measure plasma levels (45). More sensitive radioimmunoassays for PF4 have been reported by Bolton *et al.* (46), Handin *et al.* (47), Kaplan *et al.* (35), and Chesterman *et al.* (48). These radioimmunoassays are capable of detecting picogram quantities of PF4. Assays for heparin-neutralizing activity have been thought to measure PF4 in human plasma (49); however, careful correlations of heparin-neutralizing activity and PF4 content have not been performed.

β-Thromboglobulin (βTG)

In the case of PF4, a biologic activity (heparin neutralization) was recognized and then a protein possessing that activity was isolated and characterized. In contrast, β-thromboglobulin has been purified and characterized but no clear biologic activity has been identified. A specific β-globulin in platelets was first recognized by Salmon and Bounameaux (50) and Sokal (51). It was shown to be released from platelets during clotting by Nachman (52), Davey and Luscher (53), and Dzoga *et al.* (54). Moore *et al.* (15) and Moore and Pepper (16) first isolated this platelet-specific β-globulin from the supernatant of thrombin-treated washed platelets by a series of gel filtration steps using Biogel A15M, then Sephadex G-200 and finally Sephadex G-75 in pyridine-acetic acid to separate the βTG from albumin. Kaplan *et al.* purified βTG by similar methods (35). Moore and Pepper have also reported that βTG will bind to heparin-agarose columns but less tightly than does PF4, so that the two proteins can be separated by this technique (16). Rucinski and co-workers (49) have isolated a low-affinity heparin binding protein from platelets, which they call "low-affinity PF4", which appears to be quite similar to βTG with respect to amino acid analysis and pattern of migration in SDS polyacrilamide gel electrophoresis (39). "Low affinity PF4" and βTG share antigenic determinants by immunodiffusion and by radioimmunoassay, but whether they are identical or one is a degradation product of the other will not be known until amino acid sequencing studies of both proteins are completed.

βTG has a 36,000 MW, determined in the ultracentrifuge, and dissociates at acid pH to subunits of MW 6,500 (15,16). On sodium dodecyl sulfate polyacrylamide gels the material without reduction migrates as a 10,800 MW substance and after reduction as a 5,800 MW substance, which suggests an intrachain disulfide bridge (15,16). Amino acid analyses of βTG (16,35) show similarities to those of PF4 in some residues but are quite distinct in others (32-35, 41). Both molecules are low in aromatic residues. The isoelectric point of βTG is approximately 8, perhaps reflecting the relatively high lysine content (15,16).

Specific radioimmunoassays for βTG which are sensitive to picogram quantities have been reported by the Edinburgh group (55,56) and by Kaplan *et al.* (35). The radial immunodiffusion assay for "low affinity PF4" may measure the same antigen as the βTG assays (40,57).

CHARACTERISTICS OF RELEASE OF PF4 AND βTG

In vitro release of heparin-neutralizing activity from platelets by ADP (11,58-61), epinephrine (11,58-60), collagen (11, 58-61), and thrombin (11,58,59,61) has been recognized for a number strated, as has release of βTG by the same agents (35,55,62). Both PF4 and βTG are also released by epinephrine (Kaplan, unpublished results). Release of "low-affinity PF4" by ADP, collagen, thrombin, and antigen-antibody complexes has also been reported (40,57).

When thrombin (0.05 U/ml) is used to induce the release reaction, the time course of release of PF4, βTG, and the platelet-derived growth factor is similar to that of serotonin, ADP, and ATP and release of all these materials precedes release of acid hydrolases (62,63). However, when release is examined as a function of thrombin concentration, higher concentrations of thrombin are required to cause release of serotonin, ADP, and ATP than of PF4, βTG, and the platelet-derived growth factor, and acid hydrolase release requires still higher thrombin concentrations (35,62,63). One explanation for these findings is that PF4, βTG, and the growth factor occur in a third type of granule, distinct from dense granules and from lysosomes. The finding that only one of 14 patients with storage pool disease had a decreased platelet content of PF4, βTG, and the growth factor also provides evidence that the proteins are not located in the dense granules (64).

Besides being useful in the study of the platelet release reaction, the specific assays for PF4 and βTG can be used along with the specific assay for fibrinopeptide A (FPA) (65,66), the first product of thrombin action on fibrinogen, to study the interrelationship of fibrin formation and platelet release. FPA is not cleaved during release of PF4 and βTG by ADP or collagen in citrated platelet-rich plasma (35), thus ruling out a role of thrombin in the release reaction induced by those agents. Thrombin causes both FPA cleavage and platelet release, but FPA cleavage is detectable with thrombin concentrations 100 times lower than those needed to induce platelet release (35). These studies suggest that platelet release and fibrin formation can be separated and that factors which initiate one process may be distinguishable from those which initiate the other. However, when blood is allowed to clot in a tube (Fig-

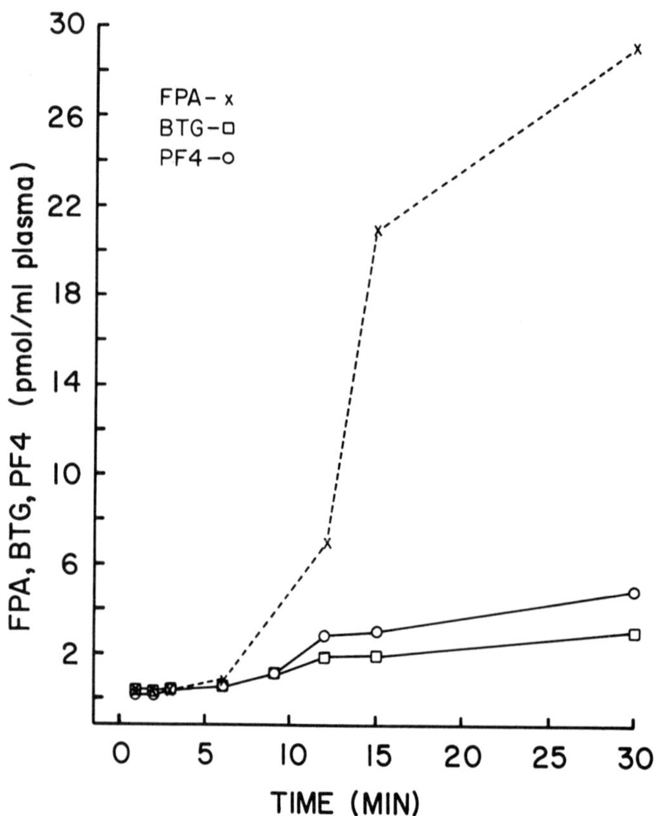

Figure 1. PF4 and βTG release and FPA cleavage in whole blood. Whole blood was incubated in plastic tubes at 37°. At 1, 2, 3, 6, 9, 12, 15 and 30 min following the beginning of blood flow into the syringe, tubes were removed from the water bath and the blood mixed with 1/10 volume of anticoagulant containing heparin, citrate, theophylline, and adenosine. Samples were prepared for assay for PF4 and βTG (35) and for FPA (66).

ures 1 and 2), release of PF4 and βTG can first be detected at the same time as FPA cleavage; following the initial slow FPA cleavage and platelet release, the rate of FPA cleavage increases rapidly while platelet release accelerates more slowly. It is possible that the rapid increase in FPA cleavage depends on initial platelet release.

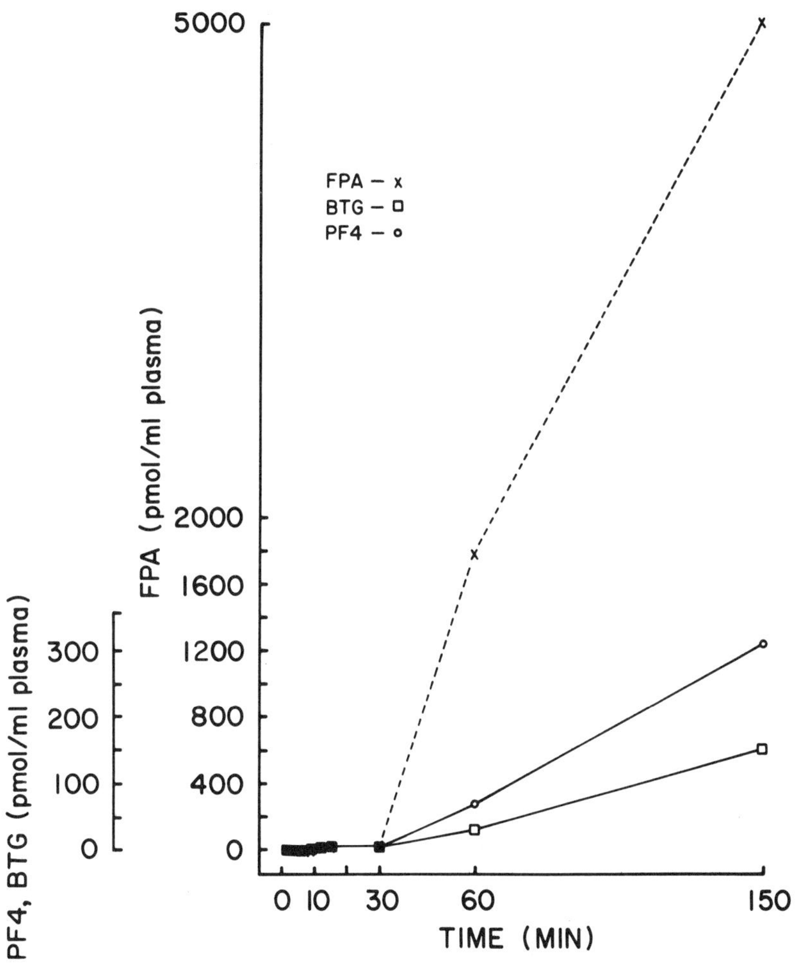

Figure 2. Same experiment as shown in Figure 1 but values at 30, 60, and 150 min are shown. The 150-min values represent 100% platelet release based on frozen and thawed blood whereas the FPA level is only 50% of that predicted from the plasma fibrinogen concentration.

CLINICAL APPLICATION

A major problem in the application of radioimmunoassays for PF4 and βTG to clinical samples has been preparation of the plasma samples in a manner that avoids artifactual elevation by *in vitro* release. Inclusion of platelet inhibitors such as theophylline and PGE_1 appears to be helpful (67), as does keeping the blood sample on ice until it is centrifuged. It is important to remove platelets from the plasma as completely as possible because as few as 500 platelets per μl can, when frozen and thawed, give rise to up to 10 ng PF4 or βTG per ml.

Plasma levels for PF4 and β-thromboglobulin measured by radioimmunoassay in normal individuals have been reported from a number of laboratories. Ludlam *et al.* initially reported a normal level for βTG of 19 ± 0.75 ng/ml (55) and later, reported 38.7 ± 9.1 (68). Smith *et al.* have stated that the normal level is 33 ± 19 ng/ml (69). Normal levels for PF4 have been reported by Bolton *et al.* as 13 ± 5.5 ng/ml (46), by Handin *et al.* as 16 ± 4 ng/ml (47), and by Chesterman *et al.* as <10 ng/ml (48).

In 1975 Ludlam *et al.* reported that 12/12 patients with clinically diagnosed thromboembolism, either venous or arterial, had elevated levels of βTG compared with normals, and 9/17 patients with prosthetic heart valves had βTG levels greater than the upper limit of the normal range (55). Later in 1975 Ludlam *et al.* reported an elevated mean level of βTG in six patients with venographic or ^{125}I-fibrinogen scanning evidence for deep venous thrombosis but not in eight patients in whom no deep venous thrombosis could be demonstrated (68).

Smith *et al.* (69) studied patients with isotopically diagnosed deep venous thrombosis or pulmonary embolism and found that 12/24 had elevated βTG levels on presentation and that nine others had elevated levels at some time during serial sampling. They also found that the onset of deep venous thrombosis as detected by ^{125}I-fibrinogen scanning was associated with a mean rise in plasma βTG but that this increase was not statistically significant. They concluded that although there appears to be an association between venous thrombosis and elevated plasma levels of βTG, current sampling techniques introduce too much variation into the results to use βTG as a diagnostic test for venous thrombosis. It is important to note that the hospital ward staff collected the blood samples for that study. Ludlam *et al.* have attempted to correlate plasma βTG levels with ^{51}Cr-labeled platelet survival (70). While there was a good correlation (r = 0.91) between the reciprocal of the plasma βTG concentration and the platelet survival in normals, such a correlation was not obtained when comparing patients with arterial thrombosis (not further defined) with normals. The patients with arterial thrombosis had a mean plasma βTG level of

108 ng/ml and a mean platelet survival of 7.4 days while the controls' mean βTG level was 30 ng/ml and mean platelet survival, 7.9 days. They concluded that plasma βTG levels provided a more sensitive index of platelet activation than did platelet survival measurements.

Bolton *et al.* (46) have reported elevated plasma levels of PF4 in 16/25 patients, elevated levels of βTG in 17/25 patients, and elevated levels of both proteins in 13/25 patients with prosthetic heart valves. Handin *et al.* (47) measured plasma PF4 levels in patients suspected of having a myocardial infarction; they found that 21 patients in whom infarction was confirmed had a mean plasma level of 95 ng/ml compared with 16 ng/ml in normal controls. The PF4 levels were also elevated 1 week after presentation in 6/8 myocardial infarction patients studied at that time.

Although technical problems still must be resolved in the clinical application of the sensitive and specific radioimmunoassays for PF4 and βTG, clinical studies summarized here suggest that such assays will be useful in studying the pathogenesis and course of thromboembolic disorders. Levels of PF4 and βTG in carefully prepared plasma samples apparently reflect *in vivo* platelet release. Also, because release of PF4 and βTG closely parallels release of platelet-derived growth factor, plasma levels of PF4 and βTG should reflect release of that protein as well. Finally, use of the assays for PF4 and βTG along with the assay for FPA in clinical samples should provide new and useful information about the relative importance of platelet release and fibrin formation in thromboembolic disorders.

REFERENCES

1. Baumgartner HR: The subendothelial surface and thrombosis. In THROMBOSIS: PATHOGENESIS AND CLINICAL TRIALS, edited by Deutsch E, Lechner K, and Brinkhous KM. Stuttgart, F. K. Schattauer Verlag, 1974, p. 91.

2. Stemerman MB: Thrombogenesis of the rabbit arterial plaque: An electron microscopic study. AM J PATHOL 73:7-26, 1973.

3. Harker LA, Slichter SJ: Platelet and fibrinogen consumption in man. N ENGL J MED 287:999-1005, 1972.

4. Weily HS, Steele PP, Davies H, Pappas G, Genton E: Platelet survival in patients with substitute heart valves. N ENGL J MED 290:534-547, 1974.

5. Steele PP, Weily HS, Davies H, Genton E: Platelet survival in patients with rheumatic heart disease. N ENGL J MED 290:

537-539, 1974.

6. Harker LA, Slichter SJ, Scott CR, Ross R: Homocystinemia: Vascular injury and arterial thrombosis. N ENGL J MED 290: 539-543, 1974.

7. Steele P, Battock D, Genton E: Effects of clofibrate and sulfinpyrazone on platelet survival time in coronary artery disease. CIRCULATION 52:473-476, 1975.

8. Harbury CB: Evidence for pre-release in circulating platelets. CLIN RES 24:310A, 1976.

9. Reimers HJ, Packham MA, Kinlough-Rathbone RL, Mustard JF: Effect of repeated treatment of rabbit platelets with low concentrations of thrombin on their function, metabolism, and survival. BR J HAEMATOL 25:675-689, 1973.

10. Reimers HJ, Kinlough-Rathbone RL, Cazenave JP, Senyi AF, Hirsh J, Packham MA, Mustard JF: *In vitro* and *in vivo* function of thrombin-treated platelets. THROMB HAEMOSTAS 35:151-166, 1976.

11. Niewiarowski S, Thomas DP: Platelet factor 4 and adenosine diphosphate release during human platelet aggregation. NATURE 222:1269-1270, 1969.

12. VanCreveld S, Paulssen MMP: Significance of clotting factors in blood platelets in normal and pathological conditions. LANCET 2:242-244, 1951.

13. VanCreveld S, Paulssen MMP: Isolation and properties of the third clotting factor in blood platelets. LANCET 1:23-25, 1952

14. Deutsch E, Johnson SA, Seegers WH: Differentiation of certain platelet factors related to blood coagulation. CIRCULATION RES 3:110-115, 1955.

15. Moore S, Pepper DS, Cash JD: The isolation and characterization of a platelet-specific β-globulin (β-thromboglobulin) and the detection of anti-urokinase and anti-plasmin released from thrombin-aggregated washed human platelets. BIOCHIM BIOPHYS ACTA 379:360-369, 1975.

16. Moore S, Pepper DS: Identification and characterization of a platelet specific release product: β-thromboglobulin. In PLATELETS IN BIOLOGY AND PATHOLOGY, edited by Gordon JL. Amsterdam, North Holland Publishing Co., 1976, p. 293.

17. Nachman RL, Weksler B, Ferris B: Increased vascular permea-

bility produced by human platelet granule cationic extract. J CLIN INVEST 49:274-281, 1970.

18. Nachman, RL, Weksler B, Ferris B: Characterization of human platelet vascular permeability-enhancing activity. J CLIN INVEST 51:549-556, 1972.

19. Weksler BB, Coupal CE: Platelet-dependent generation of chemotactic activity in serum. J EXP MED 137:1419-1430, 1973.

20. Weksler BB, Nachman RL: Rabbit platelet bactericidal protein. J EXP MED 134:1114-1130, 1971.

21. Keenan JP, Solom NO: Quantitative studies on the release of platelet fibrinogen by thrombin. BR J HAEMATOL 23:461-466, 1972.

22. Ross R, Glomset J, Kariya B, Harker L: A platelet-dependent serum factor that stimulates the proliferation of arterial smooth muscle cells *in vitro*. PROC NATL ACAD SCI USA 71:1207-1210, 1974.

23. Kohler N, Lipton A: Platelets as a source of fibroblast growth-producing activity. EXP CELL RES 87:297-301, 1974.

24. Antoniades HN, Stathakos D, Scher CD: Isolation of a cationic polypeptide from human serum that stimulates proliferation of 3T3 cells. PROC NATL ACAD SCI USA 72:2635-2639, 1975.

25. Busch C, Wasteson A, Westermark B: Release of a cell growth promoting factor from human platelets. THROMB RES 8:493-500, 1976.

26. Holmsen H: Biochemistry of the platelet release reaction. In BIOCHEMISTRY AND PHARMACOLOGY OF PLATELETS, Ciba Foundation Symposium 35. Amsterdam, Elsevier, 1975, p. 175.

27. Antoniades HN, Scher CD: Radioimmunoassay of a human serum growth factor for Balb/c-3T3 cells: Derivation from platelets. PROC NATL ACAD SCI USA 74:1973-1977, 1977.

28. Waugh TR, Ruddick DW: Studies on increased coagulability of the blood. CANAD MED ASSOC J 51:11, 1944.

29. Allen JG, Bogardus G, Jacobson LO, Spurr CL: Some observations on bleeding tendency in thrombocytopenic purpura. ANN INT MED 27:382-395, 1947.

30. Conley CL, Hartmann RC, Lalley JS: The relationship of heparin activity to platelet concentration. PROC SOC EXP BIOL MED 69:

284-287, 1948.

31. Käser-Glanzmann R, Jakabova M, Luscher EF: Isolation and some properties of the heparin-neutralizing factor (PF4) released from human blood platelets. EXPERIENTIA 28:1221-1223, 1972.

32. Moore S, Pepper DS, Cash JD: Platelet anti-heparin activity: The isolation and characterization of platelet factor 4 released from thrombin-aggregated washed human platelets and its dissociation into subunits and the isolation of membrane-bound anti-heparin activity. BIOCHIM BIOPHYS ACTA 379:370-384, 1975

33. Levine SP, Wohl H: Human platelet factor 4 (PF4): Purification and characterization by affinity chromatography. J BIOL CHEM 251:324-328, 1976.

34. Handin RI, Cohen JH: Purification and binding properties of human platelet factor 4. J BIOL CHEM 251:4273-4282, 1976.

35. Kaplan KL, Nossel HL, Drillings M, Lesznik G: Radioimmunoassay of platelet factor 4 and β-thromboglobulin: Development and application to studies of platelet release in relation to fibrinopeptide A generation. BR J HAEMATOL, 1978 (In Press).

36. Deuel TF, Keim PS, Farmer M, Heinrikson RL: Amino acid sequence of human platelet factor 4. PROC NATL ACAD SCI USA 74:2256-2258, 1977.

37. Morgan FJ, Chesterman CN, McGready JR, Begg GS. Studies on the chemistry of human platelet factor 4. HAEMOSTASIS 6:53-58, 1977.

38. Hermodsen M, Schmer G, Kurachi K: Isolation, crystallization and primary amino acid sequence of human platelet factor 4. J BIOL CHEM 252:6276-6279, 1977.

39. Nath N, Lowery CT, Niewiarowski S: Antigenic and antiheparin properties of human platelet factor 4. BLOOD 45:537-550, 1975

40. Rucinski B, Niewiarowski S, Budzynski AZ: Separation of two anti-heparin proteins secreted by human platelets. FED PROC 36:1082, 1977.

41. Käser-Glanzmann R, Jakabova M, Luscher EF: Heparin neutralizing factor (PF4) from human blood platelets and its reactivity with fibrinogen and soluble fibrin-monomer complexes. HAEMOSTASIS 1:136-147, 1972/73.

42. Barber AJ, Käser-Glanzmann R, Jakabova M, Luscher EF: Charac-

terization of a chondroitin-4-sulfate proteoglycan carrier for heparin neutralizing activity (PF4) released from human blood platelets. BIOCHIM BIOPHYS ACTA 286:312-329, 1972.

43. Morgan FJ, Begg GS, Chesterman CN: The amino acid sequence of human platelet factor 4. THROMB HAEMOSTAS (In Press).

44. Weber K, Osborn M: Proteins and sodium dodecylsulfate: Molecular weight determination on polyacrylamide gels and related procedures. Chapter 3 in THE PROTEINS, edited by Neurath H, Hill RL, Third Edition, New York, Academic Press, Inc., 1975, p. 179.

45. Gjesdahl K: An electro-immunoassay for platelet factor 4 in human plasma. SCAND J HAEMATOL 13:232-240, 1974.

46. Bolton AE, Ludlam CA, Pepper DS, Moore S, Cash JD: A radioimmunoassay for platelet factor 4. THROMB RES 8:51-58, 1976.

47. Handin RI, McDonough M, Lesch M: Elevated platelet factor 4 in plasma following myocardial infarction. CIRCULATION 54 (Suppl II):198, 1976.

48. Chesterman CN, McGready JR, Morgan FJ: Radioimmunoassay of human platelet factor 4. THROMB HAEMOSTAS 38:211, 1977.

49. O'Brien JR, Etherington M, Jamieson S, Lawford P: Heparin thrombin clotting time and platelet factor 4. LANCET 2:656-657, 1974.

50. Salmon J, Bounameaux Y: Etude des antigenes plaquettaires et, en particulier, du fibrinogene. THROMB DIATH HAEMORRH 2:93-110, 1958.

51. Sokal G: Etude methodologique des plaquettes sanguines et de la metamorphose visqueuse aux moyens d'antiserums fluorescents, antifibrinogenes et antiplaquettes. ACTA HAEMATOL (Basel) 28:313-325, 1962.

52. Nachman RL: Immunologic studies of platelet protein. BLOOD 25:703-711, 1965.

53. Davey MG, Luscher EF: Release reactions of human platelets induced by thrombin and other agents. BIOCHIM BIOPHYS ACTA 165:490-506, 1968.

54. Dzoga K, Stoltzner G, Wissler RW: The production of a highly specific antiserum to human platelets. LAB INVEST 27:351-356, 1972.

55. Ludlam CA, Moore S, Bolton AE, Pepper DS, Cash JD: The release of a human platelet specific protein measured by a radioimmunoassay. THROMB RES 6:543-548, 1975.

56. Bolton AE, Ludlam CA, Moore S, Pepper DS, Cash JD: Three approaches to the radioimmunoassay of human β-thromboglobulin. BR J HAEMATOL 33:233-238, 1976.

57. Niewiarowski S, Lowery CT, Hawiger J, Millman M, Timmons S: Immunoassay of human platelet factor 4 (PF4, antiheparin factor) by radial immunodiffusion. J LAB CLIN MED 87:720-733, 1976.

58. Youssef A, Barkhan P: Release of platelet factor 4 by adenosine diphosphate and other platelet-aggregating agents. BR MED J 1:746-747, 1968.

59. Niewiarowski S, Poplawski A, Lipinski B, Farbiszewski R: The release of platelet clotting factors during aggregation and viscous metamorphosis. EXP BIOL MED 3:121-128, 1968.

60. Harada K, Zucker MB: Simultaneous development of platelet factor 4 activity and release of ^{14}C-serotonin. THROMB DIATH HAEMORRH 25:41-46, 1971.

61. Walsh PN, Gagnatelli G: Platelet antiheparin activity: Storage sites and release mechanism. BLOOD 44:157-168, 1974.

62. Witte LD, Kaplan KL, Nossel HL, Lages BA, Weiss HJ, Goodman, DeWS: Studies of the release from human platelets of the growth factor for cultured human arterial smooth muscle cells. CIRCULATION RES, March 1978 (In Press).

63. Holmsen H, Setknowsky CA, Lages B, Day HJ, Weiss HJ, Scrutton MC: Content and thrombin-induced release of acid hydrolases in gel-filtered platelets from patients with storage pool disease. BLOOD 46:131-142, 1975.

64. Weiss HJ, Lages BA, Witte LD, Kaplan KL, Goodman DeWS, Nossel HL, Baumgartner HR: Storage pool disease: Evidence for clinical and biochemical heterogeneity. THROMB HAEMOSTAS 38:3, 1977.

65. Nossel HL, Younger LR, Wilner GD, Procupez T, Canfield RE, Butler VP Jr.: Radioimmunoassay of human fibrinopeptide A. PROC NATL ACAD SCI USA 68:2350-2353, 1971.

66. Nossel HL, Yudelman I, Canfield RE, Butler VP Jr., Spanondis K, Wilner GD, Qureshi GD: Measurement of fibrinopeptide A in human blood. J CLIN INVEST 54:43-53, 1974.

67. Ludlam CA, Cash JD: Studies on the liberation of β-thromboglobulin from human platelets *in vitro*. BR J HAEMATOL 33:239-247, 1976.

68. Ludlam CA, Bolton AE, Moore S, Cash JD: New rapid method for the diagnosis of deep venous thrombosis. LANCET 2:259-260, 1975.

69. Smith RC, Ruckley CV, Duncanson J, Allan NC, Dawes J, Pepper DS, Cash JD: β-thromboglobulin and deep vein thrombosis in surgical patients. THROMB HAEMOSTAS 38:166, 1977.

70. Ludlam CA, Davies BA, MacKay AD, Bentley NJ: β-thromboglobulin and platelet survival in patients with arterial thromboembolic disease. THROMB HAEMOSTAS 38:124, 1977.

SUMMARY OF DISCUSSION BY PARTICIPANTS

Dr. Harker asked how the samples were prepared. Dr. Kaplan replied that blood was collected in a mixture of citrate, adenosine, and theophylline. Blood samples were kept on ice until they were first centrifuged. The first centrifugation was at 3,000 *g* at 4°C for 15-20 min. The platelet-poor plasma was recentrifuged at 48,000 *g* at 4°C and the supernatant kept frozen until it was assayed.

Dr. Smith commented that it might be valuable to examine the levels of these proteins (PF4 and βTG) in platelets from patients with storage pool disease because there is a possibility of an acquired defect.

Dr. Hoak asked if studies were done on blood samples that were allowed to clot while being stirred in which fibrinopeptide A release and PF4 release were compared. Dr. Kaplan said that they have looked at non-stirred blood, and that they are planning a study in which blood is agitated or stirred.

Dr. Mustard inquired if Dr. Kaplan or anyone else has data on the release of PF4 with ADP from human platelets in the presence of citrate when the release reaction occurs. He referred to the data from Dr. Packham's laboratory[1] on the loss of proteoglycan during ADP-induced aggregation of rabbit platelets where release did not occur. He also wondered if there would be an increase in PF4 or βTG in inflammation induced by bacteria or by trauma following accidents or surgery where platelets might be involved in some reactions. Dr. Kaplan replied that she had no other data than

[1]Ward JV *et al.*: LAB INVEST 35:337-342, 1976.

those she mentioned. Dr. Packham commented on Dr. Niewiarowski's work which indicated that with washed platelets PF4 was not released during ADP-induced aggregation when no release reaction occurred.

Dr. H. J. Day thought that there might have been a flurry of publications on a correlation of PF4 and βTG with arterial thrombosis following the reports of Dr. Ludlam's group [reference 55 in Dr. Kaplan's paper] and Dr. Handin's group [reference 47 in Dr. Kaplan's paper], but such has not come to pass. Dr. Kaplan thinks that this might be because the changes seen in atherosclerosis are small. Furthermore many investigators are not completely convinced that the levels they are measuring in normal plasma are the levels that are circulating in blood. Dr. Day thought that the measurement of βTG would be more relevant than the measurement of PF4. He also wondered about the measurement of the mitogenic factor and its relationship to arterial disease. Dr. Kaplan said that they have looked at the mitogenic factor with gel-filtered and sonicated washed platelets. However, because of technical difficulties with the 3T3 assay in plasma, only limited studies of mitogenic factor release in plasma have been performed.

Dr. Packham wondered what the t1/2 of PF4 in circulation was. According to the Edinburgh group, when a high level of purified PF4 or βTG was injected, the t1/2 for βTG was 20 min[2] and that for PF4 was about 10 min.[3] However, as the normal levels of PF4 and βTG were approached, the t1/2 was about 20 min for PF4[3] and about 100 min for βTG.[2]

---

[2]Dawes J, Hunter WH, Smith RC, Duncanson J, Ruckley CV, Allan NC, Pepper DS, Cash JD: Beta-thromboglobulin clearance. (Abstract) THROMB HAEMOSTAS 38:314, 1977.

[3]Nossel HL: Report of the workshop on secreted platelet proteins. THROMB HAEMOSTAS (In Press).

Session II

ANIMAL MODELS

R. H. Rynbrandt, Chairman

ANIMAL MODELS: IMPORTANCE IN RESEARCH ON HEMORRHAGE AND THROMBOSIS*

K. M. Brinkhous, M.D.

Department of Pathology, University of North Carolina

Chapel Hill, NC

ABSTRACT

Despite some sentiments against animal research, animal models continue to be important in studying hemorrhage and thrombosis. Examples of genetic models are dogs and pigs with von Willebrand's disease. The homozygous von Willebrand pig appears to be resistant to arteriosclerosis, presumably due to impairment of the platelet aggregating function. Among acquired models, pigs are gaining in favor, perhaps because their clotting and platelet characteristics resemble those in humans. Species vary markedly in their normal plasma levels of platelet aggregating factor/von Willebrand factor (PAF/vWF). One promising approach to the study of thrombosis is using platelet anti-aggregating drugs to inhibit PAF/vWF dependent platelet thrombus formation; a drug-induced von Willebrand state seems feasible.

INTRODUCTION

An animal model of thrombosis or hemorrhage should be as similar as possible to the counterpart disorder in man. While animal disorders may not duplicate every aspect of the human disease, once the similarities and differences are well understood, the model may contribute to our understanding of thrombo-hemorrhagic disorders.

Thrombosis is no more a single disorder than hemorrhage; many different basic biologic mechanisms are involved. Disturbances of

*This research was aided in part by grants from the National Institute of Health, HL 01648 and HL 06350.

one or more of these mechanisms can initiate or promote thrombosis. Whether probing pathophysiological pathways or testing potential new therapies, careful selection of the animal model is important. While there are a great many animal models of both hemorrhage and thrombosis, one well suited for a given set of studies may not exist. Therefore the search for new models in both naturally occurring diseases in animals and development of new induced models should be continued.

Genetically determined animal models of hemophilia have advanced the understanding of hemorrhage, the improvement of diagnostic procedures, and the development of effective replacement therapy with plasma fractions. The hemophilia models represent point mutations; only a single procoagulant of a single pathway, the intrinsic pathway of clotting, is basically altered. While derivative disturbances, such as of platelet function, do exist in the hemophilia model, it was the recognition and manipulation of the primary disturbance that made this model such a powerful asset.

In the area of thrombosis, analogous genetic models, as, for example, the counterpart of thrombophilia in man, have not been discovered. So one is left with induced models in which the investigator knows only in a limited way the primary or secondary pathogenetic pathways.

PUBLIC POLICY

To keep the use of animal models in perspective, we should remember that we can search for, develop, and use animal models because it is the consensus of society that it is important to do so for the future good. But the consensus is far from unanimous. There are really two cultures, one epitomized by a group such as is assembled at this Workshop, the other by animal rights activists, including groups whose aim is prohibition of animal experimentation. Thanks to the work of a Committee on Animal Models for Thrombosis and Hemorrhagic Diseases of the National Academy of Sciences, a rational discussion of the issues was initiated in 1975 (1), followed by a further consideration of the same topic in another Academy symposium (2). Some issues are philosophical, some are technical. All agree that humane care and good management of animals should be provided, but there are differences of opinion on many aspects. If some recommendations were adopted, dogs would not be housed in cages and would be used only for acute non-recovery studies; and even here, it is contended that animals should be used only if there are no alternative ways of obtaining information.

Suggested alternatives to the use of animals include the use of cell cultures. In our field, this procedure has already been effectively used in the study of endothelial cells in culture.

There are a number of potentially exploitable endothelial cell markers for both production and prevention of thrombosis. Markers that could contribute to prevention or resolution of thrombi are: an inhibitor of platelet aggregation as shown originally by the work of Saba and Mason (3) and possibly the same as that explored recently by Vane and associates (4) in their demonstration that the inhibitor is of prostaglandin derivation; and the proactivator of the fibrinolytic system of endothelial cell origin (5). Markers that could be thrombosis inducers are the endothelial cell tissue factor (6) and the factor VIII-related antigen closely related to the platelet aggregating factor/von Willebrand factor (PAF/vWF) (7,8). Powerful as it is, this procedure of identifying thrombosis-related factors of endothelial cell origin cannot substitute for but only complement the use of whole animals. Animal models are needed to show the pathologic and pathophysiological effects of the release of the endothelial cell products (9).

Another aspect of public policy on the use of certain animal models of potentially great importance to the thrombosis, hemorrhage, and arteriosclerosis fields is the fiscal one. This applies especially to the genetic models, including hemophilia, hemophilioid states, von Willebrand disease, and platelet abnormalities, particularly in dogs and swine. Preservation of these genetic models requires constant attention, is relatively labor-intensive, and needs long-range planning for the delivery of sufficient animals for testing and research.

One way of viewing all research, including that which uses these models, is to apply the criteria of "cost-effectiveness". In a finite period of time, like a few months or a year or two, what new findings have resulted from using such animals? Scientific progress tends to occur in catapults, with the surges characteristically separated by years depending on the state of methodologies and resources available. It is during any post-catapult era that the gene preservation is in greatest danger, and these specialized animal stocks might need protection under an extension of our "endangered species" programs. Another proposal in this era of fiscal stringencies is that the genetic animal models be put in the deep freeze through semen preservation (10) and then brought forth again when a critical need exists. While in theory this procedure seems feasible, its practicability has not been demonstrated. There would obviously be a considerable time lag before sufficient animals could be engendered for experimental studies.

Another inhibitor of the full exploitation of animal models is the view that because application of our new knowledge in biomedicine is primarily directed toward man, and because species specificity does exist, human studies should be done immediately where feasible, completely or largely bypassing animal studies. There are many ethical and practical obstacles to such a course.

The wise strategy is to use our resources well but to maintain all options in exploring the unknown. Despite sentiments against the use of animal models, society's needs seem to dictate even greater usage of them. This is exemplified by the Food and Drug Administration's increasing requirements for efficacy and toxicity studies in animals.

SELECTION OF ANIMAL MODELS

There have been several reviews of animal models available for study of hemorrhage and thrombosis (1,11-13). Newer models are continuously proposed, for example, pulmonary thrombosis in the rat (14), venous thrombosis in the dog (15), and laser injury to produce arterial thrombosis in the mouse (16). In selecting a model for thrombosis (and embolism), one should consider not only the animal species and its appropriateness and genetically impaired animals versus normal animals, but also the type of thrombosis being studied, whether of the arterial, venous, or microcirculatory system or on vascular or cardiac protheses.

GENETIC MODELS

Genetically impaired animals may be used to manipulate and study the inherited disease itself as well as to determine the influence of a specific type of deficiency, as in von Willebrand's disease, on the genesis of thrombosis. With the genetic models, ordinarily one must accept the species and the type of deficiency as they may exist, but limited manipulations are possible where different types of deficiencies exist in the same animal species. We have a long-term program to develop strains of dogs with multiple inherited deficiencies. The individual deficiencies are of factor VIII (antihemophilic factor), factor IX, and platelet aggregating factor/von Willebrand's factor (PAF/vWF). Most experience has been with the two types of hemophilia (17). All possible crosses have been obtained, including double hemophilia in both males and females. The latter have not survived. Crosses between von Willebrand's disease and both hemophilia A and B have been obtained, so that we have double carriers of von Willebrand defect and each type of hemophilia. Double homozygosity has not yet been attained. The 15 genotypes in dogs (18-21) available in our colony are shown in Table 1.

Preliminary data suggest that the homozygous von Willebrand pig is resistant to arteriosclerosis, presumably due to impairment of the platelet aggregating function (22). In our hands, the heterozygous swine with about 30-50% plasma levels of PAF/vWF are susceptible to coronary atherosclerosis induced by balloon denudation of endothelium and a high-fat, high-cholesterol diet (Griggs

TABLE 1. NATURALLY OCCURRING AND DERIVED GENOTYPES OF HEMOPHILIA A, HEMOPHILIA B AND VON WILLEBRAND'S DISEASE IN DOGS

Genotype*	Phenotype	Reference
	Naturally Occurring	
X^a Y	Hemophilia A male	18
X^a X	Hemophilia A carrier female	19
X^b Y	Hemophilia B male	20
X^b X	Hemophilia B carrier female	20
A^w A	von Willebrand heterozygotes, male and female	†
	Derived from Inbreeding and Crosses Between Strains	
X^a X^a	Hemophilia A female	21
X^a X^b	Double heterozygote, hemophilia A and B	17
X^b X^b	Hemophilia B female	17
$X^{a,b}$ X^b	Hemophilia B female, hemophilia A heterozygote	17
$X^{a,b}$ X^a	Hemophilia A female, hemophilia B heterozygote	17
$X^{a,b}$ Y	Double hemophilia AB male	17
$X^{a,b}$ $X^{a,b}$	Double hemophilia AB female	17
X^a X, A^w A	Double heterozygote, hemophilia A, von Willebrand's disease	†
X^b X, A^w A	Double heterozygote, hemophilia B, von Willebrand's disease	†
X^b X^b, A^w A	Hemophilia B, von Willebrand heterozygote	†

*a = hemophilia A gene; b = hemophilia B gene; w = von Willebrand gene. †Brinkhous KM: unpublished data.

TR, Brinkhous KM, Sultzer DL, Reddick RL, unpublished data). This suggests that the specific defect as well as gene dose are important in selection of animals for study. While the genetic inheritance of von Willebrand's disease is less clear than that of hemophilia, it is possible to use animals having different degrees of severity of a defect, either dogs or swine.

ACQUIRED MODELS

With acquired models the choice of species is enormous, ranging from marine animals and other lower forms to nonhuman primates. Didisheim (12) has provided a good review of both the animals and the methods that have been used for induction of thrombosis in normal animals. The mammals in greatest favor historically have been dogs, but rats, pigs, and rabbits are also commonly used. Pigs seem to be increasing in favor, possibly because so many of their clotting and platelet characteristics seem to be close to those of man. The use of larger animals requires detailed attention to management and animal husbandry. An excellent summation of the use of the pig in biomedical research has been provided by Bustad, McClellan, and Burns (23).

The question of whether to use random animals or inbred animals has been discussed at great length. One caution about so-called normal inbred animals: they may actually be deficient in one parameter or another as recessive traits come to the fore with close inbreeding. In one well-known beagle kennel the breeder had a highly inbred strain selected for many fine characteristics, but ended up having a large number of dogs with factor VII deficiency, not recognized until after these dogs had been used in various studies as presumably normal animals.

To aid in selecting an animal species, there is an abundance of data on normal physiological parameters of both fibrin clotting and (to a somewhat lesser extent) platelet aggregation functions. Hawkey (24) has studied clotting parameters in primates and carnivores especially, while Lewis (25,26) has reported on species seldom used as models, such as bats and wallabies. Mason (27,28) has studied several primates, particularly in relationship to platelet function. These studies demonstrate great biological variability between species, as well as the usual intraspecies variations.

PAF/vWF LEVELS IN ANIMALS

Von Willebrand factor, which is deficient in von Willebrand's disease, has only become recognized as part of the factor VIII complex since 1973, and has only been measurable in the laboratory relatively recently (29,30,31,32). We recently studied some common domestic and laboratory animals in relation to the PAF/vWF levels in plasma which may be important in thrombosis (33). We found that the chimpanzee, rhesus monkey, and pig had levels of this plasma factor very close to those of humans (Table 2). The horse had a considerably reduced plasma level which varied from animal to animal. The cow, goat, and sheep had extremely high levels. Species specificity in the platelet-plasma PAF/vWF reaction was especially marked. With the assay procedures now available for PAF/vWF, plasma levels in the rabbit and dog could not be quantitated.

TABLE 2. PLATELET AGGREGATION FACTOR-VON WILLEBRAND FACTOR PLASMA LEVELS IN DIFFERENT SPECIES (33)

Species Plasma	PAF/vWF %*
Goat	1210
Sheep	1000
Cow	660
Man	*100*
Rhesus monkey	100
Pig	100
Chimpanzee	90
Horse	60

*Percent of normal human reference plasma.

In this same study species differences were most extreme when the platelet was examined. Surprisingly, cow, horse, pig and dog platelets did not react to plasma PAF/vWF and ristocetin in the way that fixed human platelets do.

One of the goals of thrombosis research is to find animal models in which pretreatment with drugs prevents development of thrombi. The use of Coumadin-treated animals with reduced procoagulant levels (12) is well known. Other approaches include use of platelet anti-aggregating drugs. Again, because of the potential that impairment of PAF/vWF activity has in limiting the formation of thrombi, we have started a search for synthetic chemicals which inhibit the PAF/vWF dependent platelet thrombus formation. Although this research is in its early phases, we have had some success in finding inhibitors, so the potential of a drug-induced von Willebrand state seems feasible. Several compounds (benzimidazolyl derivatives) completely inhibited the reaction at concentrations of 10^{-5}M and were still inhibitory at somewhat lower levels (34).

In spite of a great array of information, no standard animal model for the testing of antithrombotic drugs has yet been recognized. Perhaps there can be no one standard model, but rather each model employed must be selected to fit the type of pathophysiologic thrombotic mechanism being modified.

REFERENCES

1. ANIMAL MODELS OF THROMBOSIS AND HEMORRHAGIC DISEASES. Co-sponsored by the National Heart and Lung Institute and the Institute of Laboratory Animal Resources, National Academy of Sciences. Washington, DC, National Institutes of Health, 1975.

2. THE FUTURE OF ANIMALS, CELLS, MODELS, AND SYSTEMS IN RESEARCH, DEVELOPMENT, EDUCATION, AND TESTING. Proceedings of a Symposium, Institute of Laboratory Animal Resources, Division of Biological Sciences, Assembly of Life Sciences. Washington, DC, National Academy of Sciences, 1977.

3. Saba SR, Mason RG: Studies of an activity from endothelial cells that inhibits platelet aggregation, serotonin release and clot retraction. THROMB RES 5:747-757, 1974.

4. Johnson RA, Morton DR, Kinner JH, Gorman RR, McGuire JC, Sun FF: The chemical structure of prostaglandin X (prostacyclin). PROSTAGLANDINS 12:915-928, 1976.

5. McDonald RI, Shepro D, Rosenthal M, Booyse FM: Properties of cultured endothelial cells. SER HAEMATOL VI, 4:469-478, 1973.

6. Zeldis SM, Nemerson Y, Pitlick FA, Lentz TL: Tissue factor (thromboplastin): Localization to plasma membranes by peroxidase-conjugated antibodies. SCIENCE 175:766-768, 1972.

7. Jaffe EA, Hoyer LW, Nachman RL: Synthesis of von Willebrand factor by cultured human endothelial cells. PROC NATL ACAD SCI USA 71:1906-1909, 1974.

8. Bloom AL, Peake IR, Giddings JC, Shearn SAM, Tuddenham EGD: Endothelial cells and factor-VIII-related protein. LANCET 1: 46, 1976.

9. Nopanitaya W, Gambill TG, Brinkhous KM: Fresh water drowning. Pulmonary ultrastructure and systemic fibrinolysis. ARCH PATHOL 98:361-366, 1974.

10. Seager SWJ: Cost-effectiveness: Utilization of a sperm bank in animal breeding colonies. In ANIMAL MODELS OF THROMBOSIS AND HEMORRHAGIC DISEASE. Co-sponsored by the National Heart and Lung Institute and the Institute of Laboratory Animal Resources, National Academy of Sciences. Washington, DC, National Institutes of Health, 1975, p. 118.

11. Henry RL: Methods for inducing experimental thrombosis. ANGIOLOGY 13:554-577, 1962.

12. Didisheim P: Animal models useful in the study of thrombosis and antithrombotic agents. PROG HEMOST THROMB 1:165-197, 1972.

13. Dodds WJ: Hereditary and acquired hemorrhagic disorders in animals. PROG HEMOST THROMB 2:215-247, 1974.

14. Tomikawa M, Ogawa H, Abiko Y: Experimental model of pulmonary thrombosis in rat. THROMB DIATH HAEMORRH 31:86-102, 1974.

15. Strachan CJL, Gaffney PJ, Scully MF, Kakkar VV: An experimental model for the study of venous thrombis *in vivo*. THROMB RES 5:235-242, 1974.

16. Chan PS, Ellenbogen L: Laser-induced injury in mouse ear arteries as a model for *in vivo* studies of arterial thrombosis. THROMB RES 5:529-537, 1974.

17. Brinkhous KM, Davis PD, Graham JB, Dodds WJ: Expression and linkage of genes for X-linked hemophilias A and B in the dog. BLOOD 41:577-585, 1973.

18. Graham JB, Buckwalter JA, Hartley LJ, Brinkhous KM: Canine hemophilia. Observations of the course, the clotting anomaly, and the effect of blood transfusions. J EXP MED 90:97-111, 1949.

19. Parks BJ, Brinkhous KM, Harris PF, Penick GD: Laboratory detection of female carriers of canine hemophilia. THROMB DIATH HAEMORRH 12:368-376, 1964.

20. Mustard JF, Rowsell HC, Robinson GA, Hoeksema TD, Downie HG: Canine hemophilia B (Christmas disease). BR J HAEMATOL 6:259-

-266, 1960.

21. Brinkhous KM, Graham JB: Hemophilia in the female dog. SCIENCE 111:723-724, 1950.

22. Fuster V, Bowie EJW, Josa M, Kaye MP: Atherosclerosis in normal and von Willebrand pigs receiving a high cholesterol diet: Control and cross-aortic transplantation studies. CIRCULATION (Suppl) (In Press).

23. Bustad LK, McClellan RO, Burns MP (editors): SWINE IN BIO-MEDICAL RESEARCH. Richland, Wash., Battelle-Northwest, 1966.

24. Hawkey CM: The relationship between blood coagulation and thrombosis and atherosclerosis in man, monkeys and carnivores. THROMB DIATH HAEMORRH 31:103-118, 1974.

25. Lewis JH: Comparative hematology: Studies on Chiroptera, Pteropus giganteous. COMP BIOCHEM PHYSIOL 58A:103-107, 1977.

26. Lewis JH, Phillips LL, Hann C: Coagulation and hematological studies in primative Australian mammals. COMP BIOCHEM PHYSIOL 25:1129-1135, 1968.

27. Mason RG, Read MS: Platelet response to six agglutinating agents: Species similarities and differences. EXP MOL PATHOL 6:370-381, 1967.

28. Mason RG, Read MS: Some species differences in fibrinolysis and blood coagulation. J BIOMED MATER RES 5:121-128, 1971.

29. Weiss HJ, Hoyer LW, Rickles FR, Varma A, Rogers J: Quantitative assay of a plasma factor deficient in von Willebrand's disease that is necessary for platelet aggregation. J CLIN INVEST 52:2708-2716, 1973.

30. Sarji KE, Stratton RD, Wagner RH, Brinkhous KM: Nature of von Willebrand factor: A new assay and a specific inhibitor. PROC NATL ACAD SCI USA 71:2937-2941, 1974.

31. Allain JP, Cooper HA, Wagner RH, Brinkhous KM: Platelets fixed with paraformaldehyde: A new reagent for assay of von Willebrand factor and platelet aggregating factor. J LAB CLIN MED 85:318-328, 1975.

32. Brinkhous KM, Graham JE, Cooper HA, Allain JP, Wagner RH: Assay of von Willebrand factor in von Willebrand's disease and hemophilia: Use of a macroscopic platelet aggregation test. THROMB RES 6:267-272, 1975.

33. Brinkhous KM, Thomas BD, Ibrahim SA, Read MS: Plasma levels of platelet aggregating factor/von Willebrand factor in various species. THROMB RES 11:345-355, 1977.

34. Geratz JD, Tidwell RR, Brinkhous KM, Mohammed SF, Dann O, Loewe H: Specific inhibition of platelet agglutination and aggregation by aromatic amidino compounds. THROMB HAEMOSTAS (In Press).

NOTE: The discussion of Dr. Brinkhous' paper follows the paper by Dr. Stemerman; three papers were discussed together.

PLATELETS, ENDOTHELIUM, AND SMOOTH MUSCLE CELLS IN ATHEROSCLEROSIS*

Russell Ross, Ph.D., and Laurence Harker, M.D.

Departments of Pathology and Medicine, University of Washington, School of Medicine, Seattle, WA

ABSTRACT

A factor derived from platelets stimulates the proliferation of smooth muscle cells in culture, and is likely important in stimulating smooth muscle proliferative lesions of atherogenesis *in vivo*. The platelet factor is produced during platelet aggregation when serum is made from whole blood. *In vitro*, smooth muscle cells are potent aggregating agents for platelets, while endothelial cells can inhibit this aggregating effect. Better understanding of the interactions of platelets, smooth muscle cells, and endothelium would facilitate developing effective means of intervening in or preventing the smooth muscle proliferative lesions of atherosclerosis.

INTRODUCTION

We have been testing a hypothesis that the response to injury of the endothelium and the proliferation of the smooth muscle cells of the artery wall are the principal factors in the etiology and pathogenesis of atherosclerotic lesions (1-3). We have been examining the response of endothelium to various forms of mechanical or chemical injury *in vivo* and in cell culture. We have also been studying the ability of arterial smooth muscle cell in culture and *in vivo* to synthesize connective tissue matrix macromolecules, metabolize lipids and lipoproteins, and in particular, to respond to various mitogenic stimuli.

---

*This research was supported in part by grants from US Public Health Service HL-18645 and HL-11775.

The lesions of atherosclerosis can be characterized by three fundamental biological properties: 1) focal proliferation within the intima of smooth muscle cells; 2) formation by these smooth muscle cells of increased amounts of connective tissue matrix macromolecules, including collagen, elastic fiber proteins, and glycosaminoglycans; and 3) deposition of lipids and lipoproteins within the cells and also extracellularly.

This paper reviews the focal accumulation of smooth muscle cells in atherosclerotic lesions, and describes evidence that a factor derived from the thrombocyte is principally responsible for the proliferation of these cells in culture as well as in atherosclerotic lesions induced in experimental animals.

THE RESPONSE-TO-INJURY HYPOTHESIS

The hypothesis being tested assumes that endothelial cells lining the vessel walls are altered in some way. This alteration may range from a minor change in the permeability characteristics of the endothelium to frank lysis of the endothelial cells from the artery wall. Endothelial desquamation, or possibly less severe forms of alteration of the endothelium, may then lead to a sequence of events that includes the focal adherence of platelets at the site of the exposed subendothelial connective tissue or altered endothelium, followed by release from the platelets of material contained within their granules, and possibly by aggregation of the platelets accompanied by additional release of platelet constituents. When the endothelium is injured, plasma constituents such as plasma lipoproteins also have access to the artery wall due to the removal of the endothelial barrier that normally controls the ingress and egress of these macromolecules.

Under these circumstances, a mitogenic factor derived from the platelets, together with plasma factors such as lipoproteins, provide a stimulus for the focal migration and proliferation of smooth muscle cells. The smooth muscle cells may be derived either from the media of the artery wall or from pre-existing cells within the intima. They proliferate focally at the site of "injury". At the same time these cells are stimulated to synthesize connective tissue matrix macromolecules and, if lipoproteins are present in increased amounts, to accumulate lipids both within their cytoplasm and in the connective tissue matrix.

The hypothesis suggests that if the "injury" responsible for this endothelial alteration is a single event, the lesions can regress and disappear. On the other hand, if the injury continues on a chronic or recurrent basis, the lesions can become progressive until they are no longer silent and they present sequelae (see Figure 1).

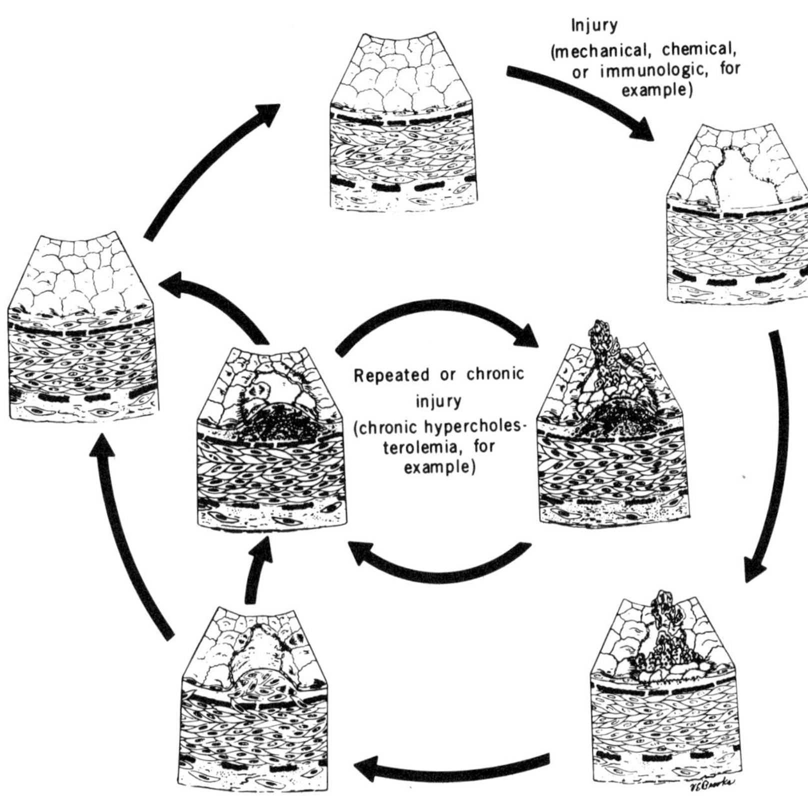

Figure 1. In the response-to-injury hypothesis, two different cyclic events may occur. The outer, or regression cycle, may represent common single occurrences in all individuals in which endothelial injury leads to desquamation, platelet adherence, aggregation, and release, followed by intimal smooth muscle proliferation and connective tissue formation. If the injury is a single event, the lesions may go on to heal and regression occur. The inner or progression cycle demonstrates the possible consequences of repeated or chronic endothelial injury as may occur in chronic hyperlipidemia. In this instance, lipid deposition as well as continued smooth muscle proliferation may occur after recurrent sequences of proliferation and regression, and these may lead to complicated lesions that calcify. Such lesions could go on to produce clinical sequelae such as thrombosis and infarction. From (3) reproduced with permission of SCIENCE: copyright 1976 by the American Association for the Advancement of Science.

IN VIVO STUDIES

We have investigated various forms of injury to the endothelium. Either mechanical denudation with an intra-arterial balloon catheter (4-6) or chemical injury as a consequence of chronic homocystinemia (7) or chronic hypercholesterolemia (3) results in platelet adherence, aggregation, and release which can be measured as decreased platelet survival. This is followed by focal accumulation of smooth muscle cells and the formation of connective tissue components by these cells.

Studies with the balloon catheter and other forms of intravascular catheterization have demonstrated a sequence of events, including focal platelet adherence, aggregation, and release, followed by smooth muscle migration and proliferation, and thus lesion formation. The endothelial injury that results from chronic homocystinemia is also associated with decreased platelet survival. This is due to the continuing adherence and degranulation of platelets at the sites of injury, return of the platelets to the circulation, and their removal by cells of the reticuloendothelial system, resulting in decreased platelet survival (7).

In studies in the pigtail monkey, we removed known amounts of endothelium with an intra-arterial balloon catheter, and demonstrated a correlation between the amount of endothelium removed and the extent of the decrease in platelet survival (Ross and Harker, unpublished observations). Furthermore, the time required for endothelial regeneration correlated with the time required for platelet survival to return to normal levels. These studies suggested that platelet survival might be used as an index of endothelial loss or "injury".

Several findings support the usefulness of this index. For example, animals that are chronically homocystinemic between 6 days and 90 days (7), or are chronically hypercholesterolemic for 9 months or longer (3), show at least 40% decrease in platelet survival. Furthermore, Ritchie and Harker (8) demonstrated that among patients with chronic angina who had angiographic evidence of atherosclerosis, >50% showed a decrease in platelet survival of >2 standard deviations below the range found in a group of individuals who had no evidence of clinical disease. To examine further the significance of these observations, a series of studies was undertaken of arterial smooth muscle cells in culture.

PLATELETS AND THE GROWTH OF CELLS IN CULTURE

Most cells in culture, except a few lines of transformed cells, require whole blood serum to proliferate or grow in culture. If serum is made from cell-free plasma, the cells can be maintained in culture for long periods of time in an apparently healthy state, but they will not proliferate (9). The principal mitogenic effect of whole blood serum that is missing from cell-free, plasma-derived serum is due to a factor derived from platelets. This factor is obtained during the process of platelet aggregation and release when serum is made from whole blood. The serum formation process involves exposing platelets to thrombin formed during the coagulation process and leads to platelet aggregation and release. The mitogenic capacity missing from serum made from cell-free plasma can be restored by adding an aliquot of purified platelets to the plasma at the time of thrombin formation. Another experiment also demonstrates that the mitogenic capacity of whole blood serum is derived from platelets. A supernatant is obtained from frozen-thawed platelets or after exposure of purified platelets to purified thrombin *in vitro*. Adding this supernatant to cell-free plasma which lacks mitogenic activity will restore all the mitogenic capacity of the serum.

These studies were confirmed by Kohler and Lipton (10), who demonstrated that freeze-thawing of a purified preparation of platelets provides a supernatant that contains mitogenic activity for 3T3 cells in culture, and by Westermark and Wasteson (11), who showed that the platelet factor will stimulate glial cells to proliferate in culture. Antoniades *et al.* (12) have looked for the growth factors in serum and demonstrated that the mitogenic factor which they isolated from whole blood serum antigenically cross-reacts with the factor derived from platelets. This implies that these two factors are identical.

In recent investigations, the platelet-derived growth factor was shown to be a basic protein with relatively low molecular weight (13,000 - 23,000) and an isolectric point of approximately 9.7 (13). It is heat stable; it has been reported to be stable at 100°C by Antoniades and coworkers and at approximately 60°C for 1/2 hour in our laboratory.

Witte *et al.* (14) demonstrated that the platelet-derived growth factor is present in the alpha granules of platelets, together with beta-thromboglobulin and platelet factor 4. These three factors appear to be released simultaneously upon exposure of platelets to thrombin. Furthermore, in unpublished observations these same investigators demonstrated that the platelets of a patient with a new form of platelet storage pool disease lack alpha granules. Serum obtained from this patient will not sustain the growth of 3T3 cells in culture. This also suggests that the alpha granule-containing fraction in which the platelet-derived growth factor is stored is responsible for the platelet-derived growth properties present in whole blood serum.

THE ROLE OF PLATELETS IN ATHEROGENESIS

Interfering with platelet function by giving pharmacologic agents such as dipyridamole (7) or sulfinpyrazone (Harker and Ross, unpublished data), or by inducing chronic thrombocytopenia with antiplatelet serum (15), prevents the intimal proliferative smooth muscle lesions of experimentally induced atherosclerosis. These studies suggest that the platelet factor that is important for the growth of cells in culture is also important for stimulating the smooth muscle proliferative lesions of atherogenesis *in vivo*. Thus, inhibition of platelet function, inhibition of the platelet-derived growth factor, and protection of the endothelium each appears to be an important approach to intervening in or preventing the process of atherogenesis.

Harker *et al.* (unpublished data) have recently demonstrated that smooth muscle cells are potent aggregating agents for platelets, and that endothelial cells can inhibit this aggregating effect. Endothelial cells appear to be able to inhibit the smooth muscle aggregating effects either directly or, when they are grown in culture, by secreting a factor into culture medium that will inhibit the aggregating properties of smooth muscle cells.

These studies all point to the platelet and its interaction with the endothelium and the smooth muscle cells as principal factors in stimulating the smooth muscle fibroproliferative lesions of atherosclerosis. A complete understanding of these interactions should permit us to develop better questions that will in turn provide answers to allow us to treat or prevent the multifactorial, complex disease entity represented by the smooth muscle proliferative lesions of atherosclerosis.

REFERENCES

1. Ross R, Glomset J: Atherosclerosis and the arterial smooth muscle cell. SCIENCE 180:1332-1339, 1973.

2. Ross R, Glomset J: The pathogenesis of atherosclerosis (Parts I and II). N ENGL J MED 295:369-377 and 420-425, 1976.

3. Ross R, Harker L: Hyperlipidemia and atherosclerosis. SCIENCE 193:1094-1100, 1976.

4. Stemerman MB, Ross R: Experimental arteriosclerosis. I. Fibrous plaque formation in primates, an electron microscope study. J EXP MED 136:769-789, 1972.

5. Bondjers G, Björkerud S: Arterial repair and atherosclerosis after mechanical injury. III. Cholesterol accumulation and

removal in morphologically defined regions of aortic atherosclerotic lesions in the rabbit. ATHEROSCLEROSIS 17:85-94, 1973.

6. Helin P. Lorenzen I, Garbarsch C, Matthiessen ME: Arteriosclerosis in rabbit aorta induced by mechanical dilatation: Biochemical and morphological studies. ATHEROSCLEROSIS 13:319-331, 1971.

7. Harker L, Ross R, Slichter S, Scott C: Homocystine-induced arteriosclerosis: The role of endothelial cell injury and platelet response in its genesis. J CLIN INVEST 58:731-741, 1976.

8. Ritchie JL, Harker L: Platelet and fibrinogen survival in coronary atherosclerosis: Response to medical and surgical therapy. AM J CARDIOLOGY 39:595-598, 1977.

9. Ross R, Glomset J, Kariya B, Harker L: A platelet-dependent serum factor that stimulates the proliferation of arterial smooth muscle cells *in vitro*. PROC NATL ACAD SCI (USA) 71: 1207-1210, 1974.

10. Kohler N, Lipton A: Platelets as a source of fibroblast growth-promoting activity. EXP CELL RES 87:297-301, 1974.

11. Westermark B, Wasteson A: A platelet factor stimulating human normal glial cells. EXP CELL RES 98:170-174, 1976.

12. Antoniades HN, Scher CD: Growth factors derived from human serum, human platelets and human pituitary: Properties and immunologic crossreactivity. J NATL CANCER INST (In Press).

13. Ross R, Glomset J, Kariya B, Raines E, Bungenberg de Jong J: The cells of the artery wall in the study of atherosclerosis. In INTERNATIONAL CELL BIOLOGY, edited by Brinkley BR, Porter KR. New York, The Rockefeller University Press, 1977, p. 629.

14. Witte LD, Kaplan KL, Nossel HL, Lages BA, Weiss HJ, Goodman DS: Studies of the release from human platelets of the growth factor for cultured human arterial smooth muscle cells. CIRC RES (In Press).

15. Moore S, Friedman RJ, Singal DP, Gauldie J, Blajchman M: Inhibition of injury-induced thromboatherosclerotic lesions by antiplatelet serum in rabbits. THROMB HAEMOSTAS 35:70-81, 1976.

SUMMARY OF DISCUSSION BY PARTICIPANTS

Dr. Bell asked Dr. Ross if in culture studies with his platelet factor he found a direct effect of platelet factor on the synthesis by the cells of protein and/or lipid. Dr. Ross replied that he has not specifically looked at lipid synthesis. The cells require plasma in order to divide, and lipoproteins are present in plasma in sufficient quantities to provide all of the cell's lipid requirements. Without plasma, incidentally, there is no cell division and no protein synthesis, merely initiation of DNA synthesis. Dr. Bell emphasized the possible role of hypercholesterolemia in modifying membrane fluidity. For example, the work of Shattil, Cooper, and colleagues shows that increases in cholesterol and phospholipid ratio modify platelet function and that hypercholesterolemia may play a very important role in this respect (J CLIN INVEST 55:636, 1975; J LAB CLIN MED 89:341, 1977). Dr. Ross noted that a cell exposed to increased lipoprotein levels is potentially capable of having more cholesterol molecules inserted in the plasma membrane. This would increase the rigidity or decrease the fluidity of the membrane and change the cell's ability to respond. In the case of endothelial cells, it would change cell-to-cell attachments. In the case of platelets, possibly it would change the cell's ability to change shape, which is necessary for its functions.

Dr. Spaet mentioned that in line with Dr. Ross' results, the platelet "may be necessary for the laying of the keel but not the launching." Work in his laboratory has demonstrated that if antiplatelet serum is going to prevent the lesion after balloon injury, it has to be given some time before the injury. If it is given immediately after the injury, so that a layer of normal platelets is allowed to deposit on the denuded epithelium, the lesion proceeds normally even though the platelet level is kept down for the next month.

Dr. Fuster asked whether the intimal thickening in the early atherosclerotic lesion is due to proliferation of smooth muscle cells, perhaps from the media of the artery, or possibly due to proliferation of endothelial cells. Dr. Ross answered that he thought smooth muscle cells already in the intima do proliferate, but a large percentage of the proliferation is of cells that have migrated from the media into the intima. He has good evidence for this in experimental animals, and it is reasonable to expect that the same applies in humans because a platelet factor will induce migration of smooth muscle cells.

In response to questions from Dr. Mustard and Dr. Didisheim about dipyridamole, Dr. Ross indicated that the drug has no effect on smooth muscle cells in his tissue culture system, and he has not determined whether monkeys given dipyridamole or other antiplatelet agents show depressant effects on release of platelet factor into the serum.

Responding to a question from Dr. H. J. Day, Dr. Ross commented that it is not clear whether his platelet factor is the same as Gospodarowicz fibroblast growth factor. Dr. Gospodarowicz thinks that the two factors are different. One piece of evidence is that the fibroblast growth factor will markedly induce endothelial cells to proliferate in culture, while the platelet factor will not. They may be homologous but different proteins.

Dr. Moore wondered if Dr. Ross' factor is the same as Dr. Antoniades' factor, and whether Dr. Ross could get an immunoassay for it. Dr. Ross discussed Dr. Antoniades' factor, which does not yet appear to be purified, and asserted that he is going to wait until he is sure he has a pure protein before he develops an immunoassay.

VESSEL INJURY AND ATHEROSCLEROSIS

Sean Moore, M.D, and Ihor O. Ihnatowycz, B.S.

Department of Pathology, McMaster University, Hamilton,

Ontario, Canada

ABSTRACT

Repeated endothelial injury causes lipid-rich lesions in animals on a normal diet. In severely thrombocytopenic animals these lesions do not form or are markedly inhibited. The occurrence of lipid in some experimental designs is related to continued or repeated deposition of thrombus. Lipid deposition occurs in areas where endothelium is repeatedly removed and regrows. Repeated deposition of thrombus may bring about changes in the metabolism of the neo-intima which favor lipid deposition.

INTRODUCTION

There is clear evidence that injury to the endothelium or intima of arteries leads to the deposition of platelets at the injury site followed by the proliferation of smooth muscle cells in the intima. This forms a plaque of smooth muscle cells lying in a matrix of collagen, elastic fibers, and glucosaminoglycans. This type of plaque is one of the lesions observed in human atherosclerosis. Many consider it an early lesion which serves as a substrate for the deposition of lipid; then calcification occurs, leading to a complicated lesion giving rise to the clinical manifestations of the disease. It is perhaps less clearly recognized that in animals maintained on a normolipemic diet, repeated experimental injury to the arterial wall causes development of the full range of atherosclerotic lesions observed in man. In this presentation we will summarize the evidence that repeated injury to the endothelium or the intima of arteries results in lipid-containing atherosclerotic lesions.

ARTERIAL WALL INJURY

Any type of injury to the arterial wall results in the development of a fibromusculo-elastic intimal plaque (1,2). This is true whether the injury is physical, chemical, or biological, and occurs if any part of the wall or the whole wall is subjected to damage. The plaque which forms shows no stainable lipid unless the injury has been accompanied by cholesterol feeding (3-16). In contrast, in response to continued or repeated injury to the intima or endothelium, lipid-containing lesions are observed in animals fed a normolipemic diet (2,17).

REPEATED INTIMAL INJURY

We have used two experimental methods, the first of which was developed by accident rather than design. During experiments examining the possible relationship between an aortic source of emboli composed of platelet aggregates and the development of vascular lesions in the kidneys of rabbits (18), we found lesions of the aortic intima (19). These were related to the presence of an indwelling polyethylene catheter. At sites where there appeared to have been repeated contact between the catheter and the aortic wall, such as at the tip of the catheter or at areas of angulation, raised lipid-containing plaques occurred. Subsequently we observed that fatty streaks and edematous plaques were present when a catheter had been in place 1 to 3 weeks. The raised lipid-containing lesions exhibited all the morphological features seen in complicated human lesions of atherosclerosis. There was a central lipid pool, cholesterol clefts were present, and calcification and eventual bone formation occurred.

These raised lesions exhibited marked accumulation of free cholesterol and cholesterol ester in comparison to intimal medial samples from normal wall or fibromusculo-elastic plaques (20). The elevation of cholesterol ester was particularly striking, being six to seven times normal at 2 weeks, and rising by 4 months to over 30 times normal intimal medial levels. As has been shown by Weigensberg, More, and Sumiyoshi (21), much of the free cholesterol is present early in the course of development of these lesions. Metabolic studies showed that the cholesterol ester accumulation resulted in part from synthesis in the arterial wall. These experiments indicated that continued or repeated injury to the endothelium of aortas of rabbits maintained on a normolipemic diet caused a spectrum of atherosclerotic lesicns similar to those occurring spontaneously in man.

Our second experimental method was developed intentionally. It seemed important to examine more closely the proposition that repeated endothelial damage could cause atherosclerotic lesions.

To do this we used human serum, which causes damage to the arterial intima of rabbits (22). However, reproducible injury could only be produced by human serum which was cytotoxic for rabbit lymphocytes. The method used was to inject a small amount of lymphocytotoxic serum into a segment of rabbit carotid artery every week for 4 weeks (23). Homologous serum, lymphocytotoxic negative serum, positive serum adsorbed against human buffy coat, or saline produced no lesion or a very minimal focal intimal thickening. When the arteries were examined 1 week following the last (4th) injection of lymphocytotoxic positive serum, raised lipid-containing lesions were found, and many showed calcification. Arteries examined after two or three injections showed edematous plaques or fatty streaks in which the lipid was mainly intracellular.

Regression of lesions induced by continued or repeated injury (24,25) occurred very rapidly following withdrawal of the injury stimulus. This was true of both the mechanical and the immunological types of injury. In both, lesions regressed to non-lipid-containing fibromusculo-elastic plaques. During this regression, the raised lipid-containing plaques appeared to pass through a stage at which fatty streaks were the predominant lesion identified. This suggests that fatty streaks might be a stage in the regression of injury-induced lipid-containing raised lesions. In a study of regression of raised lesions induced by the placement of intra-aortic catheters for 7 days followed by catheter removal, the lesions peaked at 7 days and had disappeared by 14 days after removal of the catheter.

Although the rabbits in these studies were on a normal diet, in the experiment in which immunological injury produced lipid-containing lesions in the carotid artery, a small but significant rise occurred in serum cholesterol levels (25). This elevation was maximal 1 week following the last injection of human serum. Thereafter, the serum cholesterol levels declined while the lesions regressed from lipid-containing plaques to fibromusculo-elastic plaques devoid of lipid. The elevation of serum cholesterol was not due to the operative procedure employed or to immunization, because no elevation was observed in animals receiving lymphocytotoxic negative human serum or adsorbed serum. We have no explanation for this finding.

These experiments show that repeated or continued injury to the arterial intima causes, in the absence of dietary lipid supplement, lesions similar to those seen in human atherosclerosis, including lipid-rich raised lesions and fatty streaks. They indicate the possibility that similar lesions could occur in humans as a consequence of repeated endothelial injury. However, they do not establish that endothelial injury is the mechanism involved. Electron microscopy of the lesions induced in the carotid arteries suggested that endothelial damage was the initial lesion followed by deposition of platelet-fibrin thrombus on the denuded subendothelial tissue (23).

It has been established that simple removal of the aortic endothelium by a balloon catheter in rabbits (8,26) or monkeys (27) is followed by the development of a fibromusculo-elastic intimal plaque. One of the main stimuli to proliferation of smooth muscle cells which form the plaque is a substance released from platelets (28,29), although serum factors (30) and possibly endocrine stimulation (31,32) and lipoproteins (33,35) are needed as well. From recent studies it seems that the stimulation caused by platelets acts only during the very short time when platelets adhere to the injury site (36,37).

A second injury to the neo-intima by removal of the endothelium with a balloon catheter exposes the bloodstream to a much more thrombogenic surface, with the result that the thrombus formed is much more abundant and is composed of fibrin as well as masses of platelets (26). This contrasts with the monolayer of platelets which carpets the area following the first removal of endothelium (26,39). Presumably, further episodes of removal of endothelium are also associated with more abundant thrombus deposition.

Because we had shown that continued or repeated damage to the arterial intima leads to the development of lipid-rich lesions, we decided to see if this would happen with the lesser injury to the intima caused by repeated removal of the endothelium using a balloon catheter. In order to determine how many balloon removals of the endothelium were needed to induce lesions in the intimal thickenings, we "ballooned" rabbit aortas two, three, and four times at intervals of 3 days to 1 week. In five of 27 rabbits ballooned four times, lipid was found in areas around branch vessels. In a definitive experiment, ballooning was done six times at intervals of 2 weeks and the animals killed 1, 3, and 7 weeks, 6 months, and 1 year following the last ballooning. Evans blue dye was injected intravenously half an hour before killing. This outlined areas covered by endothelium, which retained their normal (white) appearance; areas where endothelium had not regenerated were blue.

Intracellular and perifibrous lipid was found in white areas at all time periods. In a few animals small amounts of lipid were present in blue areas at 1, 3, and 7 weeks, but not in animals killed 6 months or 1 year after the last ballooning. In the latter the lesions resembled human fatty streaks in some instances but the majority closely resembled human fibro-fatty plaques.

Electron microscopy showed abundant lipid vacuoles in smooth muscle cells in white areas covered by endothelium. Cholesterol clefts and extracellular lipid droplets as well as calcium deposition were also seen. At 6 months and 1 year, lipid deposition tended to be greater and plaque thickness more marked in white areas around branch vessels.

If platelets furnish a substance required for smooth muscle cell proliferation in the arterial intima which forms the cellular substrate of the atherosclerotic plaque, removal or severe depletion of platelets in a living animal should inhibit the development of lesions in response to injury. We examined this in rabbits with an indwelling aortic catheter (39). Thrombocytopenia was produced by injections of antiserum to rabbit platelets raised in sheep. Catheters were placed in the aorta for 2 weeks. Animals that had not received antiplatelet serum or which received normal sheep serum showed extensive lipid-rich thrombo-atherosclerotic plaques. The surface area involved by the lipid-rich raised lesions was between five- and seven-fold less in groups of rabbits made thrombocytopenic by antiplatelet serum. In animals in which very low platelet counts were achieved ($\leq$1000 per mm^3), lesions were completely inhibited.

In these experiments normal sheep serum and antiplatelet serum exhibited some cross reactivity with smooth muscle cells and endothelial cells, as examined by indirect immunofluorescence. Antiplatelet serum or normal sheep serum showed equivalent anti-smooth muscle cell activity. Antiplatelet serum showed 16 times the activity of normal sheep serum against endothelium, so, in the experiment (39) comparing the effects of antiplatelet serum against normal sheep serum, the antiplatelet serum was diluted to 1:16. In subsequent experiments we have used highly purified antiplatelet serum which showed no cross reactivity with endothelium or smooth muscle cells. Because this highly purified antiplatelet serum proved to be extremely toxic for rabbits, the experiments with the indwelling aortic catheter have been repeated using busulfan in combination with smaller doses of antiplatelet serum (40). Lesions were quantitated by weighing and by planimetry. Weight and surface area of lesions were significantly less in the experimental group than in the control groups, and in many animals the lesions were virtually absent. Similarly, Friedman and his colleagues have shown marked suppression of the intimal smooth muscle cell proliferation following a single episode of ballooning using purified antiplatelet serum (41). These experiments indicate that removing most of the platelets from the animal markedly inhibits or prevents both the smooth muscle cell proliferation after a single removal of aortic endothelium and the development of raised lipid-rich lesions after repeated intimal injury.

SYNERGY OF INJURY AND HYPERCHOLESTEROLEMIA

Many experiments show that the combination of a single injury together with dietary induced hypercholesterolemia leads to the development of lipid-containing plaques in the arterial intima (3-16). The observations of Minick and his colleagues (42,43) using relatively low levels of diet-induced hypercholesterolemia combined with immunological injury are of particular interest in relation to possible mechanisms of atherogenesis in man. Fatty proliferative lesions very similar to fibrous plaques in man were produced after hyperlipemia was induced and immunological damage was caused by repeated injections of bovine serum albumin. Dietary hyperlipemia induced after an immunological injury had caused plaque formation also led to lipid accumulation in the lesions (44). Lamberson and Fritz have shown a similarly enhanced susceptibility to diet-induced atherosclerosis in rabbits following a single injection of highly purified bovine serum albumin (45). It has recently been shown by Sharma and Geer (46) that the early aortic lesions due to serum sickness in rabbits are characterized by endothelial damage followed by deposition of platelets. This suggests that antigen-antibody complexes could damage the endothelium, thus providing an initial step in plaque formation.

DRUGS INHIBITING PLATELET FUNCTION

Because a platelet factor has an essential role in the smooth muscle cell proliferative response to injury (23,39), we examined the effect of drugs inhibiting platelet function. When rabbits were treated with sulfinpyrazone for 2 weeks following balloon removal of the aortic endothelium, no difference was observed in the thickness of the neo-intima in experimental and control groups (47). Clowes and Karnowsky (48) have shown a similar lack of effect on intimal proliferation following endothelial injury in the rat carotid artery in animals exposed to aspirin, reserpine, and flurbiprofen.

In recent experiments employing tissue culture of rabbit aorta-derived smooth muscle cells, we have shown that although indomethacin or sulfinpyrazone blocked the formation of malondialdehyde when platelets were exposed to thrombin, they did not inhibit the release of the factor causing smooth muscle cell proliferation (49). Therefore, one would not expect these drugs to influence the proliferation of smooth muscle cells in the aortic wall.

In a study of the uptake of ^{51}Cr-labeled platelets following balloon removal of the aortic endothelium in rabbits, sulfinpyrazone had little effect, aspirin-treated rabbits showed an enhanced platelet uptake, and dipyridamole showed some inhibition of uptake (50). If substantiated, the increased effect with aspirin may be due to inhibition of prostacyclin production by the arterial wall (51). The result with dipyridamole is congruent with the findings of Harker and his colleagues on inhibition of lesion development caused by homocystine in baboons (52).

Clowes and Karnowsky have shown that heparin inhibits the intimal proliferation following air drying injury to the rabbit carotid artery (53). If this effect is not mediated by heparin inhibition of smooth muscle cell proliferation, it is more likely that thrombin is involved in causing the release of smooth muscle cell stimulating factor from platelets when they adhere to the damaged subendothelial structures.

RELEVANCE OF THE INJURY HYPOTHESIS TO HUMAN DISEASE

Although it now seems clear that repeated endothelial injury in animals can cause the full spectrum of atherosclerotic lesions observed in man, it is pertinent to inquire if there is any evidence that such a mechanism is important in the genesis of the human disease (54). Much of the available evidence is indirect and relates to the potential for recognized risk factors to cause endothelial injury or to modify the response of smooth muscle cells to injury. Other evidence comes from metabolic derangements in which atherosclerosis tends to appear precociously or to be more severe. Perhaps the most convincing evidence comes from a number of clinical settings where injury mechanisms can be specifically invoked.

One of the latter situations in which we have had an opportunity to examine the lesions in human material is very similar to the experiments in which catheters were inserted into the rabbit aortas. It is common practice in neonatal units to place a catheter in the aorta by way of the umbilical artery in order to monitor blood gases. The contact between catheter and the aortic wall causes thrombi with diverse clinical effects resulting from embolism. Raised thrombo-atherosclerotic lesions containing lipid are also observed (55). Electron microscopy of some of these lesions shows lipid inclusions within smooth muscle cells of the thickened intima. There are some edematous plaques, and in older lesions calcification is prominent.

Arteriovenous shunts established in patients undergoing chronic hemodialysis for kidney failure frequently occlude because of buildup of thrombus material in the vein immediately distal to the shunt (56). Venous segments removed at the time of shunt revision show marked intimal thickening with fresh luminal thrombus. Many also show lipid in the thickened intima and underlying media. In some there are collections of foam cells and (rarely) cholesterol clefts (54). Stehbens reported lipid deposition in vein walls of experimentally constructed carotid-jugular arteriovenous aneurysms in sheep (57). He and Karmody also described changes similar to those outlined above in the veins of arteriovenous fistulas in hemodialysis patients (58).

Atherosclerosis has also been described in the venous wall of aortocoronary bypass grafts (59).

Atherosclerotic change occurring in the arteries of transplanted organs may be due to immunological damage (60). Bieber and colleagues (61) find no correlation between the severity of atherosclerosis developing in the coronary arteries of transplanted hearts and serum lipid levels, although clearly a synergy between endothelial damage and hypercholesterolemia may exist in this situation analogous to that in Minick's experiments. Minick's group has provided evidence that endothelial injury may be important in the pathogenesis of arterial lesions (62).

Homocystinuria is an inborn error of metabolism associated with arterial and venous thromboses and precocious development of atherosclerosis. Harker and colleagues showed patchy endothelial loss in baboons chronically infused with homocystine (52,63). Decreased platelet survival was taken as evidence of platelet consumption in areas of endothelial damage. Plaques composed of smooth muscle cells developed after 60 days of infusion of homocystine and were inhibited by dipyridamole; this drug was also associated with a return of platelet survival to normal. Some plaques showed lipid inclusions in the smooth muscle cells.

RISK FACTORS IN ENDOTHELIAL INJURY

With the acquisition of new knowledge about the response of the vessel wall to repeated injury, it becomes important to examine how some of the risk factors for atherosclerosis might influence the process of atherogenesis. There has been recent interest in the possibility that diet-induced hypercholesterolemia may cause endothelial injury. Thus, Ross and Harker have shown that in monkeys on a hyperlipemic diet, there is a 5% loss of the endothelial cells from the surface of the aorta and iliac arteries, and that this is accompanied by a decrease of platelet survival (16) It is difficult to reconcile a decrease of platelet survival in response to such a small loss of endothelial cover with the recent experiments by Rathbone and her colleagues; in those studies no change in platelet survival was demonstrated following aortic de-endothelialization with a balloon catheter (64). However, there is evidence that in atherosclerosis induced by hyperlipemia in monkeys (65), swine (66), and rabbits (67,68), and in spontaneous atherosclerosis occurring in white Carneau pigeons (69), there are areas of endothelial damage, and platelet and leukocyte adherence in the areas of endothelial injury. Furthermore, thrombocytes in white Carneau pigeons which are susceptible to atherosclerosis are apparently altered in that they do not adhere as readily to glass or form aggregates as do thrombocytes from atherosclerosis resistant Show Racer pigeons (70). At an age when spontaneous atherosclerosis develops, White Carneau pigeons have higher levels of platelet factor 4-like activity than Show Racer pigeons (71).

LIPID ACCUMULATION AND ENDOTHELIAL INJURY

Leaving aside the question of whether hypercholesterolemia can cause endothelial damage, there is also the problem of how lipid accumulates when the endothelium is damaged by other agents in the presence or absence of hyperlipemia. When endothelium is damaged or removed under the influence of hypercholesterolemia, the intimal plaque which forms is lipid-rich with many cells containing lipid in their cytoplasm. There is little evidence that the induction of hyperlipemia augments the thickness of the plaque formed (16,72). However, the process of regression appears to be retarded (15,16,73).

Accumulation of lipid in the intima following removal of the endothelium in the presence of hyperlipemia occurs only when smooth muscle cells have proliferated on the luminal side of the internal elastic lamina (74). Similarly, cortisone is thought to inhibit the development of diet-induced atherosclerosis by preventing proliferation of cells in the intima (75). Enhanced deposition of lipid in the presence of mechanical or immunological injury suggests that the main reason for lipid accumulation is loss of the so-called "barrier function" of the endothelium (76-78). Such a mechanism is even more strongly indicated by the evidence that large deposits of lipid occur in response to repeated endothelial injury in the absence of dietary lipid supplement.

Results of recent experiments pose problems in accepting this simplistic explanation. In our experiments in which aortas were examined at intervals of 1 week to 1 year after the endothelium had been removed six times at 2-week intervals, lipid accumulated preferentially or exclusively in the areas covered by regenerated endothelium. This suggests that lipid is either being synthesized in these areas by smooth muscle cells (20) or being trapped, possibly by binding to proteoglycans. In a similar experiment recently reported by Minick, Stemerman, and Insull (79), lipid feeding, commenced 28 days after a single balloon removal of endothelium, caused lipid accumulation in areas of endothelial regeneration, examined at 13 and 15 weeks following endothelial denudation. More recently, Minick and his colleagues (80) have found an increase in Alcian-blue positive material in areas covered by endothelium in animals on either cholesterol-supplemented or lipid-poor diets. This supports the idea of lipid trapping in the lesions covered by endothelium, and suggests that lipid accumulates preferentially in areas covered with endothelium because more proteoglycan is produced in these areas than in the areas where endothelial cover has not occurred.

Alteration in proteoglycan metabolism could probably affect the processing of lipoprotein by the artery wall in a number of ways. An increase in the ratio of sulfated to nonsulfated glucosaminoglycans would be associated with an increase in permeability (81). Glucosaminoglycans produced by the smooth muscle cells could bind lipoproteins as proposed by Iverius (82). Recently it has been shown that aortic glucosaminoglycans are altered in structure and increased in amount in areas of the aortic wall of pigeons susceptible to spontaneous atherosclerosis (83).

The association of lipids and of lipoproteins with various structural elements such as the internal elastic lamina and collagen has long been recognized (84-86). Hollander has recently reviewed the evidence that plaque lipid exists as complexes of lipoprotein, acid mucopolysaccharide, and calcium (87).

Work with bovine aorta suggests that proteoglycans have an important role in the regulation of smooth muscle cell proliferation (88).

The new findings on lipid deposition in areas of endothelial regrowth strongly suggest that alterations in the neo-intima produce conditions favoring lipid deposition. In a hyperlipemic situation such deposition may occur following one removal of the endothelium. In normolipemic rabbits multiple removals of the endothelium are needed for lipid accumulation to occur. This suggests that thrombus formation in these areas may influence the changes in the neo-intima which in turn facilitate lipid deposition.

A corollary to this is that repeated injury to areas not covered by endothelium apparently does not induce thrombus formation. In recent experiments aortas which were ballooned, then left *in situ* for several days showed less uptake of ^{51}Cr-labeled platelets than did aortas removed 1 hour after ballooning (89). This suggests that areas not covered by endothelium do not support platelet or thrombus adherence and so repeated ballooning would not cause new thrombus formation in these areas.

REFERENCES

1. Hoff HF: Vascular Injury: A review. THROMB HAEMOSTAS (Suppl.)40:121-136, 1970.

2. Moore S: Atherosclerosis. In ANIMAL MODELS OF THROMBOSIS AND HEMORRHAGIC DISEASES. DHEW Publication No. (NIH) 76-962, Washington, DC, 1976, pp. 132-143.

3. Schlichter JGL, Katz LN, Myers J: The occurrence of atheromatous lesions after cauterization of the aorta followed by

cholesterol administration. AM J MED SCI 218:603-609, 1949.

4. Prior JT, Hartman WH: The effect of hypercholesterolemia upon intimal repair of the aorta of the rabbit following experimental trauma. AM J PATHOL 31:417-424, 1955.

5. Constantinides P, Gutmann-Auersperg N, Hospes D: Acceleration of intimal atherogenesis through prior medial injury. ARCH PATHOL LAB MED 66:247-254, 1958.

6. Friedman M, Byers SO: Experimental thrombo-atherosclerosis. J CLIN INVEST 40:1139-1152, 1961.

7. Courtice FC, Schmidt-Diedrichs A: Lipid deposition in injured wall of carotid artery in hypercholesterolemic and hyperlipemic rabbits. J EXP PHYSIOL 47:228-237, 1962.

8. Baumgartner HR, Studer A: Gezielte Überdehnung der aorta abdominalis am normo-und hypercholesterinaemischen kanninchen. PATHOL MICROBIOL (Basel) 26:129-148, 1963.

9. Gutstein WH, Lazzarini-Robertson A, LaTaillade JN: The role of local arterial irritability in the development of arterio-atherosclerosis. AM J PATHOL 42:61-71, 1963.

10. Friedman M, Felton L, Byers SO: Anti-atherogenic effect of iridium^{192} upon cholesterol fed rabbits. J CLIN INVEST 43:185-192, 1964.

11. Amronim GD, Gildenhorn HL, Solomon RD, Nadkarni BB, Jacobs ML: The synergism of x-irradiation and cholesterol-fat feeding on the development of coronary artery lesions. J ATHEROSCLER RES 4:325-334, 1964.

12. Friedman M, Byers SO: Aortic atherosclerosis intensification by prior endothelial denudation. ARCH PATHOL LAB MED 79:345-356, 1965.

13. Constantinides P: Lipid deposition in injured arteries. Electron microscopic study. ARCH PATHOL LAB MED 85:280-297, 1968.

14. Julian M, Pieraggi M-Th, Bouissou M: Lathyrisme et regime atherogene chez le rat. PATHOL BIOL (Paris) 20:951-959, 1972.

15. Nam GC, Lee WM, Jarmolych J, Lee KT, Thomas WA: Rapid production of advanced atherosclerosis in swine by a combination of endothelial injury and cholesterol feeding. EXP MOL PATHOL 18:369-373, 1973.

16. Ross R, Harker L: Hyperlipidemia and atherosclerosis. SCIENCE 193:1094-1100, 1976.

17. Moore S: Thrombosis and atherosclerosis. THROMB HAEMOSTAS (Suppl)60:205-212, 1974.

18. Moore S, Mersereau WA: Micro-embolic renal ischemia, hypertension and nephrosclerosis. ARCH PATHOL LAB MED 85:623-630, 1968.

19. Moore S: Thromboatherosclerosis in normolipemic rabbits: A result of continued endothelial damage. LAB INVEST 29:478-487, 1973.

20. Day AJ, Bell FP, Moore S, Friedman RJ: Lipid composition and metabolism of thrombo-atherosclerotic lesions produced by continued endothelial damage in normal rabbits. CIRC RES 29:467-476, 1974.

21. Weigensberg BI, More RH, Sumiyoshi A: Lipid profile in the evolution of experimental atherosclerotic plaques from thrombus. LAB INVEST 33:43-50, 1975.

22. O'Connell TX, Mowbray JF: Effects of humoral transplantation antibody on the arterial intima of rabbits. SURGERY 74:145-152, 1973.

23. Friedman RJ, Moore S, Singal DP: Repeated endothelial injury and induction of atherosclerosis in normolipemic rabbits by human serum. LAB INVEST 30:404-415, 1975.

24. Moore S, Friedman RJ, Gent M: Resolution of lipid-containing atherosclerotic lesions induced by injury. BLOOD VESSELS 14:193-203, 1977.

25. Friedman RJ, Moore S, Singal DP, Gent M: Regression of injury-induced atheromatous lesions in rabbits. ARCH PATHOL LAB MED 100:189-195, 1976.

26. Stemerman MB: Thrombogenesis of the rabbit arterial plaque: An electron microscopic study. AM J PATHOL 73:7-18, 1973.

27. Stemerman MB, Ross R: Experimental arteriosclerosis. I. Fibrous plaque formation in primates, an electron microscopic study. J EXP MED 136:769-789, 1972.

28. Ross R, Glomset JA, Kariya B, Harker LA: A platelet-dependent serum factor that stimulates the proliferation of arterial smooth muscle cells *in vitro*. PROC NATL ACAD SCI USA 71:1207-1210, 1974.

29. Rutherford BA, Ross R: Platelet factors stimulate fibroblasts and smooth muscle cells quiescent in plasma serum to proliferate. J CELL BIOL 69:196-204, 1976.

30. Ihnatowycz I, Moore S, Mustard JF: Platelet growth factor (PGF) stimulation of DNA synthesis in smooth muscle cells (SMC) *in vitro*. FED PROC 36:351, Abst. No. 430, 1977.

31. Stout, RW, Bierman EL, Ross R: The effect of insulin on the proliferation of cultured primate arterial smooth muscle cells. CIRC RES 36:319-327, 1975.

32. Fritz KE, Augustyn JM, Daoud AS, Jarmolych J: Effect of insulin on DNA synthesis of aortic explants in culture. FED PROC 36:401, Abst No. 698, 1977.

33. Ross R, Glomsett JA: Atherosclerosis and the arterial smooth muscle cell. SCIENCE 180:1332-1339, 1973.

34. Brown BG, Mahley R, Assman G: Swine aortic smooth muscle in tissue culture: Some effects of purified swine lipoproteins on cell growth and morphology. CIRC RES 39:415-424, 1976.

35. Augustyn JM, Fritz KE, Daoud AS, Jarmolych J: Effect of lipoprotein on *in vitro* synthesis of DNA in aortic tissue. ATHEROSCLEROSIS 27:179-188, 1977.

36. Spaet TH: Personal communication.

37. Groves HM, Kinlough-Rathbone RL: Personal communication.

38. Baumgartner HR: Platelet interaction with vascular structures. THROMB HAEMOSTAS (Suppl)51:161-176, 1972.

39. Moore S, Friedman RJ, Singal DP, Gauldie J, Blajchman MA, Roberts RS: Inhibition of injury induced thrombo-atherosclerotic lesions by anti-platelet serum in rabbits. THROMB HAEMOSTAS 35:70-81, 1976.

40. Moore S: Lipid containing fibrous plaques induced by repeated endothelial injury: Unpublished observations. Abstracts of 31st Annual Meeting Council on Arteriosclerosis. American Society for the Study of Atherosclerosis, Miami Beach, Nov. 28-30, 1977.

41. Friedman RJ, Stemerman MB, Wenz B, Moore S, Gauldie J, Gent R, Tiell ML, Spaet TH: The effect of thrombocytopenia on experimental arteriosclerotic lesion formation in rabbits. I. Smooth muscle cell proliferation and re-endothelialization. J CLIN INVEST 60:1191-1201, 1977.

42. Minick CR, Murphy GE, Campbell WG Jr: Experimental induction of athero-arteriosclerosis by the synergy of allergic injury to arteries and lipid rich diet. I. Effect of repeated injections of horse serum in rabbits fed a dietary cholesterol supplement. J EXP MED 124:635-652, 1966.

43. Minick CR, Murphy GE: Experimental induction of athero-arteriosclerosis by the synergy of allergic injury to arteries and lipid rich diet. II. Effect of repeatedly injected foreign protein in rabbits fed a lipid-rich, cholesterol-poor diet. AM J PATHOL 73:265-300, 1973.

44. Hardin NJ, Minick CR, Murphy GE: Experimental induction of athero-arteriosclerosis by the synergy of allergic injury to arteries and lipid rich diet. III. The role of earlier acquired fibromuscular intimal thickening in the pathogenesis of later developing atherosclerosis. AM J PATHOL 73:301-327, 1973.

45. Lamberson NV Jr, Fritz KE: Immunological enhancement of atherogenesis in rabbits: Persistent susceptibility to atherogenic diet following experimentally induced serum sickness. ARCH PATHOL LAB MED 98:9-16, 1974.

46. Sharma HM, Geer JC: Experimental aortic lesions of acute serum sickness in rabbits. AM J PATHOL 88:255-266, 1977.

47. Moore S, Belbeck LW, Kinlough-Rathbone RL, Packham MA, Richardson M, Mustard JF: Unpublished observations.

48. Clowes AW, Karnovsky MJ: Failure of certain anti-platelet drugs to affect myointimal thickening following arterial endothelial injury in the rat. LAB INVEST 36:452-464, 1977.

49. Ihnatowycz IO, Cazenave J-P, Moore S, Mustard JF: Platelet derived growth factor production during platelet release reaction independent of the endoperoxide pathway. VI. International Congress on Thrombosis and Haemostasis, Philadelphia 1977. (Abstract).

50. Groves HM, Kinlough-Rathbone R, Belbeck LW, Richardson M, Moore S: Unpublished observations.

51. Gryglewski RJ, Bunting S, Moncada S, Flower RJ, Vane JR: Arterial walls are protected against deposition of platelet thrombi by a substance (prostaglandin X) which they make from prostaglandin endoperoxides. PROSTAGLANDINS 12:685-713, 1976.

52. Harker LA, Slichter SJ, Scott CR, Ross R: Homocystinuria: Vascular injury and arterial thrombosis. N ENGL J MED 291:537-

543, 1974.

53. Clowes AC, Karnovsky MJ: Suppression by heparin of smooth muscle cell proliferation in injured arteries. NATURE 265: 625-626, 1977.

54. Moore S: Clinical correlations. THROMB HAEMOSTAS 33:417-425, 1975.

55. Tyson JE, deS DJ, Moore S: Thrombo-atheromatous complications of umbilical arterial catheterization in the newborn period. Clinico-pathological study. ARCH DIS CHILD 51:744-754, 1976.

56. Kaegi A, Pineo GF, Shimazu A, Trivedi H, Hirsh J, Gent M: Arteriovenous shunt thrombosis; prevention by sulfinpyrazone. N ENGL J MED 290:304-306, 1974.

57. Stehbens WE: Haemodynamic production of lipid deposition, intimal tears, mural dissection and thrombosis in the blood vessel wall. PROC R SOC LONDON [BIOL] 185:357-373, 1974.

58. Stehbens WE, Karmody AM: Venous atherosclerosis associated with arteriovenous fistulas for hemodialysis. ARCH SURG 110:176-180, 1975.

59. Barboriak JJ, Pintar K, Korns ME: Atherosclerosis in aorto-coronary vein grafts. LANCET II:621-624, 1974.

60. Minick CR: Immunologic arterial injury in atherogenesis. ANN N Y ACAD SCI 275:210-227, 1976.

61. Bieber CP, Stinson EB, Shumway NE, Payne R, Kosek J: Cardiac transplantation in man: Cardiac allograft pathology. CIRCULATION 41:753-772, 1970.

62. Alonso DR, Starek PK, Minick CR: Studies on the pathogenesis of atheroarteriosclerosis induced in rabbit cardiac allografts by the synergy of graft rejection and hypercholesterolemia. AM J PATHOL 87:415-442, 1977.

63. Harker LA, Ross R, Slichter J, Scott CR: Homocystine induced arteriosclerosis. J CLIN INVEST 58:763-741, 1976.

64. Groves HM, Kinlough-Rathbone RL, Richardson M, Mustard JF: Platelet survival and interaction with damaged rabbit aorta. Unpublished observations.

65. Wu KK, Armstrong ML, Hoak JC, Megan MB: Platelet aggregates in hypercholesterolemic rhesus monkeys. THROMB RES 7:917-924, 1975.

66. Nelson E, Gertz SD, Rennels ML, Forbes MS, Kahn MA, Farber TJ, Heald FP, Earl FL: Endothelial lesions in the aorta of egg-yolk fed miniature swine; scanning and transmission electron microscopy. CIRCULATION 51-52 (Suppl II):II-103, 1975.

67. Svendsen E, Jorgensen L: Loss of endothelium in rabbit aortas following short term cholesterol feeding. IVth International symposium on Atherosclerosis (Abs. F-81) Tokyo, Japan, Aug. 24-28, 1976.

68. Davies PF, Reidy MA, Goode TB, Bowyer DE: Scanning electron microscopy in the evaluation of endothelial integrity of fatty lesions in atherosclerosis. ATHEROSCLEROSIS 25:125-130, 1976.

69. Lewis JC, Kottke BA: Endothelial damage and thrombocyte adhesion in pigeon atherosclerosis. SCIENCE 196:1007-1009, 1977.

70. Lewis JC, Fuster V, Kottke B: Thrombocytes in atherosclerosis susceptible breeds of pigeon: A comparative ultrastructural study. EXP MOL PATHOL 25:332-343, 1976.

71. Fuster V, Lewis JC, Kottke BA, Ruiz CE, Bowie WA: Platelet factor 4-like activity in the initial stages of atherosclerosis in pigeons. THROMB RES 10:169-172, 1977.

72. Clowes AW, Ryan GB, Breslow JL, Karnovsky MJ: Absence of enhanced intimal thickening in the response of the carotid arterial wall to endothelial injury in hypercholesterolemic rats. LAB INVEST 35:6-17, 1976.

73. Daoud AS, Jarmolych J, Augustyn JM, Fritz KE, Singh KH, Lee KT: Regression of advanced atherosclerosis in swine. ARCH PATHOL LAB MED 100:372-379, 1974.

74. Katocs AS, Largis EE, Will LW, McClintock DK, Riggi SJ: Sterol deposition in the aortae of normocholesteremic- and hyper-cholesteremic rabbits subjected to aortic de-endothelialization. ARTERY 2:38-52, 1976.

75. Friedman M, Byers SO, St. George S: Cortisone and experimental atherosclerosis. ARCH PATHOL 77:142-158, 1964.

76. Bjorkerud S: Endothelial permeability interpretation from experimental lesions. In ATHEROSCLEROSIS III. PROCEEDINGS OF THE THIRD INTERNATIONAL SYMPOSIUM, edited by Schetten G, Weizel A, Berlin, Springer-Verlag, 1974, pp. 14-20.

77. Bondjers G, Bjorkerud S: Cholesterol accumulation and content in regions with defined endothelial integrity in the normal rabbit aorta. ATHEROSCLEROSIS 17:71-83, 1971.

78. Bjorkerud S, Bondjers G: Uptake, accumulation and removal of cholesterol from the normal and atherosclerotic arterial wall. NUTR METAB 15:27-36, 1973.

79. Minick CR, Stemerman MB, Insull W: Effect of regenerated endothelium on lipid accumulation in the arterial wall. PROC NATL ACAD SCI USA 74:1724-1728, 1977.

80. Minick CR, Alonso DR, Litrenta MM, Silane MF, Stemerman MB: Regenerated endothelium and intimal proteoglycan accumulation. Abstracts of the 31st Annual Meeting of council on Arteriosclerosis November 28-30, 1977, Miami Beach.

81. Glatz CE, Massaro TA: Influence of glycosaminoglycan content on mass transfer behaviour of porcine artery wall. Part 2. Differences in mass transfer rates related to variation in glycosaminoglycan content. ATHEROSCLEROSIS 25:165-173, 1976.

82. Iverius PH: The interaction between human plasma lipoprotein and connective tissue glucosaminoglycans. J BIOL CHEM 247:2607-2613, 1972.

83. Curwen KD, Smith SC: Aortic glucosaminoglycans in atherosclerosis susceptible and resistant pigeons. EXP MOL PATHOL 27:121-133, 1977.

84. Curran RC, Crane WAJ: Mucopolysaccharides in the atheromatous aorta. J PATHOL 84:405-412, 1962.

85. Walton KW, Williamson N: Histological and immunofluorescent studies on the human atheromatous plaque. J ATHEROSCLER RES 8:599-624, 1968.

86. Hoff HF, Lie TT, Titus JL, Bajardo RJ, Jackson RL, DeBakey ME, Gotto AM: Lipoproteins in atherosclerotic lesions. Investigation by immunofluorescence of APO-low density lipoproteins in human atherosclerotic arteries from normal and hyperlipoproteinemics. ARCH PATHOL LAB MED 99:253-258, 1975.

87. Hollander W: Unified concept on the role of acid mucopolysaccharides and connective tissue proteins in the accumulation of lipids, lipoproteins and calcium in the atherosclerotic plaque. EXP MOL ATHOL 25:106-120, 1976.

88. Eisenstein R, Larsson SE, Kuettner KE, Sorgente N, Hascall VC: The ground substance of the arterial wall. Part I: Extractability of glycosaminoglycans and the isolation of a proteoglycan from bovine aorta. ATHEROSCLEROSIS 22:147, 1975.

89. Cazenave J-P: Personal communication.

SUMMARY OF DISCUSSION BY PARTICIPANTS

Dr. Spittell asked Dr. Moore if repeated serum injury does the same thing as ballooning. Dr. Moore replied that it is not quite the same. Giving serum into a segment of the carotid artery of rabbits every week for 4 weeks causes raised lipid-rich lesions with an enormous amount of calcium degeneration within the 4-week period. The ballooning injury takes longer to evolve. Ballooning six times at 2-week intervals produces fairly spectacular lipid-containing lesions which seem to increase for up to 6 months and perhaps for even up to a year.

Dr. Grabowski asked if, after balloon injury, the platelets are singly adherent. Dr. Moore responded that morphologically you have a monolayer of spread platelets. He also noted that what Dr. Cazenave did was to balloon the aorta in the rabbit, then take the aorta out immediately and study the uptake of platelets. This produces a big uptake of platelets. When the aorta is left in the animal for 4 days before it is removed, the platelet uptake is very much less.

Dr. Grabowski asked Dr. Cazenave if in his experiments platelets adhered to undamaged rabbit aorta. Dr. Cazenave pointed out that what he calls undamaged aorta is aorta which has not been deliberately damaged by a balloon catheter. When the aorta is everted on the probe to expose the endothelium, some damage may result. Under the scanning electron microscope, you can see platelets adhering where there is damage.

Dr. Ross commented that Dr. Moore's slides of the gross specimen of an aorta subjected to six balloonings showed lots of areas that were not re-endothelialized, and wondered if the endothelial cells had stopped doubling by 6 months. Dr. Moore did not think so, although the process seems to be more rapid at first and slows down. About a week after ballooning there is a small circle of re-endothelialization around each branch vessel; 3 weeks later there is coverage of a few millimeters, and after 7 weeks a bit more than that. In the specimen used as an example, after 6 months only about 38% had not been re-endothelialized. After a year, the uncovered area is only 5 to 10% or approaches zero.

Dr. Bell asked whether Dr. Moore had analyzed tissues from re-endothelialized areas to see whether they actually contain more mucopolysaccharide than the surrounding blue-stained [uncovered] areas. Dr. Moore said he hadn't, but noted that Dr. Minick has shown an increase in the Alcian blue-stained areas and will be reporting this at the American Heart meeting in November, 1977.

Dr. Stemerman commented that after the balloon injury, when a certain amount of time had elapsed for endothelial regrowth, in the areas underneath the regenerated endothelium there is Alcian blue-positive staining material. Digestions with mucopolysaccharidases of different types will readily remove this Alcian blue-staining material. This seems to be the specific area in which lipid accumulates.

DELAYED CONSEQUENCES OF ENDOTHELIAL REMOVAL FROM RABBIT AORTAE*

Theodore H. Spaet, M.D., Choo Rhee, M.D., and
Charlene Geiger, B.A.

Hematology Division, Department of Medicine, Montefiore
Hospital and Medical Center, and the Albert Einstein
College of Medicine, Bronx, NY

ABSTRACT

One year after de-endothelialization of rabbit aorta by a balloon catheter, the damaged areas show arteriosclerotic thickening. In the study described here, aortae from six rabbits were examined 2 years after the single injury. Three had advanced atherosclerotic lesions. All the animals had been fed standard rabbit chow, and the five tested did not have hypercholesterolemia when they were sacrificed. Apparently vascular injury alone is sufficient basis for development of atherosclerotic disease in the rabbit.

INTRODUCTION

The sequence of events that follows selective removal of endothelium from the rabbit aorta by a balloon catheter has been described in detail in earlier publications (1,2). In brief, there is progressive re-endothelialization by direct spread of cells from undamaged endothelium; these cells originate from branches that have escaped injury. Concurrently, smooth muscle cells migrate lumenally from the media, and they proliferate to produce marked intimal thickening. A year after injury the damaged areas present the typical picture of arteriosclerotic thickening with almost all animals presenting an intact endothelial cell cover.

*Supported by U.S. Public Health Service Grant #HL 16387.

In the present studies, six rabbits were sacrificed 2 years after aortic de-endothelialization. Three of these had advanced atherosclerotic lesions with a histological picture typical of cholesterol deposits; the remainder had pathology similar to that seen a year after injury. The animals had been kept on standard rabbit chow, and had no evidence of hypercholesterolemia.

METHODS

Experimental animals were male New Zealand rabbits about 6 months of age which weighed about 2 kg at the time of initial aortic balloon injury. 2 years after the procedure they were in good health and weighed about 4 kg. Throughout this period they were kept singly caged, and were fed standard rabbit chow (Ralston Purina Rabbit chow) and water *ad libitum*. Nine animals comprised the group, and seven of these had passage of the balloon catheter to the level of the diaphragm; two others were de-endothelialized through the entire length of the aorta, to the arch. One additional rabbit was housed for the same period without ever having been subjected to vessel trauma or any other experimental procedure. He served as an age control, as did the thoracic aortae and the untouched iliac arteries on the non-ballooned side of the experimental animals.

The method of balloon catheter de-endothelialization and the processing of tissues have been described in previous publications (1,2). Serum cholesterol levels were measured by the standard AutoAnalyzer technique. Quantitation of intimal thickening was performed on tracings of histological sections as before (2), except that weighing of the cutouts was used instead of planimetry.

30 min prior to sacrifice, each animal was given 4 ml of Evans blue dye to mark possible areas which were free of endothelial cover. In most of the animals there was no vessel staining, but two showed small regions, remote from branches, which were distinctly blue.

RESULTS

All aortae showed intimal thickening in the portion of the vessel that had been subjected to balloon injury 2 years previously. The degree of thickening was irregularly distributed, and did not appear to be related to any observable anatomical landmarks. Compared to animals 6 months after injury, these animals showed no further hyperplasia or any evidence of lesion regression (Table 1).

Five animals showed arteriosclerotic vessels almost indistinguishable from those described previously, and characterized by a

TABLE 1. DEGREE OF INTIMAL THICKENING EXPRESSED AS INTIMA MEDIA (I/M) RATIO

Time After Ballooning	Number of Animals	Number of Areas Examined	Mean I/M Ratio
6 months	4	20	1.12
2 years	9	39	1.03

fibromuscular plaque. The one difference seen in these aortae and also those of the entire group was the presence of what appeared to be a reconstituted internal elastic lamina (RIEL) upon which rested a single layer of endothelial cells. These findings are illustrated in Figure 1.

The abdominal aorta of one animal showed a single area with scattered foam cells (Figures 2a and 2b). Such cells were occasionally present in several of the other animals, but they were sparser than in the one illustrated, and not located in any specific region.

Three animals had typical atherosclerotic lesions, with characteristic clefts representing sites where cholesterol had been deposited. These were usually in areas where Evans blue dye had been excluded, and where there was histological evidence of endothelial cover. In one animal, the entire ballooned abdominal aorta was involved with these deposits; in one they were seen only in the thoracic aorta; in the third, they were encountered at several unrelated loci. In none of the animals did the atherosclerotic lesions extend into the ballooned iliac arteries, which presented only the arteriosclerotic fibromuscular plaque.

Except for one area in one rabbit, there was no evidence of unusual injury to the aortae; the internal elastic lamina was intact and the underlying media was normal by both light and electron microscopy. In one animal, there was an area of disrupted internal elastic lamina, suggesting that the initial balloon trauma had been excessive. In general, atherosclerotic deposits were present throughout the thickened intima. However, the picture varied, so that there were regions in which the most lumenal part of the intima was spared, and others in which the deeper layers were not visibly laden with lipid. Typically, the cholesterol was present only in the intima, with only occasional deposits present on the medial side of the internal elastic lamina. When medial cholesterol was encountered, it was always in close apposition to the internal elastic lamina. Electron micrographs of atherosclerotic lesions showed the cholesterol spaces to be among evidently intact smooth muscle cells. Other lipid deposits were not evident. These find-

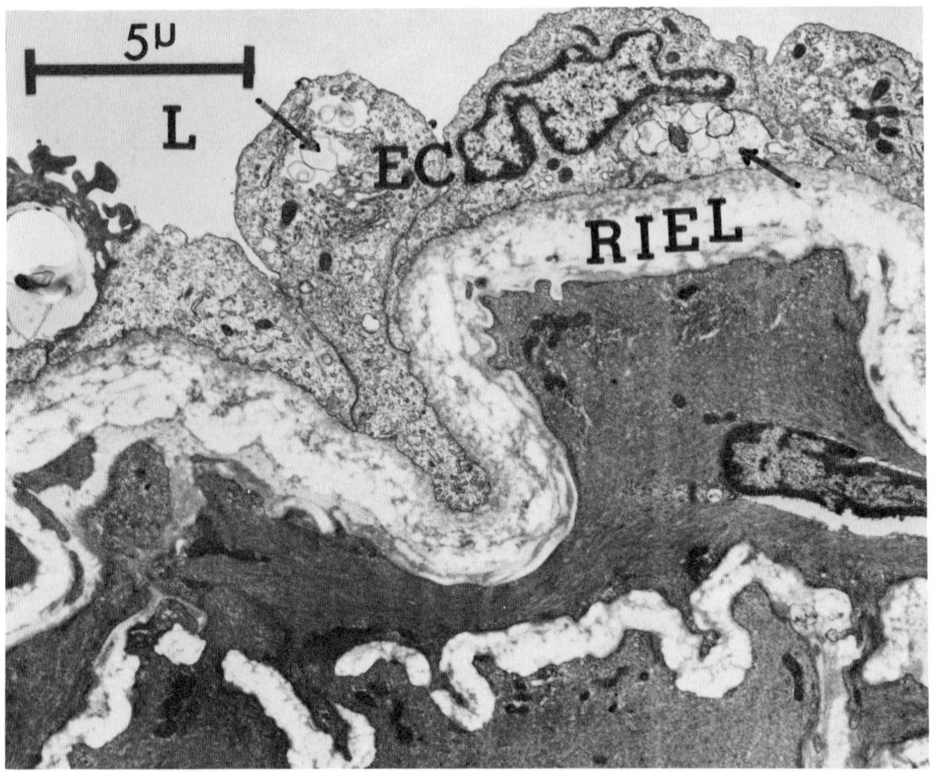

Figure 1. Electron micrograph of arteriosclerotic lesion in abdominal aorta of rabbit 2 yr after balloon de-endothelialization (TYA). Endothelial cells (EC) show possible degenerative changes (arrows). Note the presence of a reconstituted internal elastic lamina (RIEL). L = lumen.

ings are shown in Figures 3a, b, c.

Serum cholesterol levels were determined before sacrifice in five animals, two of which had atherosclerotic lesions. All had between 26 and 35 mg/dl, levels that are normal for this species.

The thoracic aortae which had not been de-endothelialized, as well as iliac arteries from the intact, non-ballooned side, showed histology normal for rabbits. There was no intimal thickening: the endothelium formed a monolayer on the internal elastic lamina. In all vessels, except as noted above, the media was of normal dimensions and was free of visible pathology. Although these vessels served as internal controls, an additional animal of similar age and weight but which had no induced vessel damage was studied. Its vessels were free of lesions.

Figure 2a

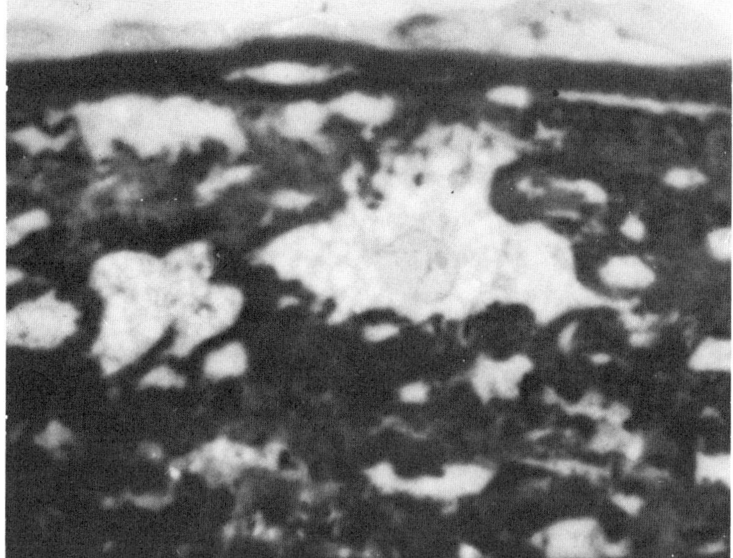

Figure 2b

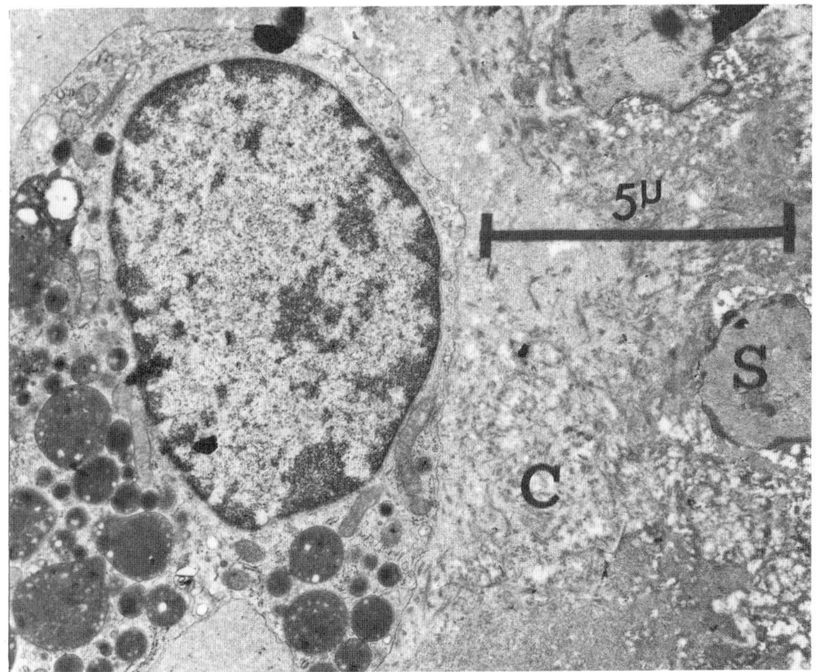

Figure 2. Foam cells seen in a rabbit aorta 2 yr after de-endothelialization. a) Light micrograph (original magnification 1400 X); b) Electron micrograph. S = smooth muscle cell; C = collagen fibrils.

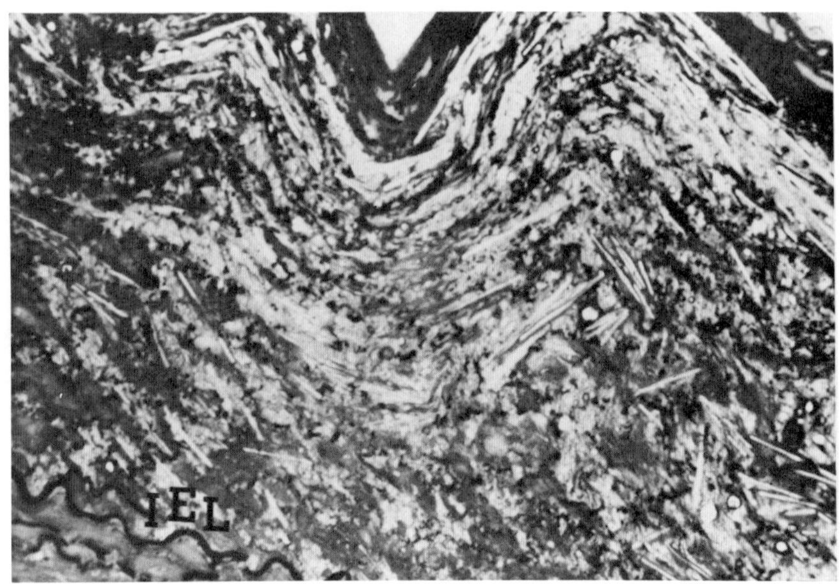

Figure 3a (see legend next page)

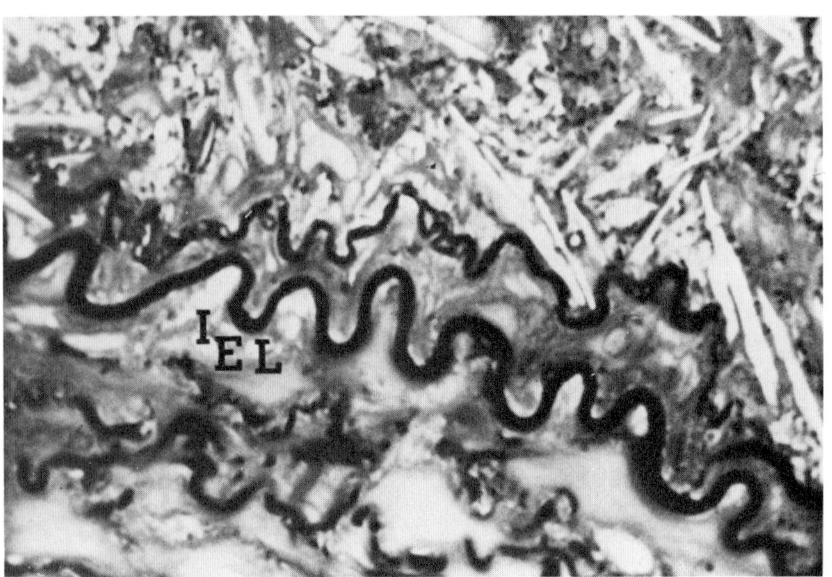

Figure 3b (see legend next page)

Figure 3c

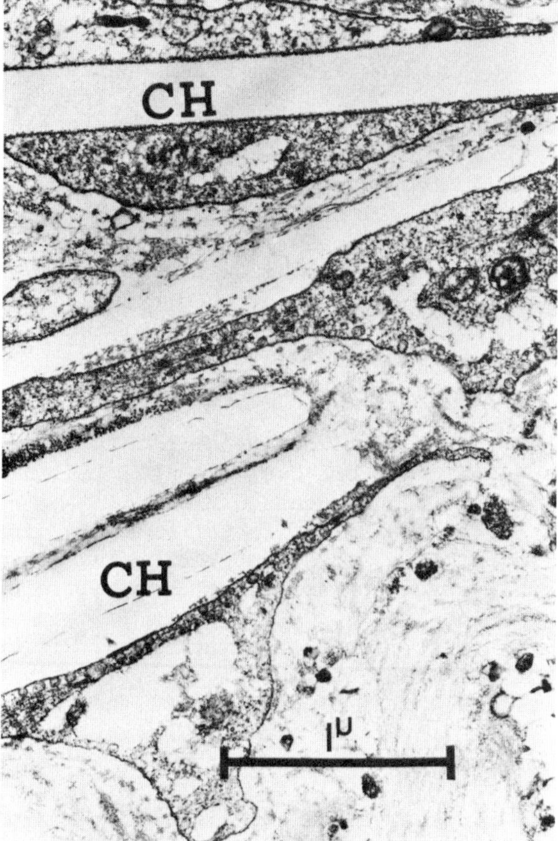

Figure 3. Atherosclerotic lesions in a rabbit aorta 2 yr after de-endothelialization. a) Low power light micrograph of entire intima (original magnification 500 X). b) Higher magnification, which demonstrates the internal elastic lamina (IEL) as a relative barrier to lesion formation (original magnification 1400 X). c) Electron micrograph showing the presence of intimal extracellular deposits characteristic of cholesterol (CH), and corresponding to those shown in Figure 3A.

DISCUSSION

The present observations show that vascular injury alone is evidently a sufficient basis for the development of atherosclerotic disease in the rabbit. The animals which presented this pathology had been given a low-cholesterol diet, and did not have evidence of hypercholesterolemia, at least at the time of sacrifice. Unfortunately, serum cholesterol measurements were not obtained on all animals because the atherosclerotic lesion was wholly unexpected. In fact, the study was originally intended to evaluate regression.

There is some evidence that repeated vascular insults may be followed by atherosclerosis and associated progressive elevation of serum cholesterol in rabbits (3), but this change has not been observed following a single de-endothelialization procedure. Additionally, rabbit atherosclerotic lesions have been produced by the continuous trauma incident to placement of an indwelling catheter, again in the absence of dietary hypercholesterolemia (4).

The source of the deposited lipid is not evident from the available data. The time-course of the lesions suggests that excessive exposure to unprocessed plasma in the absence of endothelial cover was not a significant factor. Atherosclerotic lesions were not seen in any of a large number of rabbits examined in the first year after injury (1), and intact endothelium characterized the vessels in which lipid deposits were maximal. These findings are in conformity with recent observations of Minick *et al.* (5), who showed that the major accumulation of lipid in the balloon de-endothelialized aortas of cholesterol-fed rabbits was in regions recently covered by endothelium. Whether the need for endothelial cover to favor atherosclerosis provides evidence against a blood-borne origin of the lipid remains to be demonstrated. Were the source of lipid the vessel wall itself, the material might come from increased synthesis by the intimal smooth muscle cells, or membrane material resulting from accelerated destruction of these cells.

Other interesting aspects of the study include confinement of atherosclerosis essentially to the intima in our rabbit model as in human disease; the erratic distribution of the atherosclerotic changes within a relatively uniform arteriosclerotic vessel; the increased thickening of the most lumenal internal elastic layer to create a "neo-internal elastic lamina"; and the appearance of the atherosclerotic lesions in only some animals which otherwise showed no difference from their purely arteriosclerotic colleagues.

One obvious characteristic that differed between the animals sacrificed within 1 year after trauma and those examined after 2 years was their age. It is not unreasonable to speculate that the healing response in older organisms will have its own properties. Experiments are typically performed upon young and even not fully grown animals; perhaps these are not fully relevant to diseases of aging.

REFERENCES

1. Spaet TH, Stemerman MB, Veith FJ, Lejnieks I: Intimal injury and regrowth in the rabbit aorta: Medial smooth muscle cells as a source of neointima. CIRC RES 36:58-70, 1975.

2. Stemerman MB, Spaet TH, Pitlick F, Cintron J, Lejnieks I, Tiell ML: Intimal healing. The pattern of reendothelialization and intimal thickening. AM J PATHOL 87:125-137, 1977.

3. Friedman RJ, Moore S, Singal DP, Gent M: Regression of injury-induced atheromatous lesions in rabbits. ARCH PATHOL LAB MED 100:189-195, 1976.

4. Moore S, Friedman RJ, Gent M: Resolution of lipid-containing atherosclerotic lesions induced by injury. BLOOD VESSELS 14:193-203, 1977.

5. Minick CR, Stemerman MB, Insull W: Effect of regenerated endothelium accumulation in the arterial wall. PROC NATL ACAD SCI USA 74:1724-1728, 1977.

NOTE: The discussion of Dr. Spaet's paper follows the paper by Dr. Stemerman; three papers were discussed together.

THE ROLES OF ENDOTHELIUM, PLATELETS, AND SMOOTH MUSCLE CELLS IN INTIMAL HEALING

Michael B. Stemerman, M.D.

Beth Israel Hospital, Boston MA

ABSTRACT

The continual remodeling of the artery wall significantly narrows the lumen. It contributes to the development of atherosclerotic plaque through the incorporation of lipid into the arterial intima. The steps in the repair of arterial intima include platelet accumulation followed by leukocyte attachment to denuded areas, smooth muscle migration from the media, deposition of extracellular connective tissue components, and endothelial proliferation from undamaged artery branches. Intimal growth and regression seem related to re-endothelialization, platelets, the pituitary, and unidentified factors.

INTRODUCTION

Until now methods to control atherosclerosis have emphasized the lowering of serum lipid levels (1). However, recent advances concentrating on the cell biology of the arteriosclerotic plaque and observations in tissue culture have indicated that a component of the intimal thickening is related to luminal injury (2). Therapy for recurrent intimal injury combined with dietary change may eventually result in better atherosclerosis control.

Arteries as conduits of blood contact a wide variety of substances in high concentration. This constant exposure to different chemicals and the mechanical changes of arterial pulsation lead to continual remodeling of the arterial wall (3,4). This remodeling, which eventually narrows the luminal caliber of the vessel significantly, is part of the atherosclerotic process and a phenomenon of aging. Several additional factors appear to be linked clinically to exacerbation of arterial disease. They include cigarette smoking, hypertension, hypercholesterolemia, and diabetes (4).

A major focus of the remodeling is the arterial intima. The incorporation of lipid into the thickening intima forms the characteristic lipid-rich lesion of the complicated atherosclerotic plaque. This gradual narrowing resulting from the aging process and the incorporation of lipids produces the symptoms and complications of arteriosclerosis, the major cause of death in the western world. Factors that influence this process have recently been closely scrutinized in tissue culture and in *in vivo* animal experiments. To understand the atherosclerosis that accompanies aging and the intimal incorporation of lipids requires some knowledge of the components of the vessel wall and an understanding of the arterial response to injury.

ARCHITECTURE OF THE ARTERIAL WALL

The major arteries are divided into three layers (2, 5). The innermost, the *intima*, in its formative stage is a single layer of endothelial cells resting upon the internal elastic lamina (5) to form a continuous, nonthrombogenic surface. Platelets accumulate on the endothelial surface only when the endothelial cells' integrity is compromised (6). During this early stage, scattered collagen fibers, elastin microfibrils, glycosaminoglycans, and the elastin of the internal elastic lamina can be found beneath the endothelium. Sometimes even during this early stage of vascular development, pericytes or smooth muscle cells can be found on the abluminal side of the endothelium.

The middle layer or *media* is bounded by the internal elastic lamina and external elastic lamina, the outermost elastic layer of the artery (2). Only the medias of the large elastic arteries include large lamellar units of concentric layers of elastic tissue. The vasa vasorum nourish the outer layers of the media and are found only in the outermost layers with more than 29 layers of musculoelastic units (7).

The only cell normally found in mammalian media is the vascular smooth muscle cell (SMC). These cells are aligned in a spiral around the long axis of the vessel together with extracellular connective tissue, elastin, collagen, and glycosaminoglycans (2). SMC may be readily cultured from the innermost layer of the media (8).

The outer layer or *adventitia* is composed of connective tissue, fibroblasts, and veil cells, which are probably phagocytic (9), and nerve endings.

CHANGES IN THE ARTERIAL WALL

How the various portions of the vessel wall change with age and stress has been outlined elsewhere (10). Briefly, during the aging process, the entire media and segments of the intima thicken (11). The basic cellular component of arterial growth and remodeling is the SMC. It is the major architect for rebuilding damaged arterial wall, replicating and synthesizing all the necessary connective tissue needed for wall modification. In many respects, growth and development of the arterial wall appear to be the products of the natural activities of the SMC (11).

Arteries are susceptible to many kinds of manipulations (12-14). As a result arteries isolated to study normal vascular physiology under rigidly controlled conditions quickly and irreversibly deteriorate.

The response to many kinds of vascular injury seems to be very consistent, involving endothelial detachment or dysfunction. Various physical and chemical agents injure the arterial wall (15), either initiating or accelerating the remodeling process which normally occurs with age. The hypothesis that describes injury as the progenitor of vascular change has been described in detail (2). Several experimental models ranging from immunologic injury (16) to mechanical trauma produce similar smooth muscle cell proliferation. By studying this accelerated remodeling process, some of the basic pathophysiology underlying vascular disease may be identified.

EFFECTS OF ENDOTHELIAL REMOVAL

The endothelium normally functions as a permeability barrier producing a cholesterol concentration difference between the plasma and the vessel wall (17). Therefore, the endothelium is a critical site for the entrance of lipid into the arterial wall. When this barrier is removed or impaired, even for a short time, the vessel wall may be bathed by concentrations of plasma components normally screened out by the properly functioning endothelium.

In our experiments, we have removed the endothelium with the balloon catheter first described by Baumgartner (18). This procedure is convenient, highly reproducible, and seems to damage and remove only the endothelial layer. Following this procedure, we have observed similar intimal healing in rabbits (19), monkeys (20), and rats (14). Although we do not consider widespread endothelial removal with a balloon catheter a physiologic injury, close examination of the processes following the procedure will allow a step-by-step analysis.

The first event we observed after endothelial detachment was platelet adherence to areas denuded of endothelium exposing subendothelial connective tissues to the blood. After platelet attachment, leukocytes attach to the denuded endothelium for 3 to 4 days. SMC migration appears to occur, and occasionally platelets appear at the intimal surface by approximately the fourth or fifth day after injury when the SMC begin to grow out over the denuded intima.

Detailed autoradiographic studies have been made of this phase of intimal remodeling (21). Rabbit arteries were injured by passage of balloon catheters. Each rabbit had received 4 mCi of ^{3}H-thymidine intravenously 1 hour before sacrifice to label SMC for grain counts over the nuclei. Activity was first seen on about the third day after injury and peaked between the third and fourth day. This response tapered quickly; and by approximately the 14th day, little ^{3}H-thymidine uptake was noted. The intima continued to thicken during this period by the proliferation of smooth muscle cells and by the accumulation of extracellular connective tissue components.

After 1 month, the intimal hyperplasia of the rabbit abdominal aorta had become approximately 20 cell layers thick, as thick as the media. Tissue culture experiments suggest that smooth muscle cells generate most extracellular material (22) although endothelial cells may form a type of collagen (23). In this process, fibrin formation only appears to occur in previously injured or remodeled vessels (19), where fibrin forms at the denuded surface and may even enter the vessel wall.

REGROWTH OF THE ENDOTHELIUM

A series of techniques have been developed to identify the various vessel wall cells and to follow the endothelial regrowth following denudation and the fibromusculoelastic plaque formation. A specific antibody marker for endothelial cells allows identification of endothelial cells after removal (24). This marker, adsorbed antitissue factor antibody (thromboplastin), has also been used in tissue culture to identify rabbit endothelial cells. We have recently combined this technique with the infusion of Evans blue dye one-half hour before sacrifice of the animal (25). The Evans blue dye complexes with albumin and apparently cannot permeate the vessel where it is lined with endothelium. With these techniques, we have followed re-endothelialization and examined the healed vessel where endothelium had not proliferated. We now have a highly reproducible picture of the stages of vascular healing after removal of the endothelium.

Endothelial outgrowth begins from sites in arterial branches the balloon cannot reach. Regrowth of the endothelium over the entire surface of the aorta requires approximately 9 to 14 months and involves a wide degree of unexplained biologic variability. In the areas stained by the Evans blue dye, smooth muscle cells remained at the luminal surface for prolonged periods.

The SMC ultrastructural characteristics as shown by electron microscopy were typical. The cells contained the arrays of myofilament and typical pinocytotic vesicles which appear in rows in smooth muscle cells from uninjured rabbit arteries (26). SMC extracellular basement membrane is moderately electron dense, amphorous and intermittent along the luminal surface. This membrane appears to extend into the lumen of the vessel and seems to attract platelets (25). Platelets accumulate on the smooth muscle cell basement membrane surface, spread, and presumably release their intercytoplasmic constituents. Neither the basement membrane or platelets attach to newly formed endothelium.

Morphometric measurements of the thickened intima show that the blued regions are thicker than the re-endothelialized areas. This indicates that regression of the fibromusculoelastic plaque is related in part to re-endothelialization and the presence of platelets at the surface. However, more than 4 months after injury, the plaque had gradually regressed even in blued areas not covered by endothelium. Therefore, although platelets may influence plaque formation, other important factors must further influence the process.

PLATELET, PITUITARY, AND OTHER INFLUENCES ON PROLIFERATION

Experiments in tissue culture have revealed the presence of a *platelet* component that influences the proliferation of smooth muscle cells and fibroblasts. This component may be related to the fibroblast growth factors derived from bovine pituitary glands or bovine brain (27). Whether the platelet carries this low molecular weight, cationic protein is not certain (28,29). Friedman *et al.* (30) have shown that thrombocytopenia caused by sheep antirabbit platelet serum inhibits arteriosclerotic plaque formation following balloon injury. In addition, profound thrombocytopenia may inhibit atherosclerotic plaque formation following repeated intimal injury by an indwelling aortic polyethylene catheter. These *in vivo* findings support the contention that platelets are involved in SMC proliferation.

The *pituitary* may also influence proliferation. Tiell and Stemerman (31) have demonstrated that in hypophysectomized rats, smooth muscle cells do not proliferate in animals with normal platelet counts. The rat pituitary glands were removed, and approximately 7 to 10 days later the endothelium was removed with a balloon catheter (18). Endothelial regrowth and SMC proliferation were measured in control and hypophysectomized animals. Removal of the pituitary gland markedly suppressed smooth muscle cell hyperplasia but did not affect endothelial regrowth. If the endothelium was removed less than 7 days after hypophysectomy, SMC plaque formation did not differ from that in control animals. Rat platelets survive approximately 5 days. Whether this observation is coincidental or not is unclear now but does suggest a link between the platelets and the pituitary.

Other agents influence the proliferative process. Rhee *et al.* (32) have demonstrated that estradiol suppresses the intimal thickening of resutured arteries *in vivo*. Fischer-Dzoga and Wissler (33) have demonstrated in tissue culture that serum lipoproteins enhance SMC proliferation. The proliferation also appears to be influenced by unidentified factors. Burns, Spaet, and Stemerman (21) have demonstrated that SMC proliferation greatly diminished after 14 days although platelets were still adhering to the luminal smooth muscle cells. This confirmed the observation that although regrowth of endothelial cells appears to enhance intimal regression, it begins after a time even in the absence of an endothelial cover. The factor or factors that govern regression are unknown. Whether this effect is local or systemic or whether hyperlipidemia and high blood pressure may specifically stimulate smooth muscle proliferation is not clear.

In contrast to smooth muscle cells, endothelial cells seem to proliferate even in the absence of pituitary or platelet factors *in vivo*. Therefore, endothelial proliferation may involve mechanisms markedly different from that controlling smooth muscle cell proliferation.

CONCLUSION

Even though regression of arteriosclerosis may be stimulated by dietary change (1,34,35), dietary restriction requires prudence not palatable to western man. Therefore, investigation of the pathobiology of vascular healing should continue.

REFERENCES

1. Ahrens EH: Drugs spotlight program: The management of hyperlipidemia: Whether, rather than how. ANN INTERN MED 85:87-93, 1976.

2. Ross R, Glomset JA: The pathogenesis of atherosclerosis. N ENGL J MED 295:369-377, 1976.

3. Geer JC, Haust MD: SMOOTH MUSCLE CELLS IN ATHEROSCLEROSIS. MONOGRAPH ON ATHEROSCLEROSIS, Vol. 2. Basel, S. Karger, 1972.

4. Arteriosclerosis. Report by National Heart and Lung Institute Task Force on Arteriosclerosis. 1972. DHEW Publication No. 72-219, 13.

5. French JE: Atherosclerosis in relation to the structure and function of the arterial intima, with special reference to the endothelium. INT REV EXP PATHOL 5:253-353, 1966.

6. Stemerman MB: Vascular intimal components: Precursors of thrombosis. PROG HEMOSTASIS THROMBO 2:1-47, 1974.

7. Wolinsky H, Galgov S: Nature of species differences in the medial distribution of aortic vasa vasorum in mammals. CIRC RES 20:409-421, 1967.

8. Ross R: The smooth muscle cell, II. Growth of smooth muscle in culture and formation of elastic fibers. J CELL BIOL 50: 172-186, 1971.

9. Jorres I, Majno G: Cellular breakdown within the arterial wall. An ultrastructural study of the coronary artery in young and aging rats. VIRCHOWS ARCH [PATHOL ANAT] 364:111-127, 1974.

10. Frist S, Stemerman MB: Arterial Growth and Development, In VASCULAR NEUROEFFECTOR SYSTEMS, edited by Bevan JA. S.J. Karger, 1977, pp. 19-27.

11. Haust MD, More RH: Development of modern theories on the pathogenesis of atherosclerosis. In THE PATHOGENESIS OF ATHEROSCLEROSIS, edited by Wissler RW, Geer JG. Baltimore, Williams and Wilkins Co., 1972, pp. 1-29.

12. Schwartz SM, Stemerman MB, Benditt EP: The aortic intima. II. Repair of the aortic lining after mechanical denudation. AM J PATHOL 81:15-48, 1975.

13. Poole JCF, Cromwell SB, Benditt EP: Behavior of smooth muscle cells and formation of extracellular structures in the reaction of arterial walls to injury. AM J PATHOL 62:391-414, 1971.

14. Mustard JF, Packham MA: The role of blood and platelets in atherosclerosis and complications of atherosclerosis. THROMB DIATH HAEMORRH 33:444-456, 1975.

15. Stemerman MB: Factors governing the healing response of injured arteries. ANN N Y ACAD SCI 283:310-316, 1977.

16. Minick CR, Murphy GE: Experimental induction of atheroarteriosclerosis by the synergy of allergic injury to arteries and lipid-rich diet. II. Effect of repeatedly injected foreign proteins in rabbits fed a lipid-rich, cholesterol-poor diet. AM J PATHOL 73:265-300, 1973.

17. Reichl D, Simons LA, Myant NB, Pflug JJ, Mills GL: The lipids and lipoproteins of human peripheral lymph, with observations on the transport of cholesterol from plasma and tissue into lymph. CLIN SCI MOL MED 45:313-329, 1973.

18. Baumgartner HR, Studer A: Folgen des Gefässkatheterismus am normo- und hypercholesterinaemischen Kaninchen. PATHOL MICROBIOL 29:393-405, 1966.

19. Stemerman MB: Thrombogenesis of the rabbit arterial plaque: An electron microscopic study. AM J PATHOL 73:7-26, 1973.

20. Stemerman MB, Ross R: Experimental arteriosclerosis. 1. Fibrous plaque formation in primates, an electron microscopic study. J EXP MED 136:769-789, 1972.

21. Burns ER, Spaet RH, Stemerman MB: Intimal cell proliferation following de-endothelialization of the rabbit aorta: A self-limiting process. CLIN RES 24:437A, 1976. [Abstract].

22. Wight TN, Ross R: Proteoglycans in primate arteries. II. Synthesis and secretion of glycosaminoglycans by arterial smooth muscle cells in culture. J CELL BIOL 67:675-686, 1975.

23. Jaffe EA, Minick CR, Adelman B, Becker CG, Nachman R: Synthesis of basement membrane collagen by cultured human endothelial cells. J EXP MED 144:209-225, 1976.

24. Stemerman MB, Pitlick FA, Dembitzer HB: Electron microscopic immunohistochemical identification of endothelial cells in the rabbit. CIRC RES 38:146-156, 1976.

25. Stemerman MB, Spaet TH, Pitlick FA, Cintron J, Lejnieks I, Tiell ML: Intimal healing: The pattern of reendothelialization and intimal thickening. AM J PATHOL 87:125-137, 1977.

26. Muggli R, Baumgartner HR: Pattern of membrane invaginations at the surface of smooth muscle cells of rabbit arteries. EXPERIENTIA 28:1212-1214, 1972.

27. Gospodarowicz D, Moran JS: Mitogenic effect of fibroblast growth factor on early passage cultures of human and murine fibroblasts. J CELL BIOL 66:451-456, 1975.

28. Antoniades HN, Scher CD: Radioimmunoassay of a human growth factor for Balb/C-3T3 cells: Derivation from platelets. PROC NATL ACAD SCI 74:1973-1977, 1977.

29. Antoniades HN, Scher CD: Growth factors derived from human serum, human platelets and human pituitary; properties and immunologic cross-reactivity. NATL CANCER INST MONOGRAPH No. 48 (In Press).

30. Friedman RJ, Stemerman MB, Wenz B, Moore S, Gauldie J, Gent M, Tiell ML, Spaet TH: The effect of thrombocytopenia on experimental arteriosclerotic lesion formation in rabbits. Smooth muscle cell proliferation and re-endothelialization. J CLIN INVEST 60:1191-1201, 1977.

31. Tiell ML, Stemerman MB: Inhibition of aortic intimal hyperplasia by hypophysectomy in rats. CLIN RES 24:321A, 1976. [Abstract].

32. Rhee CY, Spaet TH, Stemerman MB, Lajam F, Shiang HH, Caruso E, Litwak RS: Estrogen suppression of surgically induced vascular intimal hyperplasia in rabbits. J LAB CLIN MED 90:77-84, 1977.

33. Fisher-Dzoga K, Wissler RW: Stimulation of proliferation in stationary primary cultures of monkey aortic smooth muscle cells. Part 2. Effect of varying concentrations of hyperlipidemic serum and low density lipoproteins of varying dietary fat origins. ATHEROSCLEROSIS 24:515-525, 1976.

34. Armstrong ML, Megan MB: Arterial fibrous proteins in cynomolgus monkeys after atherogenic and regression diets. CIRC RES 36:256-261, 1975.

35. Mann GV: Current concepts. Diet-Heart: End of an era. N ENGL J MED 297:644-650, 1977.

SUMMARY OF DISCUSSION BY PARTICIPANTS

Papers by Drs. Brinkhous, Spaet, and Stemerman were discussed together.

Dr. Spittell, as a clinician, asked how the balloon injury model relates to spontaneous atherosclerosis in humans. Dr. Moore pointed out that there is definitely evidence of endothelial damage in humans as in other species. Areas around branch vessels show endothelial loss and increased endothelial turnover, as demonstrated by Helen Payling Wright, Stary and McMillan, Caplan and Schwartz, and many other workers. Increased turnover implies endothelial damage and loss - but what is the nature of the damage? And what is the cause? There is evidence that many things can damage endothelium in humans, and, as with cancer, one need not be limited to seeking a single cause. For example, antigen-antibody complexes apparently damage endothelium. And tying in with the concept of immunological injury is old autopsy work, largely forgotten now: good observers used to comment that children who had rheumatic fever attacks and various kinds of infections had more fatty streaks in their aortas than children who didn't. Papers at this Workshop presented evidence that hypercholesterolemia itself can damage endothelium. Another finding that intrigues Dr. Moore is recent work in Dr. Carl Becker's laboratory showing that an allergen in tobacco can damage endothelium.

Dr. Spaet drew attention to renewed interest in circulating endothelial cells and described his recent studies in the fawn-hooded rat, which has a platelet storage defect. One week after balloon injury, there was normal platelet adhesion reaction despite the fact that the release reaction is knocked out in these animals; possibly this could occur because the mitogen is carried by mechanisms other than the storage granules.

Dr. Kaplan noted that she has looked at sonicated platelets from patients with storage pool disease. These patients' platelets contained normal amounts of platelet factor 4 (PF4), β-thromboglobulin (βTG), and growth factor. Therefore, it is not surprising that the fawn-hooded rats produce a normal proliferative response. They may have normal levels of PF4, βTG, and growth factor that they can release even though they don't have dense granule components.

Dr. Spaet described what happens after balloon injury in the hypophysectomized animal: Dr. Melvin Tiell in his laboratory has shown that there is only a transient depression of the lesion, which starts to return to normal after a month.[1] To test the hypothesis that the lesion could be restored by a nonspecific inflammatory reaction, they gave subcutaneous turpentine or the oil which was the medium for injecting turpentine. The endothelium in nonhypophysectomized, balloon-injured controls was 6 cell layers thick (average maximal thickness). When hypophysectomized animals subjected to balloon injury were injected with turpentine, the average thickness was close to 4 cell layers, while in 12 animals injected with oil medium, the average thickness in 50 areas was only 0.17. Thus, apparently the lesion can be restored with a nonspecific inflammatory reaction. This finding further complicates the picture by implicating macrophages and leukocytes.

[1]Tiell ML, Sussman II, Moss R, Spaet TH: Arteriosclerotic plaque formation in de-endothelialized hypophysectomized rats: Restoration by nonspecific inflammatory states. FED PROC, 1978 (In Press).

Dr. Moore asked Dr. Stemerman whether it is the drop in growth hormone after hypophysectomy that explains his results, whether growth hormone might be the factor needed in addition to platelet factor. This would be analogous to the situation in which serum from diabetics is much more supportive of smooth muscle cell growth than serum from nondiabetics. Dr. Stemerman replied that giving growth hormone did not restore the lesion; but the growth hormone preparation he worked with was not pure. His approach now is to see if growth hormone is a platelet mediator.

Dr. Ross cautioned 1) that the terms "serum" and "plasma" are not interchangeable and 2) that Dr. Stemerman's model is very complicated because of various pituitary factors and cofactors, and also because of species differences. The fact that re-endothelialization occurs in hypophysectomized animals suggests that hormones are not involved. In this connection, Bob Wall in Dr. Harker's laboratory has shown that endothelial cells do not require the platelet factor to proliferate in culture. But they will respond to fibroblast growth factor; adding this will produce a response over and above the response with either whole blood serum or plasma-derived serum. The growth curves of endothelial cells in culture indicate that the cells reach the same density in the same period of time whether platelet factor is present or absent. If fibroblast growth factor is added, the cells reach a higher density. The fact that smooth muscle cells require platelet factor, while endothelial cells do not, suggests that there are differences in the molecules. An example of the problems that must be filtered out to get the answers is the concept of pituitary cofactors vs. that of pituitary hormones being picked up by platelets and carried to the sites where they are needed. Dr. Stemerman responded that the problem is even more complicated than that, as exemplified by Dr. Spaet's allusion to a macrophage factor. There may be other factors which no one has even begun to explore yet.

Dr. Spaet emphasized that any hypothesis must cover the finding that the lesion is restored in hypophysectomized animals — rapidly with turpentine, slowly without it — but in the absence of pituitary function. Dr. Stemerman responded that part of the posterior pituitary remains, or at least the pituitary blood supply from the hypothalamus is there, and it is conceivable that the material in question is actually from the hypothalamus, coming down via the blood vessels remaining in that region. Like Dr. Spaet, he sees recurrence of the lesion after 4 weeks in this model. He is considering using more completely ablated animals, but these are even more difficult to maintain than hypophysectomized animals.

INTERACTION OF PLATELETS WITH THE ENDOTHELIUM IN NORMAL AND VON WILLEBRAND PIGS*

V.D. Fuster, M.D., and E.J.W. Bowie

Department of Cardiovascular Diseases and Hematology Research, Mayo Clinic and Mayo Foundation, Rochester, MN

ABSTRACT

In order to evaluate the possible role of platelets in the development of atherosclerosis, the aortas of 11 control pigs and 11 homozygous von Willebrand (vWD) pigs were examined for spontaneous atherosclerosis. Of the 11 normal pigs, six showed multiple atherosclerotic plaques with an intimal thickening of 63 to 130 μm. In contrast, none of the von Willebrand pigs had multiple plaques and only one showed a single lesion of more than 2 mm in diameter.

In a prospective study, 11 control pigs and seven vWD pigs were given a high (2%) cholesterol diet from the age of 3 to 9 months. All of the controls developed atherosclerotic plaques; in nine the plaques exceeded 12% of the aortic surface with an intimal thickening of up to 390 μm. In contrast, four of the vWD pigs did not develop such lesions, and the lesions in two of the other pigs covered less than 8% of the aortic surface. Most of the vWD pigs did, however, develop nonatherosclerotic flat fatty lesions.

These findings, together with some preliminary findings on aortic cross-transplantation studies between control and vWD pigs, suggest the possibility of a relationship between the circulating platelet, the endothelial cell von Willebrand factor, and the reactivity of the arterial wall in the process of atherosclerosis.

*This investigation was supported by Research Grant HL-19001 and HL-17430 from the National Institute of Health, Public Health Services.

INTRODUCTION

It has been suggested that platelets, by adhering to a damaged endothelial surface and releasing platelet factors, may play a role in the initiation of atherosclerosis (1,2,3). This led us to consider that a good deal of information might be obtained by investigating whether experimental animals known to have an impairment in platelet function are less prone to the development of atherosclerosis.

A colony of pigs with homozygous severe von Willebrand's disease (vWD) has been maintained at the Mayo Clinic at Mayo Institute Hills Farm. These animals share the observed impairment in platelet function and hemostatic abnormalities of the severe form of the same disease in humans (4). In order to evaluate whether such von Willebrand (vWD) pigs are less prone to the development of atherosclerosis, we studied the incidence, quantitation, and structural characterization of spontaneous atherosclerosis and of atherosclerosis induced by a high-cholesterol diet in homozygous vWD pigs and in normal control pigs.

METHODS AND RESULTS

Spontaneous Atherosclerosis Study

We studied the aortas of 11 pigs with homozygous vWD, seven males and four females, which had died of nasal or gastrointestinal bleeding between January 1970 and December 1974. At the time of death the pigs were 1 to 3 years old and weighed an average of 150 kg (± 85 SD). Eleven control pigs of the same breed, all males, were obtained at one time, in August 1974, from a slaughterhouse. They were about 1 to 3 years old and their body weights averaged 216 kg (± 61 SD). The 11 vWD pigs had received a mixed ground meal, approximately 500 g per 40 kg body weight. The diet of the 11 control animals is unknown because they were raised on farms not under our supervision.

Seven of the 11 control pigs had multiple or single raised fatty arteriosclerotic plaques of more than 2 mm in diameter, with an intimal thickening ranging from 63 to 130 μm (Table 1). In contrast, only one of the vWD pigs had a significant single plaque of more than 2 mm in diameter. The lesser incidence and extent of atherosclerotic plaques in the vWD pigs were statistically significant ($p < 0.01$, rank Σ test).

In seven of the 11 vWD pigs, the macroscopically normal aortas, completely free of atherosclerotic plaques, showed extensive fat deposition after staining with Sudan IV. These nonatherosclerotic, so-called flat fatty lesions (5), covered 5 to 30% of the aortic surface and microscopically showed subendothelial infiltration of fat without significant intimal thickening (intimal thickness 27 to 81 μm).

TABLE 1. SPONTANEOUS DEVELOPMENT OF ATHEROSCLEROTIC PLAQUES AND FLAT FATTY LESIONS

Lesions (Area, Intimal Thickening)	Control (N=11)	vWD (N=11)
Fibrous plaques (>2 mm, >150 μm)	0	0
Raised fatty plaques (>2 mm, 63-130 μm)	7	1
Flat fatty lesions (>1%; 27-81 μm)	1	7

Induced Atherosclerosis Study

Eighteen pigs were subjected to an atherogenic diet for 6 months, beginning at the age of 3 months. Seven pigs, four males and three females, suffered from homozygous von Willebrand's disease, while eleven, five males and six females, were normal control pigs of the same breed. At autopsy mean body weights were 94 kg (± 21 SD) for the vWD pigs and 105 kg (± 30 SD) for the controls. All pigs were housed at Mayo Institute Hills Farm and were fed approximately 500 g per 40 kg body weight of a diet containing cholesterol 2%, tallow 20%, and hog bile extract 1%.

All 11 control pigs on the high-cholesterol diet developed raised fatty atherosclerotic plaques and 10 of them developed raised fibrous atherosclerotic plaques (Table 2). In nine of the pigs the aortic arteriosclerotic plaques exceeded 12% of the entire surface, with an intimal thickening ranging from 50 to 390 μm. In contrast, only three of the vWD pigs developed significant raised fatty atherosclerotic plaques and in two of them this involved only 7% of the aortic surface. The lesser incidence and extent of induced atherosclerotic plaques in the vWD pigs were statistically significant ($p < 0.01$, rank Σ test).

Despite the low incidence and small extent of atherosclerotic plaques, the aortas of six vWD pigs showed fatty lesions involving

2 to 23% of the total aortic surface area. As in the spontaneous atherosclerosis study, these nonatherosclerotic lesions were characterized microscopically by subendothelial infiltration of fat without intimal thickening (intimal thickness 12 to 50 μm).

TABLE 2. HIGH CHOLESTEROL DIET INDUCED ATHEROSCLEROTIC PLAQUES AND FLAT FATTY LESIONS

Lesions (Area, Intimal Thickening)	Control (N=11)	vWD (N=7)
Fibrous plaques (>1%, >300 μm)	10	2
Raised fatty plaques (>1%, 50-300 μm)	11	3
Flat fatty lesions (>1%, 12-50 μm)	4	6

DISCUSSION

The difference between atherosclerotic lesions in the aorta of normal pigs and those with homozygous von Willebrand's disease was striking. This was true of pigs on ordinary diets or on a high-cholesterol diet. One obvious explanation is that the impairment in platelet function in vWD (4, 6-10) may have protected them from spontaneous or induced arteriosclerosis.

It has been suggested that the physiological bonding of platelets to subendothelial surfaces to staunch bleeding (7,11,12) may be the first step in the generation of atherosclerosis (1-3). Our results indeed suggest that pigs with vWD are resistant to the development of spontaneous atherosclerosis and of atherosclerosis induced by a high-cholesterol diet; however, these pigs are prone to develop nonproliferative, nonatherosclerotic intimal fat infiltration.

A conceivable explanation of our findings is illustrated in the diagram. In normal pigs, endothelial injury caused by hemodynamic and rheological factors (13-17) and also by a high-cholesterol diet (17-20) might attract platelets to adhere to the arterial surface. As suggested by others (1-3,22), platelets may then promote the initiation of the intimal hyperplasia seen in the early atherosclerotic plaques. Moreover, the adherence of the platelet to the arterial surface in the normal animal may help to repair the endothelium and reduce its permeability (23-26). On the other hand, in the vWD pig, because the platelets do not adhere (27), intimal hyperplasia or atherosclerotic plaques would not develop. In addition, because of the lack of platelet-arterial wall interaction, endothelial integrity might not be restored and permeability might be increased allowing the fat to accumulate in the intima.

WORKING HYPOTHESIS FOR AORTIC LESIONS IN PIGS

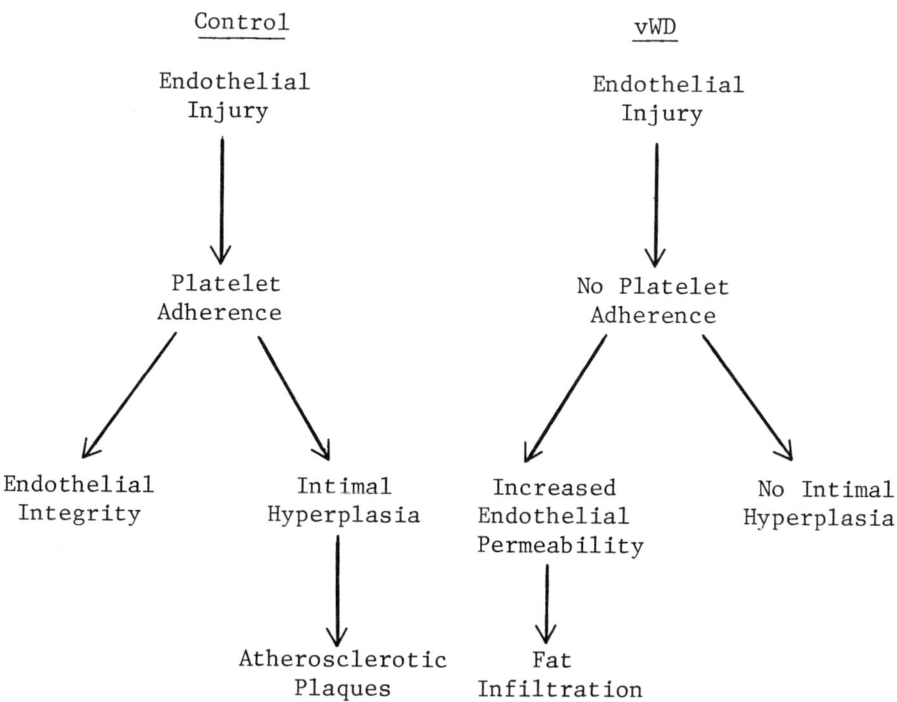

We recognize that other as yet undiscovered attributes of vWD pigs may be responsible for their resistance to arteriosclerosis. It is possible that the aortic wall of the vWD pig is genetically resistant to the development of atherosclerosis. To investigate this, we have initiated a series of aortic cross-transplantation studies between normal and vWD animals.

As a preliminary study, a 5-cm aortic segment proximal to the aortic bifurcation was resected in a control pig and in a vWD pig. The segments were cross-transplanted and a high-cholesterol diet was given for 6 months. The vWD aortic segment in the control pig developed atherosclerosis and the endothelium demonstrated reactive von Willebrand factor. On the other hand, the control aortic segment in the vWD pig did not show atherosclerosis and was devoid of reactive von Willebrand factor. These findings suggest the possibility of a relationship between the circulating platelet, the endothelial cell von Willebrand factor, and the reactivity of the arterial wall in the process of atherosclerosis (28).

An important question arising from our study in pigs is whether humans with vWD are protected from the development of atherosclerosis. Silwer *et al.* (29) reported that necropsy on three patients with vWD revealed atherosclerosis. However, in analyzing their report it becomes apparent that one of the patients showed only minute arterial yellow deposits; a second patient with a mild form of vWD (according to the laboratory data) was severely hypertensive for 10 years prior to death; and the third patient, although he had a family history of vWD, had no laboratory documentation of von Willebrand's disease.

It is important to emphasize that our pigs with vWD are homozygous with very severe disease (1). They appear to be an ideal model in the investigation of the initial mechanisms of atherosclerosis (3).

REFERENCES

1. Stemerman MB, Ross R: Experimental arteriosclerosis. I. Fibrous plaque formation in primates, an electron microscope study. J EXP MED 136:769-789, 1972.

2. Ross R, Glomset J, Kariya B, Harker L: A platelet-dependent serum factor that stimulates the proliferation of arterial smooth muscle cells *in vitro*. PROC NAT ACAD SCI USA 71:1207-1210, 1974.

3. Harker LA, Ross R, Slichter SJ, Scott CR: Homocystine-induced arteriosclerosis: The role of endothelial cell injury and platelet response to its genesis. J CLIN INVEST 58:731-741, 1976.

4. Bowie EJW, Owen CA, Jr., Zollman PE, Thompson JH, Jr., Fass DN: Tests of hemostasis in swine: Normal values and values in pigs affected with von Willebrand's disease. AM J VET RES 34:1405-1407, 1973.

5. Mitchell JRA, Schwartz CJ: The morphology of arterial plaques. In: ARTERIAL DISEASE, Philadelphia, FA Davis Co., 1965, pp. 15-67.

6. Bowie EJW, Owen CA, Jr.: The value of measuring platelet "adhesiveness" in the diagosis of bleeding diseases. AM J CLIN PATHOL 60:302-308, 1973.

7. Borchgrevink CF: Platelet adhesion *in vivo* in patients with bleeding disorders. ACTA MED SCAND 170:231-243, 1961.

8. Zimmerman TS, Ratnoff OD, Powell AE: Immunologic differentiation of classic hemophilia (Factor VIII deficiency) and von Willebrand's disease: With observations on combined deficiencies of antihemophilic factor and proaccelerin (Factor V) and on acquired circulating anticoagulant against antihemophilic factor. J CLIN INVEST 50:244-254, 1971.

9. Weiss HJ, Hoyer LW, Rickles FR, Varma A, Rogers J: Quantitative assay of plasma factor deficient in von Willebrand's disease that is necessary for platelet aggregation: Relationship to Factor VIII procoagulant activity and antigen content. J CLIN INVEST 52:2708-2716, 1973.

10. Fass DN, Brockway WJ, Owen CA, Jr., Bowie EJW: Factor VIII (Willebrand) antigen and ristocetin-Willebrand factor in pigs with von Willebrand's disease. THROMB RES 8:319-327, 1976.

11. Weiss HJ, Tschopp TB, Baumgartner HR: Impaired interaction (adhesion-aggregation) of platelets with the subendothelium in storage-pool disease and after aspirin ingestion: A comparison with von Willebrand's disease. N ENGL J MED 293: 619-623, 1975.

12. Baumgartner HR, Tschopp TB, Meyer D: Shear rate dependance of platelet adhesion to collagenous surfaces in Willebrand factor-depleted blood. THROMB HAEMOSTAS (Abstract) 38:50, 1977.

13. Fry DL: Certain chemorheologic considerations regarding the blood vascular interface with particular reference to coronary artery disease. CIRCULATION (Suppl) 39-40:IV-38-57, 1969.

14. Texon M: The hemodynamic concept of atherosclerosis. BULL NY ACAD MED 36:263-274, 1960.

15. Glagov S: Mechanical stresses on vessels and the non-uniform distribution of atherosclerosis. MED CLIN NORTH AM 57:63-77, 1973.

16. Wesolowski SA, Fries CC, Sabini AM, Sawyer PN: The significance of turbulence in hemic systems and in the distribution of the atherosclerotic lesion. SURGERY 57:155-161, 1965.

17. Somer JB, Evans G, Schwartz CJ: Influence of experimental aortic coarctation on the pattern of aortic Evans blue uptake *in vivo*. ATHEROSCLEROSIS 16:127-133, 1972.

18. Florentin RA, Nam SC: Dietary-induced atherosclerosis in miniature swine. I. Gross and light microscopy observations: Time of development and morphological characteristics of lesions. EXP MOL PATHOL 8:263-301, 1968.

19. Frost H: Study of the pathogenesis of obliterating arterial disease by means of tarter electron microscope technique. In: PLATELETS AND THE VESSEL WALL-FIBRIN DEPOSITION; Symposium of the European Atherosclerosis Group, June 15-17, 1969, edited by Schettler G. Stuttgart, Georg Thieme Verlag, 1970, p. 124.

20. Ross R, Harker L: Hyperlipidemia and atherosclerosis: Chronic hyperlipidemia initiates and maintains lesions by endothelial cell disquamation and lipid accumulation. SCIENCE 193:1094-1100, 1976.

21. Sunaga T, Yamashita Y, Numan F, Shimamoto T: Luminal surface of normal and atherosclerotic arteries observed by scanning electron microscope. In: SCANNING ELECTRON MICROSCOPY/1970, (Proceedings of the Third Annual Scanning Electron Microscope Symp. held at ITT Res. Inst, Chicago, IL) pp. 243-248.

22. Mustard JF: Platelets, drugs, and thrombosis, the problem. In: PLATELETS, DRUGS AND THROMBOSIS: Proceedings of a Symposium held at McMaster University, Hamilton, Ontario, October 16-18, 1972, edited by Hirsch J, Cade JF, Gallus AS, Schönbaum E. New York, S. Karger, 1975, pp. 1-14.

23. Fry GL, Maca RD, Hoak JC: Enhancement of endothelial contiguity by human platelets (Abstract). CLIN RES 24:570, 1976.

24. Gimbrone MA, Aster RH, Cotran RS, Corkery J, Jandl JH, Folkman J: Preservation of vascular integrity in organs perfused *in vitro* with a platelet-rich medium. NATURE 222:33-36, 1969.

25. Wojcik JD, Van Horn DL, Webber AJ, Johnson SA: Mechanism whereby platelets support the endothelium. TRANSFUSION 9:324-335, 1969.

26. Roskam J: Du rôle de la paroi vasculaire dans l'hémostase spontanée et la pathogénie des éstats hémorragiques. THROMB DIATH HAEMORRH 12:338-352, 1964.

27. Fass DN, Didisheim P, Lewis JC, Grabowski EF: Adhesion of porcine von Willebrand (vWD) platelets (Abstract). CIRCULATION (Suppl) 54:II-116, 1976.

28. Booyse FM, Quarfoot AJ, Bell S, Fass DN, Lewis JC, Mann KG, Bowie EJW: Cultured von Willebrand porcine aortic endothelial cells: An *in vitro* model for studying the molecular defect(s) of the disease. PROC NATL ACAD SCI USA 74:5702, 1977.

29. Silwer J, Cronberg S, Nilsson IM: Occurrence of arteriosclerosis in von Willebrand's disease. ACTA MED SCAND 180:475-484, 1966.

30. Fuster V, Bowie EJW, Lewis JC, Fass DN, Owen CA Jr, Brown AL: Arteriosclerosis in von Willebrand and normal pigs: Spontaneous and high cholesterol diet induced. J CLIN INVEST, 1978 (In Press).

SUMMARY OF DISCUSSION BY PARTICIPANTS

Dr. Hoak wondered if the endothelium survives the transplant. Dr. Fuster responded that he thinks the endothelium one sees has been replaced, that when the von Willebrand segment is transplanted into the normal aorta, the recipient aorta replaces the von Willebrand endothelium with normal endothelium. Dr. Harker asked if this exchange is postulated to result from endothelial cell injury induced by the transplantation procedure, and Dr. Fuster said yes.

Dr. Harker also expressed concern that the fixation procedure for the electron micrographs (EMs) might have produced artifacts. Dr. Fuster explained that the aorta is perfused *in vivo* for half an hour with fixative before the pig is sacrificed. Then the aorta is removed and opened and a picture taken before the section is removed for the EM, but done very rapidly to prevent drying.

Dr. Bell commented that lipid deposition in an artery is usually associated with increases in endogenous lipid synthesis; he wondered whether the lipid deposition Dr. Fuster sees is entirely exogenous or whether there is some contribution from endogenous synthesis. Dr. Fuster said that they are looking at the biochemical nature of the fat but have no results yet.

Dr. Moore noted that one of Dr. Fuster's slides showed a fatty streak lesion in which the lipid seemed to be at least partly within the cells of the intima, but Dr. Fuster assured him that the fat is mainly extracellular. Dr. Moore also commented on an apparent intimal thickening at lesion site and wondered if the pig has a lot of myointimal cells. Dr. Fuster said no, and explained that in the section in question, the intimal thickness was 65 microns, which is within the normal range of 15 to 75 microns for their pigs. He went on to comment that the key question is whether the flat fatty lesion seen in the von Willebrand pig is the precursor of athero-sclerosis or a different type of lesion. He is approaching this problem by sacrificing pigs at different intervals - 3 months, 6 months, and so on - to see the progression of the different types of lesions.

VESSEL INJURY, THROMBOSIS, AND PLATELET SURVIVAL*

Laurence A. Harker, M.D., and Russell Ross, Ph.D.

Harborview Medical Center and the School of Medicine

University of Washington, Seattle, WA

ABSTRACT

Vascular injury triggers platelet reactions of adhesion, aggregation, and release, and these reactions play important roles in hemostasis, thrombosis and thromboembolism, and atherogenesis. Measurement of platelet and fibrinogen turnover rates are indicators of the relative involvement of platelets and fibrin in the thrombotic process, and also provide an objective means of assessing antithrombotic therapy. Isotopic methods are preferred over chemical methods to measure platelet survival time; ^{51}Cr is used most widely to label platelets. Problems of analysis and interpretation of platelet disappearance curves are reviewed briefly.

INTRODUCTION

Platelet reactions of adhesion, aggregation, and release are initiated by vascular injury and have important roles in the mechanisms of hemostasis, arterial thrombosis and thromboembolism, wound healing, and atherogenesis (1-5). Normal endothelium presents a nonreactive surface to circulating blood, but subendothelial connective tissue initiates platelet and coagulation reactions that result in thrombosis (1-3). This process initially involves platelet ad-

*Supported by research grant HL-11775 and HL-18645 from the U.S. Public Health Service. A portion of this work was conducted through the Clinical Research Center's facility of the University of Washington with the support of grants (FR-37 and FR-133) from the National Institutes of Health.

hesion to nonendothelialized surfaces, release of constituents, and aggregation of ambient platelets to form an enlarging platelet mass. Under low shear flow conditions, as found in the venous system, the coagulation system becomes fully activated and fibrin forms in the thrombus (6).

In arteries, thrombus is composed primarily of platelets (white thrombus), because rapid blood flow promotes platelet diffusivity and adhesion to thrombogenic surfaces (7) while minimizing activation of the coagulation system. Furthermore, arterial blood flow tends to disrupt the platelet mass into microembolic fragments (8). Microembolization of such fragments from strategically placed thrombogenic foci into vulnerable microcirculatory beds may contribute to the pathogenesis of coronary insufficiency or transient ischemic attacks (9-11). Conversely, the low shear blood flow in the venous system allows clotting to become fully activated, so that the principal process involves fibrin deposition (6) with secondary involvement of platelets and the entrapment of red cells (red thrombus).

In the steady state, measurement of platelet and fibrinogen turnover rates are useful indicators of the relative involvement of platelets and fibrin in the ongoing thrombogenic process (12-14). Moreover, selective platelet consumption in the arterial system may be a potential *in vivo* indicator of endothelial loss. Because there are significant limitations to the use of platelet survival measurements in the latter regard, this discussion will focus on some of these problems regarding techniques, analysis, sensitivity, and specificity.

PLATELET LIFESPAN

In thrombocytopenia the disappearance of transfused platelets can be approximated by direct counting. This approach is inaccurate and not suitable for normal subjects; it is therapeutic as well as investigative, and this affects the validity of the results. More accurate methods have been developed that permit assessment of the rates at which platelets are removed from the circulation.

Recently a chemical method has been developed (15) that is based upon measuring the progressive normalization of the platelet's capacity to form malondialdehyde (MDA) following a single oral dose of acetylsalicyclic acid (ASA). The drug inhibits the cyclooxygenase activity in platelets which is required for synthesis of MDA from arachidonate. This approach assumes that ASA-mediated inhibition is irreversible for the life of the platelet and that normalization reflects the entry of new platelets into the circulation from the marrow. This method has a number of problems including: 1) the technical difficulties of measuring small amounts of MDA reliably; 2) the wide variability in the time for normalization

OF MDA synthesis in normal subjects; and 3) the nonlinear rate at which normalization occurs. Even if the basic assumption is verified that ASA inhibition is permanent, poor resolving power of the MDA method currently limits its use to epidemiological studies. A more basic question relates to the sigmoid shape of returning enzyme activity, because this nonlinear rate of normalization challenges the premise of irreversible enzyme inhibition by ASA and compromises objective comparisons. Moreover, it is not suitable for testing the effects of other drug therapy. Therefore, isotopic methods continue to be the preferred approach to measure platelet survival time for most purposes.

The determination of platelet survival is useful in the characterization of: 1) the mechanisms of thrombocytopenia; 2) pathogenetic involvement of platelets in disease and the effects of various therapies; 3) platelet collection, storage, and transfusion; 4) extrinsic factors affecting the efficacy of platelet transfusions.

Two isotopic approaches have been employed to study platelet survival. In one, a cohort of platelets is labeled; in the other, a population of circulating platelets is labeled; this is called "random" or "population" label.

Cohort Labeling

Although the cohort data are theoretically more readily and accurately analyzed, there is no satisfactory cohort label for platelets at the present time. So far attempts at cohort labeling with ^{32}P, $DF^{32}P$, ^{35}S, or ^{75}S-methionine have not proven satisfactory, largely because the period for which they remain available for labeling megakaryocytes or platelets is long compared with the mean platelet survival time (16-18).

Random Labeling

^{32}P-orthophosphate has proven unsatisfactory as a random label due to rapid exchange or elution and is no longer used (19). However, diisopropylfluorophosphate (DFP) labeled with ^{32}P, ^{3}H, or ^{14}C has been used widely (12,20), but its use as a platelet label is currently not recommended for two reasons. The DFP survival curve does not reach zero, but shows a plateau or even a secondary peak of radioactivity which amounts to 10 to 15% of the initial value and persists for 2 or more weeks. It is not clear whether the secondary peak is due to labeling of megakaryocytes or to reutilization of label or to both (21,22). Furthermore, when DFP is injected, red and white cells take up the label to a greater extent than platelets do. Isolation of the platelets from the blood samples with its associated variability becomes necessary.

Since platelets will bind serotonin by active uptake into intracellular granules, they can be easily and specifically labeled with ^{14}C-serotonin in whole blood or platelet-rich plasma. There is a prolonged disappearance of the platelet label implying about 10% reutilization, presumably due to serotonin exchange with the body pool (23); hence this label is not presently used for platelet survival measurements.

In view of the above shortcomings, platelets are usually labeled *in vitro* with ^{51}Cr. Since ^{51}Cr was first used for this purpose in man (24), a number of technical improvements relating to the use of ^{51}Cr have been introduced. These include: acidification of the acid citrate dextrose anticoagulant to pH 6.5 (25); processing at room temperature (26); use of newer plastic bags (26); minimal centrifugation and manipulation (27,28); and removal of nonplatelet ^{51}Cr (in free plasma or bound to cells) by centrifugation before injection (13, 29). These improvements reduce damage to the cells, increase the efficiency of labeling, and make it possible to apply the method to study the fate of autologous platelets even when the count is 50,000 per microliter or less.

It would be of considerable clinical interest to be able to localize vascular sites of platelet accumulation. While ^{51}Cr-labeling is not suitable for such imaging, platelet labeling with ^{111}In-hydroxyquinolone is attractive for use with modern imaging techniques. Development in this regard has been promising (30,31).

Platelet Survival Measurements

The recycling of the radioactive labels $DF^{32}P$ and ^{14}C-serotonin make a rectilinear survival curve appear exponential (20,21,23), but the ^{51}Cr-platelet disappearance pattern in normal individuals is linear (26,29,32). These results are most consistent with the concept that platelet removal in normal individuals is predominantly an age-related (senescent) mechanism (33,34). On the other hand, exponential disappearance curves reflect random platelet removal as occurs with severe immune or consumptive processes. Curvilinear platelet disappearance patterns result when senescence and consumption are combined. The importance of senescent platelet removal in normal man is further supported by the observations that neither anticoagulants (heparin or coumarin) nor antiplatelet agents (aspirin, dipyridamole, or sulfinpyrazone) affect the survival time of ^{51}Cr-platelets in normal man (13,29,35). Platelet disappearance becomes increasingly curvilinear with advancing age, perhaps due to the development of vascular disease (29). It should be noted, however, that a platelet population having great variation in the intrinsic lifespan of individual platelets also approximates exponential disappearance (36,37).

Analysis of Platelet Survival Data

Platelet population disappearance curves may vary in different patients between linear and exponential functions, so an objective system of analysis free from observer bias is essential for meaningful comparisons. This is particularly important when differences are modest, as observed in some vascular abnormalities and with some therapies. The complex theoretical considerations have been recently reviewed (34,36,37) and an adaptation of the Mills-Dornhorst equation has been recommended (38). In this system of cell survival analysis, the initial slope of the disappearance curve intercepts the time axis at a distance equal to the mean platelet lifespan. In applying this approach, precision and reliability depend largely on the quality of the initial portion of the disappearance curve. Unfortunately, this part of the curve is subject to both error and "noise" because of variable initial recoveries associated with uncontrolled "collection injury" associated with *in vitro* labeling.

An alternative procedure depends upon the whole disappearance curve. It carries out regression analysis of nonlinear data in an objective, unbiased manner by least squares computer fitting to a gamma function (36,37). Good experience with this program has been reported in patients with coronary artery disease (39). Gamma function analysis shows that in normal individuals, autologous ^{51}Cr platelets have a lifespan of 9.5 ± 0.6 days; two-thirds of the injected ^{51}Cr-platelets circulate immediately while the remaining one-third exist as a pool in the spleen that exchanges freely with the general circulation. In asplenic individuals, nearly 100% of the labeled platelets are recovered in the general circulation. In contrast, splenomegaly is associated with a marked increase in splenic pooling of as much as 90% of the total intravascular platelets.

In estimating mean platelet survival time as an aid to practical diagnosis and prognosis in an individual patient, the disturbance of platelet survival is frequently expected to be marked. The disappearance curve can be approximated by visual fitting of the tangent to the curve at the point where it intersects the vertical axis, although this is imprecise and subject to observer bias. Where the survival time disappearance is exponential, the mean may also be calculated by finding the length of time required for radioactivity to be reduced by 50% (T_{50}) and using the formula: Mean survival = 1.443 (T_{50}). In order to make objective use of curvilinear data in the absence of computer facilities, calculations of weighted means may be a useful compromise.

Platelet turnover, calculated from platelet count divided by platelet survival, reflects the rate of platelet removal (destruction) from circulation. In normal subjects (32) turnover is 35,000 ± 4,300 platelets per microliter per day (calculated by dividing the platelet count by platelet survival and correcting for splenic pooling).

Factors Affecting Platelet Survival

Platelet survival is reduced by either intrinsic or extrinsic mechanisms of removal.

Experimentally produced intrinsic platelet defects that compromise platelet viability include various physical, chemical, microbiologic, or enzyme alterations. For example, marked reduction in platelet survival follows 4°C storage *in vitro* for 24 hours or longer, whereas platelets stored at room temperature survive normally when reinfused (26,28). Similarly, exposure to elevated or reduced oxygen tension *in vivo* causes a shortening in platelet survival through an intrinsic modification (40). Virus also impairs platelet survival (41). Treatment with some enzymes also produces intrinsic platelet alterations that compromise viability as shown by the effects of *in vitro* incubation with trypsin, chymotrypsin, or plasmin (42). Of particular importance are the effects of changing platelet membrane glycoproteins on platelet survival. *In vitro* removal of surface sialic acid by neuraminidase treatment (43) or glycoprotein modification by exposure to sodium periodate (44) greatly reduces platelet survival. These data are in accord with the hypothesis that platelet reactions *in vivo* are related to surface glycoprotein and that physiological removal of platelets, i.e., platelet senescence results from progressive depletion of surface glycoproteins (45). Conversely, however, repeated *in vitro* platelet aggregative events induced by ADP or thrombin are not associated with a reduction in platelet survival despite degranulation unless there is concomitant fibrin formation (46).

Experimental extrinsic mechanisms of platelet destruction include immune, infectious, coagulation-mediated, and surface-related processes (13). Platelet removal by nonendothelialized surfaces resulting in a measurable increase in platelet consumption is of particular interest. Four examples follow.

1) Recent studies in primates demonstrate the quantitative relationship between platelet consumption and the amount of de-endothelized surface exposed to circulating blood. When polymeric biomaterials are incorporated into the circulation of baboons as an arteriovenous shunt, platelet consumption by the prosthetic surface is directly related to the exposed area (47). A similar relationship is reported in man (48).

2) Implantation into baboons of aortic velour fabric grafts of constant area produces marked platelet consumption which normalizes in direct relationship to the rate at which endothelialization

of the luminal graft surface occurs (49). Analogous observations are found in man.

3) Balloon desquamation of the aorta of monkeys (*M. nemestrina*) shortens platelet survival in direct relationship to the amount of de-endothelialized surface produced, and normalization of platelet survival is directly related to the process of endothelialization (50).

4) Homocystinemic baboons develop a patchy loss of endothelium that is proportional to the plasma homocystine concentration and the resultant shortening in platelet survival is related to the amount of lost aortic endothelium (4).

The evidence relating nonendothelized vascular surfaces to shortened platelet survival is used to implicate cardiovascular disease as the possible cause of platelet consumption in man (13, 29,39,51).

Mechanisms of Platelet Destruction in Man

In man increased destruction of platelets is almost always due to an extrinsic mechanism. Intrinsic genetic defects that are associated with platelet destruction are rare.

Extrinsic platelet destruction is immunologic or consumptive.

Immune injury to platelets due to antigen-antibody reactions produces patterns of destruction resembling those of red cells in immune hemolytic anemia. Autoimmune platelet destruction may be unaccompanied by other disease, i.e., idopathic thrombocytopenic purpura (ITP), but it may also occur as a manifestation of lymphoproliferative disease (lymphomas, chronic lymphatic leukemia) or lupus erythematosus, or occasionally with some infectious disorders such as infectious mononucleosis. Maternal alloantibodies due to multiple pregnancies may produce temporary thrombocytopenia in the newborn, and alloantibody formation against platelets is induced by multiple random donor blood transfusions. Occasionally, a precipitous fall in circulating platelets follows ingestion of quinidine, quinine, sulfonamides, or other medications as the result of immunologic interaction of drug, platelets, and antibodies induced by the specific drug.

Platelet consumption is either thrombin-mediated as part of the process of intravascular coagulation, or surface-mediated as a reaction to nonendothelialized surfaces.

Entry of procoagulant material into circulating blood activates the coagulation system, and in the process of fibrin formation, there is consumption of platelets, fibrinogen, prothrombin, factor V, factor VIII, and factor XIII. Involvement of the coagulation system is evidenced by the increased turnover of radioiodine-labeled fibrinogen. With thrombin-mediated destruction, platelets and fibrinogen are consumed at comparable rates.

Tissue injury such as trauma or surgery produces combined destruction of platelets and fibrinogen localized at the site of injury; the amount and duration are related to the extent of tissue injury, e.g., with severe injury consumption increases five to six times normal and disappears gradually over 2 weeks. Intravascular activation of clotting is also associated with obstetrical complications (dead fetus syndrome, abruptio placenta, and amniotic fluid infusion); intravascular hemolysis; malignancy (acute myelocytic leukemia, carcinoma of the prostate, lung, gastrointestinal tract, gall bladder, or ovary); viral diseases (varicella, vaccinia, variola, rubella, rubeola, and arboviruses); bacteremia (meningococcus, pyogenic and gram-negative bacilli, and malaria)(13,34).

With widespread vascular injury, i.e., vasculitis, thrombocytopenia is produced by the direct consumption of platelets at sites of endothelial loss without appreciable depletion of clotting factors such as fibrinogen. This mechanism operates in patients who have thrombotic thrombocytopenic purpura, hemolytic-uremic syndrome, and vasculitis induced by immunologic, toxic, or metabolic factors, or by prosthetic surfaces, such as the extracorporeal pump oxygenator. Modestly increased platelet consumption is also observed with artificial heart valves, Silastic arteriovenous cannulae, or aortofemoral artery prosthesis, and in arterial thromboembolism. Vascular consumption may coexist with intravascular coagulation in patients with infection, e.g., Rocky Mountain spotted fever, or when vascular injury is extensive and involves stasis.

THROMBOGENESIS AND ITS PREVENTION

Measurements of ^{51}Cr-platelet and ^{125}I-fibrinogen survival and turnover reflect the basic difference between arterial and venous thrombus formation. Arterial thrombosis is characterized by platelet consumption that can be interrupted by some inhibitors of platelet function but not by heparin. In contrast, venous thrombosis involves combined and equivalent consumption of both platelets and fibrinogen. This process is blocked by anticoagulation but not by drugs that inhibit platelet function.

In vivo kinetic measurements such as ^{51}Cr-platelet and ^{125}I-fibrinogen survival and turnover are indirect but useful indicators of the relative contributions of platelets and fibrinogen in thrombus formation *in vivo* and provide an objective means of assessing antithrombotic therapy (13). The use of platelet survival measurements to predict antithrombotic efficacy is illustrated by the capacity of dipyridamole to interrupt both platelet consumption and arterial thromboembolic events (48,52).

ATHEROGENESIS

Atherosclerotic lesions represent proliferative lesions of smooth muscle cells together with their connective tissue secretory products and accumulated lipid (4,5). The genesis of these lesions appears to involve: 1) endothelial cell injury leading to focal desquamation of cells; 2) adherence and aggregation of platelets to exposed subendothelial connective tissue; 3) local release of platelet constituents and passage of platelet and plasma constituents into the underlying artery wall; 4) migration of smooth muscle cells into the intima and platelet-mediated intimal proliferation of smooth muscle cells; 5) formation of connective tissue matrix by the smooth muscle cells through synthesis and secretion of collagen and elastic fiber proteins and proteoglycans; and 6) intracellular and extracellular lipid accumulation.

This formulation suggests that repeated chronic endothelial cell loss is the first event leading to atherosclerosis and that the reaction of platelets to exposed subendothelial connective tissue is required to induce the proliferative smooth muscle cell response. During the release reaction platelets provide a mitogen not present in plasma that mediates the intimal proliferative response of smooth muscle cells (53). Platelets are consumed in this process of adhesion, aggregation, and release on exposed subendothelial connective tissue surfaces to form platelet thrombi. In experimental animals both platelet consumption and lesion formation are interrupted by some inhibitors of platelet function.

The role of platelets in atherogenesis is illustrated by *in vivo* studies of homocystinemic baboons (5). Experimental homocystinemia causes patchy endothelial desquamation comprising approximately 10% of the aortic surface that produces a three-fold increase in platelet consumption. Endothelial cell sloughing induces a compensatory increase in endothelial cell regeneration as shown by a marked increase in thymidine uptake by arterial endothelium. After 3 months of homocystinemia, these animals show typical atherosclerotic intimal lesions composed of proliferating smooth muscle cells and connective tissue matrix components. The lesions are morphologically characteristic of arteriosclerosis. Intra- and extracellular accumulation of lipid by intimal smooth muscle cells also occurs. In these animals, platelet consumption and intimal lesion formation are prevented by dipryridamole's inhibition of platelet function.

Platelet survival studies in patients with vascular disease

(13,29,39,51) suggest that the mechanism of clinical atherogenesis is similar and imply that pharmacologic prevention may be possible.

REFERENCES

1. Baumgartner HR: The subendothelial surface and thrombosis. In THROMBOSIS; PATHOGENESIS AND CLINICAL TRIALS, edited by Deutsch E, Brinkhous KM, Lechner K, Hinnom S. Stuttgart-New York, FK Schattauer Verlag, 1974, p. 91.

2. Mustard JF, Kinlough-Rathbone RL, Packham MA: Recent status of research in the pathogenesis of thrombosis. THROMB DIATH HAEMORRH (Suppl) 59:157-188, 1974.

3. Weiss HJ: Platelet physiology and abnormalities of platelet function. N ENGL J MED 293:531-541, 1975.

4. Harker LA, Ross R, Slichter SJ, Scott CR: Homocystine-induced arteriosclerosis: The role of endothelial cell injury and platelet response in its genesis. J CLIN INVEST 58:731-741, 1976.

5. Ross R, Harker LA: Hyperlipidemia and atherosclerosis: Chronic hyperlipidemia induces lesion initiation and progression by endothelial cell desquamation and lipid accumulation. SCIENCE 193:1094-1100, 1976.

6. Baumgartner HR: Platelet and fibrin deposition of subendothelium: Opposite dependence on blood shear rate. THROMB HAEMOSTAS 38:133, 1977.

7. Goldsmith HL: The flow of model particles and blood cells and its relation to thrombogenesis. In PROGRESS IN HEMOSTASIS AND THROMBOSIS, edited by Spaet TH, New York, Grune and Stratton, Inc., 1972, p. 97.

8. Jorgenson L: The role of platelet embolism from crumbling thrombi and of platelet aggregates arising in flowing blood. In THROMBOSIS, edited by Sherry S, Brinkhous KM, Genton E. Washington, National Academy of Sciences, 1969, p. 506.

9. Honour AJ, Russel RW: Experimental platelet embolism. BR J EXP PATHOL 43:350-362, 1962.

10. Gunning AJ, Pickering GW, Robb-Smith AHT, Russell RR: Mural thrombosis of the internal carotid artery and subsequent embolism. Q J MED 33:155-195, 1964.

11. Haerem JW: Mural platelet microthrombi and major acute lesions

of main epicardial arteries in sudden coronary death. ATHEROSCLEROSIS 19:529-541, 1974.

12. Adelson E, Rheingold JJ, Parker O, Beunaventure A, Crosby WH: Platelet and fibrinogen survival in normal and abnormal states of coagulation. BLOOD 17:267-281, 1961.

13. Harker LA, Slichter SJ: Platelet and fibrinogen consumption in man. N ENGL J MED 287:999-1005, 1972.

14. Harker LA, Slichter SJ: Arterial and venous thromboembolism: Kinetic characterization and evaluation of therapy. THROMB DIATH HAEMORRH 31:188-203, 1974.

15. Stuart MJ, Murphy S, Oski FA: A simple nonradioisotope technique for the determination of platelet life-span. N ENGL J MED 292:1310-1313, 1975.

16. Leeksman CHW, Cohen JA: Determination of the lifespan of human blood platelets using diisopropylfluorophosphonate. J CLIN INVEST 35:964-969, 1956.

17. Odell TT, Jr., Anderson B: Production of lifespan of platelets. In THE KINETICS OF CELLULAR PROLIFERATION, edited by Stohlman F, Jr. New York, Grune and Stratton, Inc., 1959, p. 278.

18. Najean Y, Ardaillou N: The use of ^{75}Se-methionin for the *in vivo* study of platelet kinetics. SCAND J HAEMATOL 6:395-401, 1969.

19. Grossman CM, Kohn R, Koch R: Possible errors in the use of P^{32} orthophosphate for the estimation of platelet life-span. BLOOD 22:9-18, 1963.

20. Mustard JF, Rowsell HC, Murphy EA: Platelet economy (platelet survival and turnover). BR J HAEMATOL 12:1-24, 1966.

21. Bithall TC, Athens JW, Cartwright GE, Wintrobe MM: Radioactive diisopropylfluorophosphate as a platelet label: An evaluation of *in vitro* and *in vivo* techniques. BLOOD 29:354-372, 1967.

22. Cooney DP, Smith BA, Fawley DE: The use of ^{32}diisopropylfluorophosphate (^{32}DFP) as a platelet label: Evidence for reutilization of this isotope in man. BLOOD 31:791-805, 1968.

23. Heysel RM: Determination of human platelet survival utilizing C^{14}-labeled serotonin. J CLIN INVEST 40:2134-2141, 1961.

24. Aas K, Gardner F: Survival of blood platelets labeled with chromium. J CLIN INVEST 37:1257-1268, 1958.

25. Aster RH, Jandl JH: Platelet sequestration in man. I. Methods. J CLIN INVEST 43:843-869, 1964.

26. Murphy S, Gardner FH: Platelet preservation. Effect of storage temperature on maintenance of platelets viability. Deleterious effect of refrigerated storage. N ENGL J MED 280:1094-1098, 1969.

27. Slichter SJ, Harker LA: Preparation and storage of platelet concentrates. I. Preparation: Factors influencing the harvest of viable platelets from whole blood. BR J HAEMATOL 34:395-402, 1976.

28. Slichter SJ, Harker LA: Preparation and storage of platelet concentrates. II. Storage variables influencing platelet viability and function. BR J HAEMATOL 34:403-419, 1976.

29. Abrahamsen AF: Platelet survival studies in man - with special reference to thrombosis and atherosclerosis. SCAND J HAEMATOL (Suppl) 3:7-53, 1968.

30. Thakur ML, Welch MJ, Joist JH, Coleman RE: Indium-111 labeled platelets. Studies on preparation and evaluation of *in vitro* and *in vivo* function. THROMB RES 9:345-357, 1976.

31. Scheffel R, McIntyre PA, Evatt B, Dvornicky JA, Jr., Natarajan TK, Bolling DR, Murphy EA: Evaluation of indium-111 as a new high photon yield gamma-emitting "physiological" platelet label. JOHNS HOPKINS MED J 140:285-293, 1977.

32. Harker LA, Finch CA: Thrombokinetics in man. J CLIN INVEST 963-974, 1969.

33. Ginsburg AD, Aster RH: Kinetic studies with ^{51}Cr-labeled platelet cohorts in rats. J LAB CLIN MED 74:138a-144, 1969.

34. Paulus JM: PLATELET KINETICS. Amsterdam, North-Holland Pub. Co., 1971, p. 360.

35. O'Neil B, Firkin B: Platelet survival studies in coagulation disorders, thrombocythemia and conditions associated with atherosclerosis. J LAB CLIN MED 64:188-201, 1964.

36. Murphy EA, Francis ME: The estimation of blood platelet survival. I. General principles of the study of cell survival. THROMB DIATH HAEMORRH 22:281-295, 1969.

37. Murphy EA, Francis ME: The estimation of blood platelet survival. II. The multiple hit model. THROMB DIATH HAEMORRH 25:53-80, 1971.

38. Dornhorst AC: The interpretation of red cell survival curves. BLOOD 6:1284-1292, 1951.

39. Ritchie JL, Harker LA: Platelet and fibrinogen survival in coronary atherosclerosis: Response to medical and surgical therapy. AM J CARDIOL 39:595-598, 1977.

40. Pflug EA: Unpublished observations.

41. Turpie AGG, Chernesky MA, Larke RPB, Moore S, Regoeczi E, Mustard JF: Thrombocytopenia and vasculitis induced in rabbits by newcastle disease virus. In THROMBOSIS AND HEMOSTASIS III CONGRESS ABSTRACTS. Durham, North Carolina, The Seeman Printery Inc., 1972, p. 344.

42. Packham MA, Greenberg JP, Scott S, Reimers HJ, Mustard JF: Modifications of rabbit platelets that shorten their survival. AM SOC OF HEMATOLOGY ABSTRACTS No. 523, 1977 (In Press).

43. Greenberg J, Packham MA, Cazenave J-P, Reimers HJ, Mustard JF: Effects on platelet function of removal of platelet sialic acid by neuraminidase. LAB INVEST 32:476-484, 1975.

44. Cazenave J-P, Reimers JH, Kinlough-Rathbone RL, Packham MA, Mustard JF: Effects of sodium periodate on platelet functions. LAB INVEST 34:471-481, 1976.

45. George JN, Lewis PC: Membrane glycoprotein loss from circulating platelets: Inhibition by dipyridamole and aspirin. THROMB HAEMOSTAS 38:111, 1977.

46. Reimers JH, Kinlough-Rathbone RL, Cazenave J-P, Senyi AF, Hirsh J, Packham MA, Mustard JF: *In vitro* and *in vivo* function of thrombin-treated platelets. THROMB HAEMOSTAS 35:151-166, 1976.

47. Harker LA, Hanson SR, Hoffman AS: Platelet kinetic evaluation of prosthetic material *in vivo*. ANN NY ACAD SCI 283:317-331, 1977.

48. Harker LA, Slichter SJ: Studies of platelet and fibrinogen kinetics in patients with prosthetic heart valves. N ENGL J MED 283:1302-1305, 1970.

49. Harker LA, Slichter SJ, Sauvage LR: Platelet consumption by arterial prostheses: The effects of endothelialization and

pharmacologic inhibition of platelet function. ANN SURG 186: 594-601, 1977.

50. Harker LA: The kinetics of platelet production and destruction in man. In CLINICS IN HEMATOLOGY, Vol. 6, No. 3, edited by Lewis SM. London, England, WB Saunders, Inc., 1977, pp. 671-693

51. Steele PP, Weily HS, Davies H, Genton E: Platelet function studies in coronary artery disease. CIRCULATION 48:1194-1200, 1973.

52. Sullivan JM, Harken DE, Gorlin R: Pharmacologic control of thromboembolic complications of cardiac-valve replacement. N ENGL J MED 284:1391-1394, 1971.

53. Ross R, Glomset J, Kariya B, Harker LA: A platelet-dependent serum factor that stimulates the proliferation of arterial smooth muscle cells *in vitro*. PROC NATL ACAD SCI USA 71:1207-1210, 1974.

SUMMARY OF DISCUSSION BY PARTICIPANTS

Dr. Didisheim wondered why Dr. Harker has found shortened platelet survival in patients with venous thrombosis and Dr. Genton has not. Dr. Harker answered that the most likely explanation is that more of Dr. Genton's patients had deep vein thrombosis, and most such patients do not demonstrate significantly shortened platelet survival. Dr. Harker's patients with ongoing venous or arterial thrombosis were selected to show what might occur under ideal experimental circumstances. Dr. Genton agreed with this interpretation of the different findings in the two studies. In the McMaster group's study, some patients had shortened platelet survival time, and the vast majority of those patients had had their first episode of venous thrombosis. The frequency of shortened platelet survival times is much higher in patients with clinically established multiple recurrences. Whether such patients would benefit from pharmacologic intervention has not yet been clearly determined by an adequate clinical trial.

Dr. Didisheim also raised questions about differences between Dr. Harker's laboratory and Dr. Shulman's laboratory at NIH in regard to platelet survival times in homocystinemic patients. Dr. Harker indicated that his group is attempting to compare results from several laboratories studying platelet survival. Analysis is an important component; he thinks that the best available method for analyzing disappearance data is with nonlinear gamma function least squares fitting procedures (N ENGL J MED 296:818, 1977).

Dr. H. J. Day asked if Dr. Harker had found increased MDA

production in any clinical models in which he feels confident. Dr. Harker reiterated that he has not had as good results with the MDA analysis method as with ^{51}Cr labeling, and asked Dr. Genton to comment on experience with the MDA method at McMaster University. Dr. Genton said that they had failed to establish the technique's usefulness, and went on to say that very few groups have been able to reproduce the results of Stuart, Murphy, and Oski [reference 15 in the Harker and Ross paper]; furthermore, Dr. Murphy himself has acknowledged that the technique has many deficiencies and that he has stopped using it. Dr. Day pointed out that a paper describing a modified method with increased sensitivity was presented at the recent meeting of the International Society of Thrombosis and Hemostasis.

Dr. Smith noted that he and Dr. Murphy are trying to develop a thromboxane radioimmunoassay as a platelet survival assay, and also pointed out that the MDA technique measures platelet production, not survival. He and Dr. Harker agreed that, although in a steady state production and survival must be equivalent, in situations where some damage results in sudden removal of platelets there may be a difference. Dr. Harker went on to say that the reappearance rate implies that acetylation of cyclo-oxygenase may not be permanent, because the MDA curve is sigmoid, not linear like the curve with the chromium technique.

Dr. Mustard commented that the data on sulfinpyrazone, the first drug found to have an effect on platelet survival, do not show much effect on platelet adhesion to the subendothelium or to collagen. In contrast, dipyridamole apparently inhibits platelet adherence to the vessel wall. In homocystinemia, sulfinpyrazone apparently acts by protecting against endothelial injury. In earlier experiments, giving animals sulfinpyrazone prevented them from developing vasculitis after infusion of Newcastle disease virus, and it was suspected at that time that the drug might have some protective effect on the endothelium. These earlier observations are in support of Dr. Harker's clear-cut demonstration that sulfinpyrazone protects the endothelium from injury.

Dr. Mustard and Dr. Harker then discussed whether in the shunt experiments in which platelet aggregates block the renal flow, it is possible to remove all fibrin. Because heparin does not block local fibrin formation, Dr. Harker doubted that the experiment could be conducted without fibrin present.

Dr. Moore asked if indium-111 labeled platelets could allow visualization of thrombosis in the coronary artery. Dr. Harker responded that in a baboon with indium-111 labeled platelets and a segment of the iliac vessel ballooned and desquamated, "it lights up rather nicely in contrast to the column of blood in the background". Thus in that experimental system the thrombus could be identified. He went on to say that the coronary artery is different, and he does not know whether one can pick out the thrombus there.

Session III

CLINICAL MODELS

B. A. Molony, Chairman

VENOUS THROMBOSIS: MECHANISMS AND TREATMENT

Michael Hume, M.D.

Tufts University School of Medicine and Lemuel Shattuck Hospital, Boston, MA

ABSTRACT

The role of Virchow's triad in the etiology and treatment of venous thrombosis, the natural history of postoperative thrombosis, and methods for monitoring venous embolism are described. In patients with hip joint replacements the effects of several drugs or drug combinations or placebos on wound hematoma and the effects of age, obesity, and activity and several drug combinations on venous embolism are reported.

INTRODUCTION

An understanding of the etiology of postoperative venous thrombosis can suggest how to prevent it and its most serious complication, pulmonary embolism. Virchow was the first to perceive that this etiology involves more than one of the following triad: a vascular factor, blood stasis, and hypercoagulability. Knowledge about these three factors has been refined considerably in the last hundred years.

THE VASCULAR FACTOR

Intimal damage, the particular vascular factor so important in arterial thrombosis, does not explain venous thrombosis since no direct evidence of any inherent abnormality of the venous endothelium has been found (1). Indwelling catheters and venipunctures can damage venous endothelium and provoke thrombosis and should be avoided below the waist, but they are not responsible for the increasing problem of venous thromboembolism.

However, vascular factors may not be wholly unrelated. In venous thrombosis, the peculiar normal anatomy of the leg veins may be a vascular factor which does not involve the endothelium. Thrombi tend to arise in the leg veins rather than in all the peripheral veins in general. The valves in the leg veins have deep cusps, and the soleal veins have inlets and outlets smaller than their capacious, reservoir-like trunks. The soleal veins appear dilated in contrast phlebograms in older subjects. This age-related dilatation may account for the greater frequency of venous thrombosis in hospitalized elderly patients. Commonly, small thrombi begin in valve cusps and soleal veins, supporting the concept that venous thrombosis as nidus thrombosis originates at such sites and may develop at several foci simultaneously. The specific anatomy of the leg veins must be considered a vascular factor contributing to the location of venous thrombosis and may be a contributing causative factor. To prevent thrombosis, appropriate physical measures may be limited to the legs rather than directed toward all the veins. For a few selected patients, interrupting the vena cava is appropriate prophylaxis against recurrent embolism.

Two other vascular factors may be involved in venous thrombosis following hip joint replacement. Torsion of the femoral vein during hip joint replacement has been demonstrated phlebographically (2). The torsion or the heat generated during polymerization of the acrylic cement used in that operation might injure the endothelium, accounting for some postoperative thrombosis. Isolated femoral vein thrombosis at the level of the lesser trochanter is said (2) to occur more commonly after hip joint replacement than after nailing of hip fractures. Nailing of hip fractures does not involve the use of acrylic cement or radical torsion of the femoral vein but is otherwise comparable to hip joint replacement in that venous thrombolism is prevalent. Direct examination of removed veins has not confirmed endothelial injury at this level in the femoral vein, but these thrombi, unlike other venous thrombi, may arise on damaged endothelium. Platelet adherence to damaged endothelium can be demonstrated in animal models, and drug therapy inhibiting platelet adherence would be rational if the hip replacement operation causes endothelial damage in many patients.

VENOUS STASIS

Although the role of a vascular factor in venous thrombosis has not been established, venous stasis is undoubtedly important and provides a rational basis for physical prevention of thromboembolism. Prevention involves early ambulation, compression by elastic stockings or pneumatic leggings or both, elevation of the foot of the bed, and electrical stimulation of the calf musculature. At least some postoperative venous thrombosis may originate during preoperative inactivity or during an elaborate and invasive diagnostic workup, arduous, at least for the elderly, and associated with fluid and dietary restriction (3). These patients' hospital routines cannot compare with their ordinary activity level at home or at work, and venous stasis is imposed to some degree. Accordingly, physical measures to minimize stasis should be applied during this period.

How effective are these measures? The simplest routines systematically studied seem only weakly effective but valuable nonetheless. Elastic stockings and early ambulation are inadequate for patients with a high risk of venous thrombosis. Flanc *et al.* (4) found that more rigorous physical measures, which included walking, in-bed exercise, stockings, and bed elevation, monitored by ^{125}I fibrinogen leg scanning were effective only for patients at least 60 years old, but their supervision was quite time-consuming. Improved stocking technology may prevent postoperative thrombosis better (5,6). After major surgery, pressure-gradient stockings significantly reduced the incidence of thrombosis detected by ^{125}I fibrinogen leg scan from 49% to 23% (5). Most hospital-issue elastic stockings do not produce graduated pressure.

More effective measures for prevention of stasis involve expensive equipment with limited patient-acceptability, and use will probably be restricted to selected patients with few or no other choices. Electrical stimulation of the calf musculature reduces the incidence of venous thrombosis demonstrated by ^{125}I fibrinogen leg scan (7) but cannot continue during a prolonged risk period. Pneumatic leggings appear to reduce stasis and effectively lower the incidence of postoperative venous thrombosis (8), but some trials of this means have not been well designed. Therefore, anticoagulant prophylaxis after hip joint replacement may be preferable (9). After neurosurgery, pneumatic calf compression significantly reduced venous thrombosis in a well-designed study reported by Turpie *et al.* (10).

Pneumatic compression does reduce stasis, but this may not be the only way it acts to reduce the incidence of vein thrombosis. Compression of the arm reduced the incidence of thrombosis in leg veins (11), which suggests that compression may release a vascular activator factor of the thrombolytic system. The attractiveness of physical measures for prevention of thromboembolism derives from their assumed lack of interference with hemostasis. If they activate thrombolysis a possible effect on hemostasis may be considered.

HYPERCOAGULABILITY

The third etiologic factor in Virchow's triad is awkwardly referred to as hypercoagulability. Anticoagulant drugs produce effective prophylaxis, but the occurrence or fear of postoperative hemorrhage has slowed their widespread use in the United States. After total hip replacement, wound hematoma is common enough to cause concern, and the consequence of wound bleeding may be serious. This problem has stimulated the search for alternative drug prophylaxis.

The effects of several drugs on the formation of wound hematomas have been compared in patients treated at New England Baptist Hospital (Table 1). The observations reported were made when total hip reconstruction served as a clinical model for investigation of various drugs proposed for prevention of postoperative venous thrombosis.

Total hip reconstruction is a useful clinical model because:

It is the commonest major joint reconstruction operation,

TABLE 1. WOUND HEMATOMA AFTER HIP RECONSTRUCTION

Drug	No. Pts.	No. Pts. with Hematomas		% Pts. with Hematomas
		Major	Minor	
None, placebo	91	2	4	6.6
ASA + hydroxy-chloroquine	44	3	3	13.6
Aspirin	21	1	1	9.5
Flurbiprofen	48	2	3	10.4
Heparin, 5000 units q 8h	18	7	3	55.6
Hydroxychloroquine	24	0	1	4.1
Sudoxicam	51	0	0	-
Warfarin	69	2	8	14.5

After hip joint reconstruction, venous thrombosis is frequent enough that small patient series may provide statistically significant results.

Pulmonary embolism is almost the only cause of death after this operation.

Orthopedic surgeons are uniformly and enthusiastically committed to embolism prevention and encourage their patients to participate in drug trials.

Untreated or placebo-treated control patients can be included ethically because venous thrombi can be detected and full-dose anticoagulant therapy can begin before major embolism results.

Since wound hematoma is not rare and its consequences may be serious, bleeding complications are a significant outcome criterion.

Drug therapy which prevents venous thrombosis after this operation without aggravating wound bleeding will be used readily after general surgical operations and when the risks of thrombosis and of bleeding are finely balanced.

THE INFLUENCE OF AGE, OBESITY, AND ACTIVITY

The incidence of thrombosis after hip joint replacement is significantly influenced by age, obesity, and the preoperative activity limitation such as that imposed by degenerative arthritis in many joints. A large group of patients had other risk factors so seldom that they did not appear as significant variables in discriminant function analysis (12). 368 patients monitored with ^{125}I fibrinogen leg scan after total hip replacement were ranked according to a discriminant function derived from these three significant variables. Analysis showed that the risk of developing venous thrombosis postoperatively varied from about 10% in the young, slender, mobile patients, to about 75% in elderly, obese, and substantially crippled patients.

This means that:

Risk factors are additive and that the individual's risk of developing venous thrombosis can be calculated from significant variables identifiable before surgery.

These factors cannot be used to categorize any patient undergoing hip replacement as not at risk, but the physician is more obligated to provide effective prophylaxis for patients at one end of the ranking than for those at the other.

METHODS OF MONITORING VENOUS EMBOLISM

Before less invasive monitoring techniques were validated, the outcome of clinical trials had to be based on phlebograms. Since ascending phlebography is uncomfortable and patients do not accept repeat studies well, some orthopedic surgeons hesitate to include all patients in a drug trial involving phlebograms. In their place, a combination of two less invasive techniques, ^{125}I fibrinogen leg scanning and cuff-occlusion impedance plethysmography (IPG), has been established as the preferred means for postoperative monitoring during drug trials (12,13). ^{125}I fibrinogen (^{125}I-FG) scanning detects calf-vein thrombi, and IPG specifically detects more proximal vein thrombosis. Each compensates for the false negatives of the other. We monitor with a leg scan every day for the first 3 days after surgery and then every other day. We use IPG before surgery to establish a baseline and then twice a week. If the results of either are abnormal, we repeat both daily.

The use of contrast phlebography may be limited to selected patients to rule out false positives and to support management decisions regarding full-dose anticoagulant therapy. Phlebograms required for these reasons are more readily accepted by the patient and the orthopedic surgeon than routine phlebograms required by rigid protocol.

Criteria in trials so monitored will then include the result of ^{125}I-FG leg scan; the result of IPG confirmed by phlebograms; and embolism if chest symptoms occur and embolism is proven by perfusion/ventilation lung scan, chest x-ray, and pulmonary angiography (if appropriate).

NATURAL HISTORY OF POSTOPERATIVE THROMBOSIS

The natural history of postoperative thrombosis and embolism has been revealed by combined monitoring techniques (12). ^{125}I-FG scanning showed that the incidence of early postoperative thrombosis is quite dramatic. In patients with normal IPG results, these thrombi remain small, and many will resolve spontaneously even without treatment. They may be nidus thrombi only. In a few patients, resolution is accompanied by small, symptomatic pulmonary embolism. Phlebograms showed moderately extensive thrombi soon after IPG results became abnormal during the first postoperative week, but more extensive and obstructive thrombosis during the second postoperative week. Embolism, if it occurs, tends to produce symptoms around the beginning of the third week. No patient we have monitored has ever developed major much less fatal embolism.

RESULTS OF DRUG TRIALS

The effects of six different drugs, placebo, and two combinations have been measured in prospective, randomized trials in patients with total hip replacements (12,14,15) (Table 2). The trials with flurbiprofen or hydroxychloroquine and placebo were double-blind. In another double-blind trial, aspirin was no more effective than placebo (16). Including this last trial, little evidence has been found that drugs affecting platelet function influence the occurrence of venous thrombosis after hip replacement. Aspirin appeared to be effective only in trials in which controls were not studied concurrently with treated patients (15,17), a flaw in trial design that has been properly criticized (18).

TABLE 2. VENOUS EMBOLISM FOLLOWING HIP RECONSTRUCTION IN PATIENTS TREATED WITH VARIOUS DRUGS, PLACEBO, OR NO DRUG

Treatment	No. of Pts.	By ^{125}I-FG Scan Yes	By ^{125}I-FG Scan No	By Phlebogram*	Reference
Warfarin	52	17	35	5	14
Sudoxicam	51	14	37	5	
Warfarin	17	10	7	3	
Heparin, 5000 units q 8h	18	6	12	3	14
No drug	19	8	11	4	
Flurbiprofen	48	23	25	8	12
Placebo	50	18	32	9	
Hydroxychloroquine	20	10	10	4	15
Placebo	20	10	10	4	
ASA + hydroxychloroquine	19	6	13	2	
ASA + hydroxychloroquine	20	5	15	1	15
ASA + placebo	21	7	14	2	

*Extensive or moderately extensive thrombus per phlebogram

THE HIP RECONSTRUCTION MODEL

The hip reconstruction model has been used in evaluations of drugs to prevent venous embolism since 1971 (Table 3). All patient monitored, but not all patients who underwent this operation, were included. The study was interrupted twice. The annual incidence of venous thrombosis varied, both in the last 3 years when ineffective, platelet-inhibiting drugs were tested, and in the first 2 years when warfarin and low-dose heparin were tested. No explanation can be offered for this annual variation, but the need to include control subjects concurrently is obvious.

TABLE 3. VENOUS THROMBOSIS (VT) AFTER HIP REPLACEMENT

Period	No. of Months	No. of Operations	No. of Pts. with VT	% of Pts. with VT
12-71 to 8-72	9	103	21	20.4
1-73 to 5-73	5	54	24	44.4
2-74 to 1-75	12	89	36	40.5
2-75 to 1-76	12	72	29	40.3
2-76 to 2-77	13	110	35	31.8
TOTAL		428	145	
			Mean %:	35.5

Annual, but not seasonal, variation in the occurrence of fatal pulmonary embolism has been reported (19), but in Australia postoperative venous thrombosis seems directly associated with cool seasons (20). Weather-related variables should be systematically evaluated to explain variations in the incidence of venous thrombosis in this model. Few attempts have been made in this country to find an answer, and the relationship of venous thrombosi to the weather has been regarded as anecdotal or even mythical. Seasonal or weather-related variables complicate the evaluation of trial results; such factors might influence the choice of therapy (20).

REFERENCES

1. Hume M, Sevitt S, Thomas DP: VENOUS THROMBOSIS AND PULMONARY EMBOLISM. Cambridge, Harvard University Press, 1970, p. 86.

2. Stamatakis JD, Kakkar VV, Sagar S, Lawrence D, Nairn D, Bentley PG: Femoral vein thrombosis and total hip replacement. BR MED J 2:223-225, 1977.

3. Heatley RV, Hughes LE, Morgan A, Okwanga W: Preoperative or postoperative deep-vein thrombosis? LANCET 1:437-439, 1976.

4. Flanc C, Kakkar VV, Clarke MB: Postoperative deep-vein thrombosis, effect of intensive prophylaxis. LANCET 1:477-478, 1969.

5. Holford CP: Graded compression for preventing deep venous thrombosis. BR MED J 2:969-970, 1976.

6. Scurr JH, Ibrahim SZ, Faber RG, LeQuesne LP: The efficacy of graduated compression stockings in the prevention of deep vein thrombosis. BR J SURG 64:371-373, 1977.

7. Rosenberg IL, Evans M, Pollock AV: Prophylaxis of postoperative leg vein thrombosis by low-dose subcutaneous heparin or preoperative calf muscle stimulation: A controlled clinical trial. BR MED J 1:649-651, 1975.

8. Madden JL, Hume M: VENOUS THROMBOEMBOLISM - PREVENTION AND TREATMENT. New York, Appleton-Century-Crofts, 1976, pp. 61-90, 173-181.

9. Salzman EW: Physical methods for prevention of venous thromboembolism. SURGERY 81:123-124, 1977.

10. Turpie AGG, Gallus AS, Beattie WS, Hirsch J: Prevention of venous thrombosis in patients with intracranial disease by intermittant pneumatic compression of the calf. NEUROLOGY 27:436-438, 1977.

11. Knight MTN, Dawson R: Effect of intermittant compression of the arms on deep venous thrombosis in the legs. LANCET 2:1265-1268, 1976.

12. Hume M, Turner RH, Kuriakose TX, Surprenant J: Venous thrombosis after total hip replacement. Combined monitoring as a guide for prophylaxis and treatment. J BONE JOINT SURG 58-A: 933-939, 1976.

13. Hull R, Hirsch J, Sackett DL, Powers P, Turpie AGG, Walker I: Combined use of leg scanning and impedance plethysmography in suspected venous thrombosis - an alternative to venography. N ENGL J MED 296:1497-1500, 1977.

14. Hume M, Kuriakose TX, Zuch L, Turner RH: ^{125}I fibrinogen and the prevention of venous thrombosis. ARCH SURG 107:803-806, 1973.

15. Hume M, Bierbaum B, Kuriakose TX, Surprenant J: Prevention of postoperative thrombosis by aspirin. AM J SURG 133:420-422, 1977.

16. Hume M: Sex, aspirin, and leg vein thrombosis after hip reconstruction. (Submitted for Publication).

17. Harris WH, Salzman EW, Athanasoulis C, Waltman C, Baum S, DeSanctis RW: Comparison of warfarin, low-molecular-weight dextran, aspirin, and subcutaneous heparin in prevention of venous thromboembolism following total hip replacement. J BONE JOINT SURG 56-A:1552-1562, 1974.

18. Genton E, Gent M, Hirsch J, Harker LA: Platelet-inhibiting drugs in the prevention of clinical thrombotic disease. N ENGL J MED 293:1174-1178; 1236-1240; 1296-1300, 1975.

19. Coon WW, Coller FA: Some epidemiologic considerations of thromboembolism. SURG GYNECOL OBSTET 109:487-501, 1959.

20. Lawrence JC, Xabregas A, Gray L, Ham JM: Seasonal variation in the incidence of deep-vein thrombosis. BR J SURG (In Press).

SUMMARY OF DISCUSSION BY PARTICIPANTS

Dr. Salzman opened the discussion by indicating that he and Dr. William Harris had a report of a larger clinical trial scheduled to appear in the December 8, 1977, issue of the NEW ENGLAND JOURNAL OF MEDICINE[1] showing favorable effects from aspirin in preventing post hip surgery venous thromboembolism. This was a double-blind, randomized, placebo-controlled, prospective study in which every patient was studied by phlebography as well as impedance plethysmography and I^{125} labeled fibrinogen. In this trial the protection

[1]Reference added in proof:
Harris WH, Salzman EW, Athanasoulis CA, Wahman AC, DeSanctis RW: Aspirin prophylaxis of venous thromboembolism after total hip replacement. N ENGL J MED 297:1246-1249, 1977.

afforded by aspirin was statistically significant, the incidence of thromboembolism being approximately twice as high in the control group as in the aspirin-treated group. Interestingly, the protection afforded by aspirin was not simply for thigh thrombi, which they thought might be the case in view of local trauma from surgery in the region of the femoral vein, but there was also significant protection against calf thrombi. An additional surprising finding was that the aspirin afforded protection only for the males. The frequency of venous thromboembolism in male patients taking aspirin was reduced from that in the control group to a highly significant degree. In the female patients, aspirin provided no significant protection. Because of this finding they reviewed their experience in earlier trials comparing aspirin with placebo; the same thing was true for the earlier studies, although it was not appreciated then. Again the protection with aspirin was entirely in males, while the women received no protection. No apparent explanation for this finding was discovered and they are still studying it. Dr. Salzman also felt that this question deserved study in other clinical settings. This observation in the postoperative total hip replacement trial may provide an explanation for some of the conflicting results with the use of aspirin that have been reported in the medical literature. The dosage of aspirin employed in the trial was 0.6 gram twice daily.

Dr. H. J. Day called attention to the fact that aspirin has different activities at various doses. For example, something like 25 micrograms is enough to inhibit the cyclo-oxygenase system in platelets. However, when the dose is increased to 0.6 gram twice a day, it may be an analgesic effect that one is encountering. And when doses of 3.2 gram are reached, the effect is probably anti-inflammatory as well. The anti-inflammatory aspect of venous thrombosis was something that Gwen Stewart had studied and called attention to in earlier trials in dogs.[2] She studied veins that were mechanically injured and found tremendous infiltration of white cells in the vein rather than finding platelets early on in the lesion as might have been anticipated. In further study,[3] she found that more white cells were present, and postulated that venous thrombosis was a white cell disease rather than a platelet disease. Other studies published about 3 or 4 years ago demonstrated that lidocaine had an effect on white cell migration, and when Gwen

---

[2] Stewart GJ, Ritchie WGM, Lynch PR: Venous endothelial damage produced by massive sticking and emigration of leucocytes. AM J PATHOL 74:507-532, 1974.

[3] Stewart GJ: The role of the vessel wall in deep vein thrombosis. In: ADVANCES IN AETIOLOGY, PREVENTION AND MANAGEMENT OF DEEP VENOUS THROMBOSIS, edited by Nicolaides AN. Lancaster, England, Medical & Technical Publishing Company, Ltd., 1975. Pages 101-135.

Stewart studied it in a dog model, she found that lidocaine also decreased the incidence of venous thrombosis in veins which were mechanically injured. These observations were in dogs and not humans. However, a study published in LANCET[4] describes a series of about 14 patients treated with lignocaine or placebo after hip surgery. The investigators were able to decrease the incidence of venous thrombosis using lignocaine; this may be a compound that warrants further study.

Dr. Mustard underscored Dr. Salzman's finding of apparent benefits of aspirin in males and not in females. He indicated that Dr. Barnett's study presented at this Workshop [pages 257 to 264] examining the value of nonsteroidal anti-inflammatory drugs in TIA prevention and stroke prevention showed that these effects were predominantly in males and not in females. Hormonal influence as opposed to a platelet effect might be involved in the male-female difference.

Dr. Molony, commenting on Dr. Harris and Salzman's study, pointed out that these patients were in the older age groups and the females beyond the menopause, so a hormonal effect might not be the explanation for the differences between male and female response. Referring to Dr. Hume's paper, he mentioned that there is confusion in the literature about the benefits of elastic stockings The apparent benefits reported in the studies from England might be explained, as Dr. Hume said, by the graded pressures produced by the stockings fitted for each patient's needs. These are graded so that the highest pressure is produced in the extremes of the lower extremity with decreasing pressure toward the thighs. The mere fact of putting on a pair of elastic stockings is apparently not enough. These must be properly fitted and so designed that the greatest pressure is exerted on the lower extremities at the toes with decreasing pressure up the leg to the thigh.

---

[4]Cooke ED, Lloyd MJ, Bowcock SA, Pilcher MF: Intravenous lignocaine in the prevention of deep venous thrombosis after elective hip surgery. LANCET 2:797-799, 1977.

CARDIAC THROMBOEMBOLISM: EVIDENCE FOR ROLE OF PLATELETS AND VALUE OF PLATELET SUPPRESSANT THERAPY

Edward Genton, M.D.

McMaster University, Hamilton, Ontario, Canada

ABSTRACT

Thromboembolism remains a frequent and serious problem in cardiac patients. Methods to identify the thrombosis prone patient and the identification of safe and effective forms of treatment would be of great value.

The accumulating evidence which indicates that abnormalities in platelet tests are often present in cardiac patients and may help identify those at greatest risk of thrombosis is encouraging. It suggests that patients with cardiac disease are desirable groups for investigation. It also indicates that the platelet survival test may be useful as a reference against which new and more practical tests can be compared, as well as a means to identify useful platelet suppressant drugs or to monitor the effects of these drugs.

INTRODUCTION

Thrombosis frequently develops in a diseased heart, and the consequences of the thrombotic lesion at the local site or from embolization into the pulmonary or systemic circulation may cause severe morbidity or mortality. The thrombotic process is important regardless of the nature of the cardiac condition and whether it involves the myocardium, cardiac valves, or coronary arterial circulation.

Degenerative or infectious processes involving the myocardium, such as those seen with primary myocardiopathy or endocarditis, are associated with intracardiac thrombi in the majority of cases, and in nearly one-third of those patients embolization becomes clinically significant. Following acute myocardial infarction (MI), mural thrombus overlying the area of infarction develops in approximately one-half of patients and emboli, often to the cerebral circulation, are seen in 5% to 10% of MI cases. Thromboembolism is common in valvular heart disease, especially in patients with mitral valve abnormalities: approximately 25% will have an embolic episode at some point in their course, and thromboembolism produces about 20% of deaths. Following removal and replacement of diseased valves, the problem persists; thrombotic complications have been the major obstacle in the development of prosthetic heart valves. Even with the present generation of valves which use low thrombogenic materials, thrombosis remains the major cause of later mortality and a persistent cause for clinicians' concern.

Conventional antithrombotic therapy with anticoagulant drugs reduces but does not eliminate the problem of cardiac thromboembolism. This indicates that a process unaffected by anticoagulants is likely involved. With appreciation of the important and often primary role played by the blood platelet in thrombosis, investigators have been encouraged to determine whether platelet abnormalities are present in patients with cardiac disorders, and whether drugs which alter platelet reactivity can influence the incidence of thromboembolic complications in patients with cardiac disease. Available information is persuasive that alteration of platelet tests is frequently present in cardiac patients and suggestive that platelet suppressant drugs may have therapeutic value.

CORONARY ARTERY DISEASE

The role of platelets in the genesis of atherosclerosis in the coronary arteries has not been precisely elucidated, but increasing evidence supports the so-called incrustation or thrombogenic hypothesis of atherosclerosis. It is now widely held that thrombi contribute to the development and course of atherosclerosis, and that the blood platelet plays a primary and probably key role in arterial thrombosis.

Regardless of platelets' role in the genesis of atherosclerosis, there seems little doubt that they are primarily involved with the thrombotic complications of atherosclerosis. The question of how frequently an extramural thrombotic occlusion is etiologic in the pathogenesis of myocardial necrosis remains controversial, but all would agree that with transmural infarction coronary thrombosis is frequent and that, again, the blood platelet plays a major role. Another question is what is the role of emboli of platelet aggregates in the microcirculation of patients with coronary disease? Such lesions are identifiable in victims of sudden death, and animal studies indicate that platelet microemboli in the coronary circulation may be produced by a number of stimuli and produce myocardial ischemia or necrosis (1).

Abnormalities of platelet reactivity have been observed in a variety of tests of "platelet function". These include increased platelet adhesion or hypersensitivity of platelets to exposure to aggregating agents such as epinephrine and ADP, spontaneous platelet aggregation in patients with coronary disease, and abnormalities in platelet survival time. A number of workers have observed that shortening of platelet survival is present in half or more of patients with angiographically demonstrated coronary disease, compared to a normal group (2). Even when age-matched controls are examined, there is significant separation between the controls and those patients with coronary atherosclerosis (3).

Shortened platelet survival and the degree of shortening do not correlate with the age or sex of the patients or the location or severity of coronary lesions. There is evidence that patients with coronary disease and hyperlipoproteinemia (Type 4) are more likely to have shortened platelet survival than those with normal lipid patterns. The possibility that platelet survival time may correlate with the clinical course of patients is indicated by the observation that the incidence of occlusion of aortocoronary bypass may be greater in patients with shortened platelet survival than in those who have normal survival time (4). In patients with saphenous vein grafts documented by angiography to be occluded, the average platelet survival time was shorter than that in a group with patent grafts. Platelet survival measured preoperatively did not change postoperatively. More than 90% who developed graft occlusion had shortened platelet survival time. If these observations are confirmed, they would suggest that the measurement of platelet survival time in patients scheduled to undergo bypass surgery may identify those at high risk of occlusion and the patients who might derive benefit from drugs which alter platelet reactivity.

Several platelet suppressant drugs have been evaluated in patients with coronary disease and shortened platelet survival. Sulfinpyrazone, clofibrate, and dipyridamole, alone or combined with aspirin, lengthen the abnormally short platelet survival time in about three-quarters of cases, and return it to normal in nearly 50% (5).

The combined evidence suggesting a role for platelets in coronary disease, documentation of altered platelet tests in these cases, and demonstration that drugs may alter these abnormalities have led to various clinical trials of platelet suppressant therapy in coronary disease.

Genton and others (6) discussed earlier trials of platelet

TABLE 1. PLATELET SUPPRESSANT THERAPY IN CORONARY ARTERY DISEASE

Study (Ref.)	Drug (g)	Years Observed	No. of Patients		% Developed M.I.		% Died	
			Control	Rx	Control	Rx	Control	Rx
Scottish 1971 (7)	Clofibrate 2.0	6	367	350	15	12	10	10
Newcastle 1971 (8)	Clofibrate 2.0	5	253	244	27	18	19	11*
C D P 1975 (9)	Clofibrate 1.8	8	2789	1103	30	28	25	25
M R C 1974 (10)	Aspirin 0.325	2.5	624	615	--	--	18	12
C D P A 1975 (11)	Aspirin 1.0	1-2	771	758	4	4	8	6
German-Austrian 1977 (12)	Aspirin 1.5	2	309	317	12	8	7	4

* $p < 0.05$

suppressive drugs in coronary artery disease. Table 1 lists six randomized controlled trials in patients with symptomatic coronary disease, in most instances following myocardial infarction, to determine the effect of clofibrate and aspirin on incidence of reinfarction or death. The Scottish (7) and Newcastle (8) multicenter trials evaluated clofibrate in patients with angina or prior myocardial infarction, or both. Both were designed to evaluate the cholesterol lowering effects of clofibrate on the course of coronary disease over a period of 5 or more years. A similar but larger study which extended follow-up for a longer period of time was included in the Coronary Drug Project (CDP) (9). While each trial was basically well designed, the two earlier trials have been criticized for imbalances in matching the control and treated groups. The CDP trial appeared to fulfill most of the criteria for an optimal clinical trial.

The aspirin trials have varied somewhat in the type of patients studied and the drug dosage. The Medical Research Council (MRC) study (10) entered patients whose mean interval from the qualifying infarction was 10 months, and used a small dose of drug. All patients admitted were several years post infarction. In contrast, the German-Austrian study (12) entered only patients who were 4 to 6 weeks post infarction and used a higher dose of aspirin.

The results in these trials are, for the most part, negative or inconclusive. In the Newcastle trial the clofibrate group had a significant overall reduction in frequency of sudden death and all deaths. This trend was most pronounced in patients who had angina alone or angina in combination with myocardial infarction. In the Scottish trial the clofibrate-treated group as a whole did not show significant overall reduction in either sudden death or all deaths. However, among patients with angina at the time of admission to the trial, the clofibrate-treated patients did show a significant reduction in both sudden death and all deaths. In both trials the incidence of nonfatal infarction was less, although not to a point of statistical significance, in the treated groups than in the placebo groups. This reduction was more pronounced when there was a previous history of angina rather than infarction. In both trials there was a highly significant reduction in all events in all the angina subcategories. However, in the Scottish trial there was no significant reduction in events in patients with a past history of myocardial infarction alone. The death rate for patients with a history of myocardial infarction and no angina was higher for clofibrate than for placebo.

In the Coronary Drug Project study, no benefit from clofibrate was found in total mortality or cause-specific mortality either for the entire group or for identified subgroups. The clofibrate group showed decreased rates of both coronary death and a combination of coronary death and definite nonfatal myocardial infarction.

On the other hand, patients receiving clofibrate showed a statistically significant excess incidence of pulmonary embolism, angina pectoris, and intermittent claudication.

In all three aspirin trials there was some reduction in the incidence of death in the treated groups, but in none did the difference reach statistical significance. Of possible importance in the Cardiff study (10) is the observation that among the patients who entered the trial within 6 weeks after the onset of their infarction, the aspirin group had a statistically significant reduction in overall mortality compared to the placebo group. In the German-Austrian trial (12), in which all patients admitted were 4 to 6 weeks post infarction, an impressive trend favoring aspirin was observed in death rate, but the number of cases in the study was small and the difference did not achieve significance.

A number of large-scale, well designed studies are underway to clarify the question of effects of platelet suppressant drugs on secondary prevention of myocardial infarction. Four of the trials will provide information concerning the effects of aspirin, and one will compare this drug alone with the combination of dipyridamole and aspirin. Effects with sulfinpyrazone are being obtained in two similar studies, and results from one will be reported soon.

One completed study compared the effects of aspirin, warfarin, and placebo on occlusion of aortocoronary bypass grafts (13). After 6 to 40 months of observation, there was some but not statistically significant reduction in occlusion rate in aspirin-treated patients compared to controls, while significant benefit was obtained from warfarin therapy (Table 2). Two current studies are evaluating bypass occlusions; one is comparing dipyridamole-aspirin against aspirin, and the other, sulfinpyrazone or dipyridamole-aspirin against control.

TABLE 2. EFFECT OF PLATELET SUPPRESSANT THERAPY ON OCCLUSION OF AORTOCORONARY BYPASS GRAFTS (13)

Drug	No. of Patients	No. of Grafts	% Grafts with Occlusion
Placebo	52	74	28%
Aspirin	47	81	20%
Warfarin	56	65	16%*

* $p < 0.1$

In conclusion, in patients with coronary artery disease the data appear persuasive that platelet abnormalities are frequently demonstrable, but the implications of these observations remain to be established. Various platelet suppressant drugs show effects on the abnormal test values, indicating that they alter platelet responsiveness or stimulus-producing platelet abnormalities in the patients studied. However, morbidity and mortality results in the clinical trials are difficult to interpret. The consistent trends suggesting benefit in aspirin-treated patients are exciting. Perhaps a particular subgroup of patients may derive benefit from this type of treatment, and if they constitute only a small percentage of the total patients, benefit may be masked. Identifying their characteristics would allow proper stratification. Conceivably, the patients with shortened platelet survival time constitute such a group.

VALVULAR HEART DISEASE

Shortened platelet survival times were found regularly in patients with older-model, highly thrombogenic prosthetic valves. With newer, less thrombogenic valves, many patients have platelet survival times within the normal range, and the mean value for groups of patients with a particular type correlates with the incidence of embolism with that valve (14). Of interest is that in each group of patients, even with low thrombogenic valves, some patients have shortened platelet survival times, and the data suggest that the survival time correlates with the incidence of thromboembolism. Patients with a history of thromboembolism have significantly shorter mean platelet survival times than those with no such history. In patients with prosthetic valves and shortened platelet survival, approximately half will give a history of embolic episodes, compared to less than 10% frequency in those with normal platelet survival. Similarly, practically all patients with a history of embolization will be found to have a shortened platelet survival time.

Such studies have been extended to non-operated patients with mitral valve disease, and results are similar. Again, there is a significant difference between patients with a history of embolism and those without, with the latter subgroup not differing from normal (15). Again, patients with shortened platelet survival will frequently have a history of embolization, compared to only about 10% frequency in those with normal platelet survival. Similarly, virtually all patients with thromboembolism are found to have shortened platelet survival, while only about half of those without embolism will have such an abnormality. This suggests that platelet survival may help identify the thrombosis prone patients with valvular heart disease, and conceivably the patients who are in particular need of antithrombotic therapy. Also, the thrombogeni-

TABLE 3. PLATELET SUPPRESSANT THERAPY IN PATIENTS WITH PROSTHETIC HEART VALVES

Study (Ref.)	Comparison		Months Observed	No. of Patients		% with Emboli		Comment
	Control	Experimental		Control	Rx	Control	Rx	
Sullivan 1971 (16)	Oral A/C*	Oral A/C + dipyridamole (400 mg)	12	84	79	14	1.3	Randomized Blinded
Arrants 1972 (17)	Oral A/C	Oral A/C + dipyridamole (200 mg)	24 vs 10	20	39	40	2.5	Sequential noncomparable groups
Taguchi 1975 (18)	Oral A/C	Dipyridamole (450 mg) + ASA (3 g)	14	34	35	14.7	2.9	Large dosage High dropout rate Nonrandomized
Altman 1976 (19)	Oral A/C	Oral A/C + ASA (0.5 g)	24	65	57	20.3	5.2	Group imbalance
Dale 1977 (20)	Oral A/C + placebo	Oral A/C + ASA (1 g)	42	73	75	13.7	2.6	Randomized Blinded High dropout rate (30%)

* A/C = anticoagulant

city of prosthetic materials to be used in substitute valves might be measured by testing their effects on platelet survival time.

In patients with prosthetic heart valves, or those with rheumatic valve disease and shortened platelet survival time, several drugs have been tested for their effects on platelet survival time. Both sulfinpyrazone and dipyridamole plus aspirin usually lengthen the shortened platelet survival time, and in about one-third of cases, return it to normal (5).

Table 3 lists five studies on the effects of platelet suppressants on the incidence of systemic embolization in patients with prosthetic heart valves. In most of these studies the drug has been combined with oral anticoagulants, regarded as a conventional form of treatment, and the combination compared with oral anticoagulants alone. In one trial an untreated group was compared. Only two of the trials (16,20) had optimal study design and conduct. Results of these studies are consistent in indicating a reduction in the incidence of embolization in patients receiving the platelet suppressant drug, and the differences between the study groups has been quite marked. One study is underway to evaluate the effects of sulfinpyrazone in patients with mitral valve disease without substitute valves. Preliminary reports from this trial again suggest reduced systemic embolization in patients receiving the platelet suppressant. There is inadequate information at this point to indicate whether the platelet suppressants alone can reduce thromboembolic complications, or whether their benefit requires oral anticoagulants as well. The one study (18) using an untreated group showed favorable results with drug, but the nonrandomized nature of that study limits the conclusions.

The available data allow the conclusion that there is promise for the use of platelet suppressants in patients with valvular heart disease or those who have prosthetic valves. It is uncertain whether the drugs will be useful when used alone, but they certainly may be indicated in combination with oral anticoagulants, especially in patients who have had an embolic episode in spite of oral anticoagulants.

REFERENCES

1. Genton E, Steele PP: Platelets, drugs and heart disease. In PLATELETS, DRUGS AND THROMBOSIS, edited by Hirsh J, Cade J, Gallus A, Schonbaum E. Basel, Karger, 1975.

2. Steele PP, Weily HS, Davies H, Genton E: Platelet function studies in coronary artery disease. CIRCULATION 48:1194-1200, 1973.

3. Ritchie JL, Harker LA: Platelet and fibrinogen survival in coronary atherosclerosis. AM J CARDIOL 39:595-598, 1977.

4. Steele PP, Battock D, Pappas G, Genton E: Correlation of platelet survival time with occlusion of saphenous vein aortocoronary bypass grafts. CIRCULATION 53:685-687, 1976.

5. Genton E, Steele PP: Platelet survival: Value for the diagnosis of thromboembolism and evaluation of antithrombotic drugs. PROCEEDINGS OF INT'L. SYMPOSIUM ON PLATELETS AND THROMBOSIS, Milan, 1976. (In Press)

6. Genton E, Gent M, Hirsh J, Harker LA: Platelet-inhibiting drugs in the prevention of clinical thrombotic disease. N ENGL J MED 293:1174-1178, 1236-1240 and 1296-1300, 1975.

7. Research Committee of the Scottish Society of Physicians: Ischaemic heart disease: A secondary prevention trial using clofibrate. BR MED J 4:775-784, 1971.

8. Group of Physicians of the Newcastle upon Tyne Region: Trial of clofibrate in the treatment of ischaemic heart disease. BR MED J 4:767-775, 1971.

9. Coronary Drug Project Research Group: Clofibrate and niacin in coronary heart disease. JAMA 231:360-381, 1975.

10. Elwood PC, Cochrane AL, Burr ML, Sweetnam PM, Williams G, Welsby E, Hughes SJ, Renton R: A randomized controlled trial of acetyl salicyclic acid in the secondary prevention of mortality from myocardial infarction. BR MED J 1:436-440, 1974.

11. Coronary Drug Project Research Group: Aspirin in coronary heart disease. J CHRONIC DIS 29:625-642, 1976.

12. Breddin K, Uberla K, Walter E: German-Austrian multicenter two-year prospective study on the prevention of secondary myocardial infarction by ASA in comparison to phenprocoumon and placebo. THROMB HAEMOSTAS 38:168, 1977 (Abstract).

13. McEnany MT, DeSanctis RW, Harthorne JW, Mundth ED, Weintraub RM, Austen WG, Salzman EW: Effect of antithrombotic therapy on aortocoronary vein graft patency rates. CIRCULATION 54 (Suppl II):II-124, 1976 (Abstract).

14. Weily H, Steele PP, Davies H, Pappas H, Genton E: Platelet survival in patients with substitute heart valves. N ENGL J MED 290:534-537, 1974.

15. Steele PP, Weily HS, Davies H, Genton E: Platelet survival in patients with rheumatic heart disease. N ENGL J MED 290: 537-539, 1974.

16. Sullivan JM, Harken DE, Gorlin R: Pharmacologic control of thromboembolic complications of cardiac-valve replacement. N ENGL J MED 284:1391-1394, 1971.

17. Arrants JE, Hairston P: Use of Persantine in preventing thromboembolism following valve replacement. AM SURG 38:432-435, 1972.

18. Taguchi K, Matsumura H, Washizu T, *et al.*: Effect of athrombogenic therapy, especially high dose therapy of dipyridamole, after prosthetic valve replacement. J CARDIOVASC SURG 16:8-15, 1975.

19. Altman R, Boullon F, Rouvier J, Raca R, Fuente L, Favaloro R: Aspirin and prophylaxis of thromboembolic complications in patients with substitute heart valves. J THORAC CARDIOVASC SURG 72:127-129, 1976.

20. Dale J, Myhre E, Storstein O, Stormorken H, Efskind L: Prevention of arterial thromboembolism with acetylsalicyclic acid. AM HEART J 94:101-111, 1977.

SUMMARY OF DISCUSSION BY PARTICIPANTS

Dr. Fuster opened the discussion by referring to the two trials of Altman and Dale [references 19 and 20 in the paper] in which they used aspirin and Coumadin and obtained good results in decreasing the incidence of thrombosis and embolism. Dr. Fuster indicated that his group had tried aspirin and Coumadin in a few patients, but that their results were not good because of bleeding. He asked if Dr. Genton had any information on the incidence of bleeding in the two trials he described. Dr. Genton replied that the dropout rate in the studies was high, but this was not so much from bleeding as from the side effects of the drugs, particularly gastrointestinal irritation. He thought that the incidence of bleeding was not much greater in patients receiving combination therapy than in patients who received oral anticoagulants alone.

Dr. Fuster went on to elaborate that they had 10 patients with mitral valve prostheses who had thromboembolic episodes while taking Coumadin; about 2 years ago they added aspirin (over 1g a day) to the regimen and three of these patients bled. At that point they decided not to use aspirin and added dipyridamole instead. Dr. Genton then asked if the patients bled while their prothrombin times were in the therapeutic range. Dr. Fuster replied that they had one patient in whom the prothrombin time was in control, and they did not know the prothrombin time in the other two at the time of bleeding.

Dr. Genton commented that there is a fair bit of experience with oral anticoagulants in patients receiving aspirin in combination with dipyridamole and that Dr. Harker has followed a group of patients using that combination. Dr. Genton further mentioned that his group had also done some similar studies and had not encountered too many problems; they had quite a number of patients taking oral anticoagulants with sulfinpyrazone. He raised this point because sulfinpyrazone is known to displace Coumadin from its protein-binding sites, and one has to anticipate this problem. Their practice is to reduce the maintenance dose of Coumadin by about 50% at the beginning of combination therapy, because sulfinpyrazone can displace Coumadin from its binding sites very rapidly. With this regimen they have not had any great difficulties. The patient will generally be on a lower maintenance dose of anticoagulant, as one might predict, and aside from that they have had no problems with combination therapy.

Dr. Genton asked Dr. Harker about his experience with aspirin plus Coumadin in patients with heart valve replacements. Dr. Harker replied that they had followed patients who were taking the combination and had not experienced any difficulties except when using a single high dose of aspirin. When a smaller amount of aspirin, namely 300 mg, is given with dipyridamole 3 times a day, things seemed to work out fine. His experience using the combination with sulfinpyrazone was similar to Dr. Genton's in that the warfarin dose must be reduced about 50%.

Dr. Genton then mentioned that it is not their practice to use combination therapy in patients with substitute heart valves; anticoagulants alone are quite effective. But in patients with embolic breakthrough in spite of anticoagulant therapy, adding another drug with an effect on platelets may prove to be beneficial. His group is actively seeking alternative therapy to oral anticoagulants because at this time clinicians essentially anticoagulate 100% of their patients, or at least those patients past age 45 who have valvular disease plus atrial fibrillation. In such patients the incidence of embolization is only around 20-25%, which means that about 75% of the patients theoretically don't need antithrombotic therapy. It is undesirable to expose them to the risk of that treatment for long periods of time. If one of the antiplatelet drugs used alone could be shown to be effective, then this would clearly be desirable therapy. He further commented that patients with nonoperative rheumatic heart disease are an attractive group to study because most of them don't get anticoagulants until they are past age 45 or 50. This clinical situation would be a nice setting in which to study single drug versus placebo in patients under age 45 or 50, because one might be able to show efficacy with an active compound.

Dr. Fuster then alluded to the problem of drug absorption and their experience with absorption of dipyridamole in different animal species and in humans. They found, for example, that pigs and pigeons do not absorb dipyridamole too well, and that humans vary tremendously in their ability to absorb the drug. And even the same human at different times may show different rates of absorption and varying blood drug levels. He cautioned that in clinical trials one must be concerned about absorption of drug and try to demonstrate adequate blood drug levels of the compound before concluding that the approach is invalid. Dr. Genton pointed out that this assumes that the effect on platelets is related to blood levels, which is still an open question.

Dr. Harker noted that not only platelet accumulation in thrombus but fibrin formation, which also involves platelet action, occurs in these states, and this has to be considered when planning therapy. In clinical situations where blood flow patterns are altered, there should be additional documentation about what kind of fibrin deposition can be monitored — by the appearance, by fibrinopeptide A measurements, or by fibrinogen turnover studies. Dr. Harker's group studied patients with rheumatic heart disease, and found in a limited number of observations a significant utilization of fibrinogen and positive fibrinopeptide A assay results. The situation is therefore complicated, because fibrin deposition (red thrombus versus white thrombus) is going on, perhaps to a variable extent in different patients. Dr. Harker is reluctant to use that model for antiplatelet therapy without having some additional documentation to unravel the problem of fibrin formation. He cautions that one has to remember these facts when studying patients with atrial fibrillation, those with a dilated left atrium due to rheumatic heart disease, and even those with mitral valve replacement, because of the alterations in hemodynamics.

Dr. Hoak then asked about the incidence of thromboembolic complications in patients with atrial fibrillation who do not have mitral valvular disease. Dr. Genton replied that a few groups feel that the incidence of embolization is about as high in patients without valvular obstructions as in those with valvular obstruction. However, this is contrary to the general experience and the opinion of most clinicians, who feel that patients with atrial fibrillation associated with atherosclerotic heart disease are not at significant risk of embolization, and that one should not treat these people for embolic complications until embolism has been documented. He realizes that some neurologists probably disagree with that viewpoint, but is not convinced that their evidence is persuasive.

Dr. Spaet then raised a point about the interesting phenomenon mentioned in the presentation, namely, that increased turnover of platelets is sometimes identified, and that this is not taking place at the site of primary pathology. This was best illustrated by the fact that when a coronary vessel is completely closed off, as Dr. Genton demonstrated, platelet survival time was still shortened. This suggests that there is increased platelet turnover at some point distant from the site of primary pathology, and raises the question as to what was going on in platelet turnover studies. Such studies identify abnormality of the total state of a patient, and this may have different therapeutic implications than active thrombosis at a particular site. Dr. Genton agreed that there are situations in which a problem which seems to be small in size is great in importance, for example, in shunts. Shunts of a certain size placed in the circulation will affect platelet survival time. A coronary lesion of a particular type could have similar effects. He noted that Dr. Harker has stated in the past that in these situations you are obviously measuring total vascular effects on the platelets and not entirely a consequence of some minor local pathology. Dr. Harker's group had looked at some patients with unstable angina and apparently felt that the platelet survival time may be changing with the changing clinical state of the patient.

Dr. Mustard added that pathologists have always found thrombi in arterial disease not located just at a specific site; they can often be found in other vessels when patients are examined post mortem. This further supports the point raised by Dr. Spaet about many sites of vascular injury affecting platelets.

Dr. Mustard then raised four additional points and asked if Drs. Genton or Harker had data relating to them. 1) Is there any sex difference in drug effects on platelet survival? 2) In the clofibrate trials was there any sex difference in the outcome? 3) If you administer dipyridamole to a patient and do not get a drug effect, and then use sulfinpyrazone, whose actions may be different, can you get an effect? 4) In view of the facts that aspirin may have a beneficial effect in the management of some forms of arterial disease, but aspirin does not affect platelet survival while the other drugs do, how important is platelet survival?

Drs. Genton and Harker responded to these four questions as follows:

1) Neither know of any sex differences in response of patients with shortened platelet survival times.

2) Regarding the clofibrate studies, Dr. Genton did not recall any sex differences in effects of the drugs on shortened platelet survival time. Dr. Harker was unimpressed with clofibrate's activity except in the management of Type IV hyperlipidemia.

3) Both Dr. Genton and Dr. Harker have seen patients who re-

spond to dipyridamole but not sulfinpyrazone or vice versa. Dr. Genton also mentioned that it takes longer to normalize a shortened platelet survival time with sulfinpyrazole than with dipyridamole, so the time that the measurements are made will affect results.

4) Dr. Genton and Dr. Harker agreed that we would learn a lot by understanding why aspirin is beneficial in clinical vascular disorders. At this time the clinical effects of aspirin or sulfinpyrazone cannot be attributed entirely to their effects on platelets.

Dr. Spittell asked whether attention was paid to the absorption of aspirin, and whether or not buffering of aspirin was studied and in turn its effects on platelet activity. Dr. Harker replied that they had tried aspirin with and without buffering and it didn't seem to make any difference. In addition, they tried the so-called delayed absorption types of aspirin and these showed absolutely no effect. In fact, they were not able to demonstrate that absorption of aspirin occurred from these delayed action aspirin tablets.

Dr. Spittell brought up the dilemma of young women who have cardiac valve prostheses and who wish to have families. The problem with oral anticoagulants is significant, because the fetal wastage in young women who conceive while on oral anticoagulant therapy seems exceedingly high. It was 50% in their experience in a group of about 43 women who conceived after they had cardiac valve prostheses.

RATIONALE FOR ANTIPLATELET AGENTS IN DIABETIC VASCULAR DISEASE*

John A. Colwell, M.D.,Ph.D., Perry V. Halushka, M.D., Ph.D., Kay E. Sarji, Ph.D., and Julius Sagel, M.B.,Ch.B.

Charleston Veterans Administration Hospital; and the Endocrinology-Metabolism-Nutrition Division and the Clinical Pharmacology Division of the Department of Medicine, and Department of Pharmacology, Medical University of South Carolina, Charleston, SC

ABSTRACT

Studies summarized in this paper indicate that some diabetics have increased sensitivity to platelet aggregating agents. The problem is in the platelet release reaction and may reflect increased synthesis of prostaglandins or their precursors. An interaction of plasma factors such as von Willebrand factor with platelets may also be involved. Based on these and other considerations, a prospective study on the use of aspirin and dipyridamole on diabetic lower extremity vascular disease is underway as a Veterans Administration Cooperative Study.

INTRODUCTION

The platelet has been ascribed an important role in the pathophysiology of atherosclerosis (1). In view of this, we have investigated platelet behavior in subjects with diabetes mellitus, a disorder with an accelerated rate of atherogenesis. A role for

*Supported by Veterans Administration Institutional Research Funds, South Carolina State Appropriation for Medical Research, and N.I.G. M.S. Grant No. 20387. Dr. Halushka is the recipient of a Pharmaceutical Manufacturer's Association Foundation Development Award in Clinical Pharmacology. Dr. Sagel is Director, Specialized Diagnostic and Therapeutic Unit, Charleston Veterans Administration Hospital.

platelets in diabetic microvascular disease has also been postulated (2).

Our studies in diabetic patients over the past few years have been directed at the following questions:

1. Are diabetics' platelets hypersensitive to aggregating agents *in vitro*? And a related question: Does the hypersensitivity precede the development of clinically apparent vascular disease?

2. Do abnormalities in diabetics' plasma contribute to abnormal platelet behavior?

3. Do diabetic patients have abnormalities in platelet prostaglandin (or precursor) production which contributes to platelet hypersensitivity?

4. Can clinical trials be based on these and similar studies?

We think that affirmative answers can be given to each of these questions, and present supporting evidence in this paper.

PLATELET HYPERSENSITIVITY IN DIABETICS WITH OR WITHOUT VASCULAR DISEASE

Early reports demonstrated increased platelet adhesiveness in diabetics (3-10). This has been most apparent in patients with established vascular disease (5,8,9-11), but has also been reported in diabetics without clinically apparent vascular disease (3-7).

As techniques for studying platelet aggregation *in vitro* improved, it also became apparent that diabetics had increased sensitivity to ADP-induced platelet aggregation (6,11-21). As was the case with platelet adhesion, the findings were usually seen in diabetics with advanced microvascular disease (6,11-19). In some series, however, hypersensitivity has been reported before the onset of clinically apparent vascular disease (13,14,18,21).

In our laboratories, hypersensitivity to ADP- and epinephrine-induced platelet aggregation in diabetics has been demonstrated (18,21,23). Our studies have been confined to males. The results are summarized in Table 1. The second phase of platelet aggregation is accentuated with these aggregating agents. A significantly greater percentage of diabetics than nondiabetics ($p < 0.01$) show hypersensitivity to these two aggregating agents. Heightened sensitivity to aggregating agents is seen in diabetics with and without clinically apparent vascular disease (Table 1). The results do not relate to duration or type of diabetes or to fasting plasma glucose, triglyceride, or cholesterol levels. Similar results are seen with collagen and arachidonic acid in frank diabetics (18,35).

TABLE 1. PERCENT PLATELET AGGREGATION* *IN VITRO* AFTER ADDITION OF ADP OR EPINEPHRINE TO PLATELET-RICH PLASMA FROM NORMAL AND DIABETIC MEN†

Type of Patient	No. Patients in Groups	ADP		Epinephrine
		0.5 μM	1.0 μM	0.5 μM
Normals	15-25	19±2	42±3	39±2
Diabetics (all)	51-67	44±5	67±5	51±5
Latent diabetes (no apparent vascular disease)	8-13	50±9	78±5	58±6
Frank diabetes (no apparent vascular disease)	21-26	44±6	63±5	40±5§
Peripheral vascular disease	12-15	39±9‡	66±6	58±6‡
Retinopathy-nephropathy	10-13	48±9	70±5	62±5

*Mean ± SEM.
†Compared with normals, values in diabetics differ significantly at the p <0.01 level except as noted.
‡p <0.05.
§Not significantly different from value in normals.

Collectively, these studies indicate that increased platelet adhesiveness and hypersensitivity to platelet aggregating agents are present in diabetics and may precede the development of clinically apparent vascular disease.

PLASMA FACTORS

Most of the studies on abnormal platelet behavior in diabetes have been performed using platelet-rich plasma. Interactions between platelets and plasma factors might then help account for the phenomena observed. We have been interested in two platelet-active factors which are elevated in patients with diabetes mellitus.

The first factor was initially described by Kwaan in 1972 (2, 22), and termed platelet aggregation enhancing factor (PAEF). This activity reflects an additive effect of plasma from diabetics on ADP-induced platelet aggregation of platelets in PRP from a nondiabetic donor. The effect is seen as an elevation of the aggregation percentage 4 minutes after adding an amount of ADP just below the threshold for the irreversible second phase reaction (22). We found PAEF activity in 55% (31 of 56) diabetics and only 16% (4 of 25) nondiabetic male controls ($p < 0.01$). The effect was seen in patients who did not yet have clinically apparent vascular disease. This activity has now been reported from three laboratories (14,22, 23), while others report negative results (16,24). Patient selection and variability of techniques may account for these differences.

A second plasma factor of importance in platelet function is von Willebrand factor; its activity is one of those associated with factor VIII. This complex has at least three separate activities: ristocetin cofactor activity (VIII R:WF), antigenic activity (VIII R:AG), and procoagulant activity (VIII:C). Elevated levels of VIII R:AG in diabetics with retinopathy have been found (25). Conflicting data on VIII:C appear in the literature (16,25). Increased plasma levels of VIII R:WF have been reported in diabetic patients with proliferative retinopathy (16).

We have studied VIII R:WF levels in 33 diabetic males and have found a mean value of 209±14% (SEM), significantly greater than the mean of 137±14% in 28 controls ($p < 0.001$). Elevated levels were seen before clinically apparent vascular disease (18,26). While the precise relationship between this observation and the previously described platelet abnormalities is not well defined, the elevated plasma VIII R:WF levels do show some correlation with hypersensitivity to aggregating agents and PAEF activity.

PLATELET PROSTAGLANDINS IN DIABETES

Platelet aggregation curves indicate that the second phase of platelet aggregation occurs at lower concentrations of aggregating agents in diabetic subjects than in normals. This finding, coupled with an explosion of information implicating prostaglandin endoperoxides in the platelet release reaction (27-33), indicated that a prostaglandin-related mechanism could help explain the findings in diabetic patients.

We were able to provide indirect evidence to support this concept by observing the effect of prostaglandin synthetase inhibitors on the hypersensitive platelet response in diabetics. The response was blocked by eicosatetraynoic acid *in vitro* (34) and by acetylsalicylic acid (21). These findings suggested that increased prostaglandin synthesis might be present in platelets from diabetics

We next studied 17 insulin-requiring diabetics, the majority of whom were free from apparent vascular disease, and 21 age- and sex-matched controls (18,35). As anticipated, the diabetics showed increased sensitivty to low concentrations of ADP (1 μM), epinephrine (1 μM), and collagen (1 μg/ml). Platelet aggregation measured 4 minutes after adding the agent was 80-82% in the diabetics, significantly greater ($p < 0.05$) than in controls for all three aggregating agents.

Table 2 shows the amount of immunoreactive prostaglandin E-like material (iPGE) synthesized in response to these concentrations of ADP, epinephrine, and collagen. Production of iPGE in diabetics was significantly greater than in controls with all three agents. Other results suggested a dose response relationship with collagen, but not with the other agents (35).

TABLE 2. PRODUCTION OF iPGE (pg/ml/500,000 PLATELETS)* IN PRP FROM DIABETICS AND NORMALS

Aggregating Agent, Conc.	Subjects	iPGE	P
ADP, 1 μM	Controls	90±35	<0.05
	Diabetics	269±78	
Epinephrine, 1 μM	Controls	190±49	<0.05
	Diabetics	689±250	
Collagen, 1 μg/ml	Controls	504±71	<0.05
	Diabetics	800±138	

*Mean ± SEM.

In a further attempt to determine whether there was increased activity of the prostaglandin synthetase system, PRP was incubated with an excess of the substrate, arachidonic acid 0.5 mM. Platelets obtained from diabetic subjects metabolized arachidonic acid at a greater rate ($p < 0.05$) and extent ($p < 0.001$) than platelets obtained from control subjects. The addition of arachidonic acid resulted in the synthesis of nanogram quantities of iPGE (Table 3) compared to only picogram quantities induced by ADP, epinephrine, or collagen (Table 2).

The increased iPGE synthesis in PRP obtained from diabetic subjects may reflect increased activity of the system at one or more sites. There may be an increase in the absolute levels of arachidonic acid or its availability. Or there may be an increase in one or more of the metabolizing enzymes, such as platelet phospholipase A3, cyclo-oxygenase, thromboxane synthetase, or prostaglandin endoperoxide isomerase. Clearly, additional studies are required to determine the site or sites contributing to the increased activity of the system.

TABLE 3. SYNTHESIS OF iPGE (ng/ml/500,000 PLATELETS)* BY PRP AFTER ADDITION OF ARACHIDONIC ACID (0.5 mM)

	Time (minutes)				
Subjects	0.5	1.0	2.0	3.0	4.0
Controls	2.1±7	5.7±1.4	14.8±2.3	20.1±1.1	21.9±1.6
Diabetics	2.1±.5	9.7±2.5	21.9±4.1	30.0±5.4	30.8±4.2

*Mean ± SEM.

CLINICAL STUDIES

These *in vitro* findings have demonstrated abnormalities of platelet function and some possible mechanisms in diabetic patients. *In vivo* studies, however, have been few in number. Only one group has studied platelet survival in diabetic patients (36). In a small group of insulin-requiring diabetics free from apparent vascular disease, they found a decreased platelet half-life (5.2±2.3 days) in diabetics compared to controls (11.7±5.4 days, $p < 0.01$ in the t test). These authors concluded that there was an increased utilization of platelets in diabetics. Indirect evidence to support this concept has also been reported by two groups, who found an increased percentage of megathrombocytes in diabetics, usually in patients with established micro- or macrovascular disease (23,37). An excellent correlation between percentage of megathrombocytes and platelet turnover has been found (38). These findings therefore suggest an increased platelet turnover and possible increased utilization, particularly in diabetics with established vascular disease.

The abnormalities of platelet behavior in diabetics are summarized in Table 4. It appears reasonable to postulate that these abnormalities may play a role in atherosclerotic vascular disease and perhaps in microangiopathy of diabetes mellitus. Without a properly designed prospective study in diabetic patients free from apparent vascular disease, it is impossible to determine if these abnormalities precede the vascular disease, are a consequence of it, or bear no relationship to it.

TABLE 4. ABNORMAL PLATELET FUNCTION IN DIABETES MELLITUS

Increased platelet adhesiveness

Hypersensitivity to platelet aggregating agents

Elevated levels of plasma factors which interact with platelets

- Platelet aggregation enhancing factor (PAEF)
- von Willebrand ristocetin cofactor activity (VIII R:WF)

Increased iPGE production by platelets

Increased platelet turnover

One way to determine the clinical significance of abnormal platelet behavior is to perform a prospective study on the effectiveness of antiplatelet drugs on the natural course of established diabetic vascular disease. Two such drugs are aspirin, a prostaglandin synthetase inhibitor, and dipyridamole, an agent which returns the reduced platelet survival time in nondiabetics toward normal (39). A Veterans Administration Cooperative Study entitled "Antiplatelet Aggregating Agents in Diabetic Lower Extremity Vascular Disease" is now underway. The major objectives of this double-blind, placebo-controlled study are to determine whether the administration of aspirin (325 mg tid) plus dipyridamole (75 mg tid):

-Influences the acute course of gangrene in diabetic patients.

-Reduces the occurrence of gangrene of the opposite extremity in diabetic patients with recent amputation for diabetic gangrene.

Recruitment of 270 patients in the first group and 186 patients in the second group began in 10 participating V.A. Hospitals in March, 1977. Patients will be followed weekly for 6 weeks for the acute study. Serial photographs and diagrams of gangrene are used during the acute study. Both groups are followed quarterly for 3 years, with occurrence of gangrene of the opposite extremity as the major endpoint. Death from vascular causes and acute vascular events such as myocardial infarction and stroke are secondary endpoints. Serial photographs and diagrams of the feet are made at each visit, and follow-up clinical examinations and platelet aggregation tests are performed. A centralized biochemical laboratory performs serum glucose, triglyceride, and cholesterol determinations and a central hematology laboratory is responsible for quality control and interpretation of platelet aggregation and plasma salicylate and dipyridamole levels. Statistical support is provided by the Cooperative Studies Program Coordinating Center, Perry Point, Maryland. It is hoped that this study will provide definitive information on the use of antiplatelet agents in one form of diabetic vascular disease.

CONCLUSIONS

The collective evidence suggests strongly that platelet adhesion and aggregation are altered in patients with diabetes mellitus. Although abnormalities in both functions have been found before the onset of clinically apparent vascular disease, it is not possible to conclude that either or both of these abnormalities is important in the genesis of vascular disease. Clinical assessment of vascular disease is crude, and it is quite possible that all patients studied to date had apparent or inapparent vascular disease at the time of investigation of platelet function.

Although much remains to be learned about the mechanisms of abnormal platelet behavior in diabetes, it is likely that plasma factors such as PAEF and VIII R:WF play a role in accentuated platelet adhesiveness. Effects on platelet aggregation may also be present. Further, it is probable that abnormalities of the platelet prostaglandin synthetase system are involved in the increased sensitivity these platelets show to platelet aggregating agents. Although *in vivo* data from diabetics are limited, the available information suggests that platelet turnover is more rapid than normal in these patients.

These considerations have led to a therapeutic trial of antiplatelet agents in diabetes mellitus. Such a study could produce indirect information on the role of platelets in the genesis of vascular disease. A study of the potential efficacy of aspirin in preventing or reducing the incidence and severity of diabetic vascular disease is attractive because of its low incidence of toxicity, its effective inhibition of platelet prostaglandin synthesis, and its apparent salutary effect on diabetic vascular disease (40). Dipyridamole, an agent which acts to return accelerated platelet turnover towards normal *in vivo* (32), is also an attractive therapeutic agent. Accordingly, a double-blind study on the effects of aspirin and dipyridamole on vascular disease of the lower extremity in diabetics has been undertaken as a V.A. Cooperative Study. We hope that the results will provide important therapeutic information about the prevention of advanced diabetic vascular disease.

ACKNOWLEDGEMENTS

The expert technical assistance of Marta Laimins, James

Kleinfelder, and Cindy Weiser is gratefully appreciated. Statistical analyses were done with the assistance of Drs. Boyd Loadholt and Dan Lurie, Department of Biometry.

REFERENCES

1. Ross R, Glomset JA: The pathogenesis of atherosclerosis. N ENGL J MED 295:420-425, 1976.

2. Kwaan HC, Colwell JA, Cruz S, Suwanwela N, Dobbie JG: Increased platelet aggregation in diabetes mellitus. J LAB CLIN MED 80:236-246, 1972.

3. Odegaard AE, Skalhegg BA, Hellem AJ: Increased activity of "anti-Willebrand factor" in diabetic plasma. THROMB DIATH HAEMORRH 11:27-36, 1964.

4. Shaw S, Pegrum GD, Wolff S, Ashton WL: Platelet adhesiveness in diabetes mellitus. J CLIN PATHOL 20:845-847, 1967.

5. Valdorf-Hansen F: Thrombocytes and coagulability in diabetics. DAN MED BULL 14:244-248, 1967.

6. Heath H, Brigden WD, Canever JV, Pollock J, Hunter PR, Kelsey J, Bloom A: Platelet adhesiveness and aggregation in relation to diabetic retinopathy. DIABETOLOGIA 7:308-315, 1971.

7. Seth HN: Fibrinolytic response to moderate exercise and platelet adhesiveness in diabetes mellitus. ACTA DIABETOL LAT 10:306-314, 1973.

8. Badawi H, El-Sawy M, Mikhail M, Nomeir AM, Tewfik S: Platelets, coagulation, and fibrinolysis in diabetic and nondiabetic patients with quiescent coronary heart disease. ANGIOLOGY 21:511-519, 1970.

9. Hellem AJ: Adenosine diphosphate induced platelet adhesiveness in diabetes mellitus with complications. ACTA MED SCAND 190:291-295, 1971.

10. Mayne EE, Bridges JM, Weaver JA: Platelet adhesiveness, platelet fibrinogen, and factor VIII levels in diabetes mellitus. DIABETOLOGIA 6:436-440, 1970.

11. Breddin K: Experimental and clinical investigations on the adhesion and aggregation of human platelets. EXP BIOL MED 3:14-23, 1968.

12. Szirtes M: Platelet aggregation in diabetes mellitus. ADV

CARDIOL 4:179-186, 1970.

13. Hassanein AA, El-Garf TA, El-Baz Z: Platelet aggregation in diabetes mellitus and the effect of insulin *in vivo* on aggregation. THROMB DIATH HAEMORRH 27:114-120, 1972.

14. Leone G, Bizzi B, Accorra F, Boni P: Functional Aspect of Platelets in Diabetes Mellitus. In PLATELET AGGREGATION AND DRUGS, edited by Caprino L, Rossi FC. New York, Academic Press, 1974, pp. 49-61

15. Passa P, Bensoussan D, Levy-Toledano S, Caen J, Canivet J: Etude de l'agregation plaquettaire au cours de la retinopathie diabetique: Influence de L'hypophysectomie. ATHEROSCLEROSIS 19:277-285, 1974.

16. Bensoussan D, Levy-Toledano S, Passa P, Caen J, Canivet J: Platelet hyperaggregation and increased plasma level of von Willebrand factor in diabetics with retinopathy. DIABETOLOGIA 11:307-312, 1975.

17. O'Malley BC, Ward JD, Timperley WR, Porter NR, Preston FE: Platelet abnormalities in diabetic peripheral neuropathy. LANCET 2:1274-1276, 1975.

18. Colwell JA, Halushka PV, Sarji K, Levine J, Sagel J, Nair RMG: Altered platelet function in diabetes mellitus. DIABETES 25(Suppl 2):826-831, 1976.

19. Fleischman AI, Beirenbaum ML, Stier A, Somol H, Watson PB: *In vitro* platelet function in diabetes mellitus. THROMB RES 9:467-471, 1976.

20. Rathbone RL, Ardlie NG, Schwartz CJ: Platelet aggregation and thrombus formation in diabetes mellitus: An *in vitro* study. PATHOLOGY 2:307-316, 1970.

21. Sagel J, Colwell JA, Crook L, Laimins M: Increased platelet aggregation in early diabetes mellitus. ANN INTERN MED 82:733-738, 1975.

22. Kwaan HC, Colwell JA, Suwanwela N: Disseminated intravascular coagulation in diabetes mellitus with reference to the role of increased platelet aggregation. DIABETES 21:109-113, 1972.

23. Colwell JA, Sagel J, Crook L, Chambers A, Laimins M: Correlation of platelet aggregation, plasma factor activity, and megathrombocytes in diabetic subjects with and without vascular disease. METABOLISM 26:279-285, 1977.

24. Coller BS, Frank R, Gralnick HR: Correlation of hemoglobin A1C, von Willebrand factor (vWF), fibrinogen (f) and ADP-induced platelet aggregation enhancement factor (ADP-PAEF) in normals and diabetics. ANN INTERN MED 1978 (In Press).

25. Pandolfi M, Almer LO, Holmberg L: Increased von Willebrand-antihaemophilic factor A in diabetic retinopathy. ACTA OPHTHALMOL 52:823-828, 1974.

26. Sarji KE, Schraibman HB, Chambers A, Nair RMG, Colwell JA: Quantitative studies of von Willebrand factor (vWF) in normal and diabetic subjects: Role of vWF in second-phase platelet aggregation. MICROCIRCULATION II (Proceedings of the 1st World Congress for the Microcirculation, University of Toronto, Toronto, Canada, 1975), 1976, pp. 296-297.

27. Smith JB, Ingerman C, Kocsis JJ, Silver MJ: Formation of an intermediate in prostaglandin biosynthesis and its association with the platelet release reaction. J CLIN INVEST 53:1468-1472, 1974.

28. Willis AL, Vane FM, Kuhn DC, Scott CG, Petrin M: An endoperoxide aggregator (LASS) formed in platelets in response to thrombotic stimuli. PROSTAGLANDINS 8:453-507, 1974.

29. Hamberg M, Samuelsson B: Prostaglandin endoperoxides. Novel transformations of arachidonic acid in human platelets. PROC NAT ACAD SCI USA 71:3400-3404, 1974.

30. Hamberg M, Svensson J, Samuelsson B: Prostaglandin endoperoxides. A new concept concerning the mode of action and release of prostaglandins. PROC NAT ACAD SCI USA 71:3824-3828, 1974.

31. Hamberg M, Svensson J, Wakabayashi T, Samuelsson B: Isolation and structure of two prostaglandin endoperoxides that cause platelet aggregation. PROC NAT ACAD SCI USA 71:345-349, 1974.

32. Hamberg M, Svensson J, Samuelsson B: Thromboxanes: A new group of biologically active compounds derived from prostaglandin endoperoxides. PROC NAT ACAD SCI USA 72:2994-2998, 1975.

33. Smith JB, Ingerman C, Silver MJ: Persistence of thromboxane A_2-like material and platelet release-inducing activity in plasma. J CLIN INVEST 58:1119-1122, 1976.

34. Colwell JA, Chambers A, Laimins M: Inhibition of labile aggregation-stimulating substance (LASS) in platelet aggregation

in diabetes mellitus. DIABETES 24:684-687, 1975.

35. Halushka PV, Lurie D, Colwell JA: Increased synthesis of prostaglandin-E-like material by platelets from patients with diabetes mellitus. N ENGL J MED 297:1306-1310, 1977.

36. Ferguson JC, Mackay N, Philip JAD, Sumner DJ: Determination of platelet and fibrinogen half-life with [^{75}Se]seleno-methionine: Studies in normal and in diabetic subjects. CLIN SCI MOL MED 49:115-120, 1975.

37. Garg SK, Lackner H, Karpatkin S: The increased percentage of megathrombocytes in various clinical disorders. ANN INTERN MED 77:361-369, 1972.

38. Karpatkin S: Biochemical and clinical aspects of megathrombocytes. ANN NY ACAD SCI 201:262-279, 1972.

39. Harker LA, Schlichter SJ: Studies of platelet and fibrinogen kinetics in patients with prosthetic heart valves. N ENGL J MED 283:1302-1305, 1970.

40. Powell ED, Field RA: Diabetic retinopathy and rheumatoid arthritis. LANCET 2:17-18, 1964.

SUMMARY OF DISCUSSION BY PARTICIPANTS

Dr. Molony asked if the sensitivity of the platelets of diabetic subjects to aggregating stimuli could possibly be an age-related phenomenon. He also wondered whether Dr. Colwell's group included people who were age-matched with diabetics, or were the diabetic patients a more elderly group and the matched subjects younger people such as the house staff, lab technicians and the like who are commonly used as normal controls. Were the diabetic patients hospitalized and perhaps more physically inactive than the controls? His last questions were, could the abnormal platelet findings in diabetics be a consequence rather than a cause of the microvascular disease, and is there any way of getting at that question?

Dr. Colwell replied that a prospective study is needed to get at the last point; in his opinion there is no evidence at the moment which will tell us whether the platelet abnormality is a cause or an effect of the diabetic microvascular disease. His impression is that it may not be a consequence of the disease, because he has seen fairly fresh diabetics without any previous history of diabetes who show increased sensitivity of the platelets

To go back to the questions about the study groups, the hospitalized patients were a mixture. About 50% were outpatients and active and the other 50% were inpatients. Of course, a major problem in this type of study is doing platelet aggregation work in outpatients who frequently tend to take aspirin, whereas the problem of aspirin use can be controlled in inpatients. In terms of the activity of the patients, except perhaps for the amputee group most of the patients certainly were active. Concerning age, Dr. Colwell's group has not seen any age-related platelet hypersensitivity or decreased sensitivity either in the normal group up to age 55 or in the diabetics up to age 70. However, they do not have normals over age 55. They are doing glucose tolerance tests to separate chemical diabetes from normal glucose tolerance, and under those conditions they do not see any age-related phenomena, but this may be because they do not have enough elderly normal subjects.

Dr. Gorman said his group has found that very, very small amounts of prostacyclin can essentially shut down cyclo-oxygenase completely. So he was wondering if Dr. Colwell's group had measured cyclic nucleotides in platelets. The reason for his question was that thromboxane has a tendency to inhibit cyclase and prostacyclin enhances it, so if there is a loss of endothelial cell or loss of prostacyclin, the base level of cyclic nucleotides may be depressed and that could account for the enhanced aggregability. Dr. Colwell replied that Dr. Sagel worked with him on this problem. They never published the data, but they did measure about 30 resting platelet cyclic nucleotide levels in diabetics and in normal platelets and found no difference. They also measured resting serotonin levels and found no difference. Likewise, they measured ADP and ATP resting levels and found no difference. However, they never looked at these when they were stimulated.

Dr. Ross noted that he does not use aggregometry, and asked how one can relate the increased aggregability in the aggregometer with what is going on in the patient. For example, agents like dipyridamole don't affect aggregation in an aggregometer, but do affect platelet survival *in vivo*. What is the significance of these aggregometer observations and how do we use the information? Dr. Colwell agreed that this is obviously an important question, one which has bothered him and others all along, and it is difficult to answer. He didn't think that one can necessarily jump from an aggregometer observation into an *in vivo* situation at all. They have made no attempt to correlate such observations with anything other than some estimate of platelet turnover using megathrombocytes, which might give some idea about an *in vivo* parameter other than the clinical parameters discussed in the paper.

Dr. Spaet commented that with aggregometry it was probably a problem of fact versus artifact. For example, one of the major problems is that a slight change in hematocrit changes the results, and if you are making a constant citrate addition, you are going to see changes. If you have changes in the period of time that you wait from the time you collect the specimens, or if you spin the specimens differently, or if you do various other maneuvers you can affect the aggregometry. So it is extremely important to take exact measures to standardize the various conditions that the platelets are exposed to during aggregometry. Dr. Colwell agreed, and said that in their studies they consistently used platelet-rich plasma, and kept the interval between 1 and 2 hours after drawing blood, and they looked at hematocrits and found no difference. So in standardizing their studies they have tried to control all the known variables.

Dr. Spittell asked whether Dr. Colwell was aware of any studies that can give us some information on the effect of diabetes on the prognosis for graft patency, either coronary graft or peripheral graft patency. Dr. Colwell did not know of any well-controlled studies directed at this.

Dr. Harker remarked that their group had an opportunity to study long-standing juvenile diabetics and found that none of them had shortened platelet survival, whereas patients who had established clinically symptomatic vascular disease did show evidence of a shortened platelet survival. He then speculated whether glycosylation could be involved in the modification of this reaction similar to the way that glycosylation alters hemoglobin. Some more recent data from the Rockefeller Institute have also suggested that fibrinogen itself is modified by glycosylation, which impairs its capacity to circulate. Dr. Harker asked whether Dr. Colwell knew about the glycosylation of various proteins involved in the aggregation response, and whether there is information about glycoproteins and surface-related glycoprotein components.

Dr. Colwell replied that he was not sure how to answer that question. The levels of circulating glycoproteins are, of course, high in diabetics. He was interested in Dr. Harker's comments on platelet turnover rate in long-standing juvenile diabetics, and surprised that he did not find shortened survival rates in those patients. Accelerated platelet turnover rates might be expected if shortened survival is related to macrovascular disease, and the majority of patients with long-standing juvenile diabetes will show macrovascular disease after 25 to 30 years of diabetes.

THE ROLE OF PLATELETS IN TRANSIENT ISCHEMIC ATTACKS AND CEREBRAL VASCULAR ACCIDENTS*

H.J.M. Barnett, M.D.

Department of Clinical Neurological Sciences, University of Western Ontario, London, Ontario, Canada

ABSTRACT

In a 5½-year study in 585 patients, aspirin, 1200 mg/day, reduced by 50% the risk of stroke or death in men who had experienced at least one episode of neurological disability in carotid or vertebral-basilar territory. Adding sulfinpyrazone to aspirin did not improve the results, and sulfinpyrazone alone was no better than placebo. Women did not experience the same benefit; aspirin did not reduce their risk of stroke or death.

INTRODUCTION

During the period 1959 to 1968, observations recorded in thrombosis research set the stage for a possible new approach to stroke prevention. First, it was recognized that platelet reaction was closely connected to intra-arterial thrombogenesis in a significant number of patients experiencing a transient ischemic attack (TIA) or stroke (1,2). Second, there were reports that certain drugs could alter platelet function (3-5). These findings raised the exciting prospect that platelet-inhibiting drugs might prevent stroke.

During this same period a clearer understanding evolved of TIA — its pathogenesis, incidence, prognosis, and symptomatology (6-8). It became apparent that some cases of TIA were hemodynamic, some were due to emboli from the heart, and a substantial number were due to emboli from the major cerebral arteries in the neck and

*Supported by Canadian Medical Research Council Grant MA 4537.

in the cranium below the terminal branching of the major arteries. The embolic material originating from atheromatous, ulcerative, and stenotic lesions was recognized to be of two varieties: 1) primarily platelet-fibrin material or 2) cholesterol-containing atheromatous debris. Atheromatous lesions were presumed to initiate secondary platelet-induced thrombogenesis, and this has been confirmed (9).

Estimates of the incidence of TIA preceding stroke have varied considerably. In retrospective studies of patients with cerebral infarction, previous TIA has been recorded as infrequently as 10% (10) and as frequently as 79% (11). The higher figure is closer to the average from the reports available. In prospective studies, the estimates also vary, but a generally accepted conservative estimate indicates that among patients who have had their first TIA, approximately 5% per year will have a stroke; in addition, approximately 4% per year will die of vascular causes, one-third of these from stroke and two-thirds from other vascular disorders, particularly myocardial infarction (12,13). The prognosis is not significantly different between carotid and vertebral-basilar TIA cases, despite early impressions to the contrary (14,15).

The symptomatology of TIA in carotid artery territory has been more readily definable and recognizable than that in vertebral-basilar artery distribution. Ipsilateral amaurosis fugax and contralateral motor, sensory, and dysphasic disorders make up the majority of cases. There is a high correlation between these symptoms and recognizable defects in the appropriate carotid arteries (16,17). Hemodynamic (perfusion)deficits are likely to mimic artery-to-artery embolic episodes in the vertebral-basilar arterial territory; this dictates caution in classifying as TIA cases that may be of arterial embolic nature in the posterior circulation. Furthermore, certain symptoms occurring or even recurring in isolation are not now accepted as diagnostic of TIA; these include vertigo, diplopia, amnesia, loss of consciousness, drop attacks, and visual blurring other than amaurosis fugax.

Several factors – clarification of the clinical picture of "threatened stroke", recognition of a group of patients with cerebral ischemia apparently of artery-to-artery embolic origin, the knowledge that platelets play a role in some of these ischemic events, and the availability of apparently safe and effective platelet-inhibiting drugs – led to treatment of a few isolated cases and a few small series of cases of retinal and cerebral ischemia (18). These preliminary studies were not designed to establish efficacy with regard to the important endpoints of stroke and death, but suggested that two platelet-inhibiting drugs, aspirin and sulfinpyrazone, might reduce TIA recurrence. This challenged a group of Canadian investigators, as well as an American group sponsored by the NHLBI, to set up parallel collaborative, randomized studies in an attempt to settle this issue.

The more abbreviated American trial, which studied aspirin alone in a group from which a "surgical" cadre was preselected, has been concluded and reported (19).

THE CANADIAN TRIAL

Methods

A multicenter, randomized clinical trial, sponsored by the Canadian Medical Research Council, was designed in 1970-1971 (20, 21) to determine whether aspirin or sulfinpyrazone, singly or in combination, could reduce the incidence of TIA, stroke, or death to 50% or less of that among similar patients receiving placebo alone.

Patients eligible for the trial had experienced one or more episodes of neurological disability in carotid or veretebral-basilar territory during the preceding 3 months. Excluded from the trial were patients whose ischemic events were judged to be of hemodynamic origin, i.e., orthostatic hypotension, bradyarrhythmia or tachyarrhythmia, serious aortic stenosis, or polycythemia; patients who were probably experiencing their ischemic events on the basis of emboli from the heart; patients who had hypercoagulable states; or patients who had a clinical picture compatible with lacunar infarction. Patients were also excluded if they were judged to have serious co-morbid conditions which might lead to their death during the 12-month period after they entered the trial. Also excluded were patients who were unable to tolerate platelet-inhibiting drugs or who would require platelet-inhibiting drugs or anticoagulants on a long-term basis for other medical conditions.

The patients were assigned to one of four treatment categories by a predetermined randomization procedure:

Aspirin capsule 325 mg plus placebo tablet, 4 of each daily

Sulfinpyrazone tablet 200 mg plus placebo capsule, 4 of each daily

Aspirin capsule 325 mg plus sulfinpyrazone tablet 200 mg, 4 of each daily

Placebo capsule and placebo tablet, 4 of each daily

The patients were to record attacks or untoward symptoms in diaries and bring their diaries with them to their follow-up visits at 1 month, 13 weeks, and every 3 months for the next 5 years.

Details of the study design and methods have been described elsewhere (22). The endpoints counted against the therapeutic regimens were recurrent TIAs, stroke, or death.

RESULTS

Between November 1971 and June 30, 1976, 585 patients who fulfilled the study entry criteria began treatment, while 756 patients were excluded from the trial because they failed to meet the strict criteria. Results summarized here are based on follow-up information through June 30, 1977; follow-up information to that date was obtained in 99.3% of the 585 patients. Detailed results are described elsewhere (22).

The average duration of therapy was 717 days, and the average period of follow-up was 1002 days. The difference was accounted for by withdrawal of therapy for a variety of reasons, including death, stroke, or persistence of symptoms prompting the attending physician to administer nonapproved concomitant therapy or to recommend surgery.

Considering all three endpoints (continuation of TIAs; stroke; or death), the aspirin-treated group showed a 20% reduction in the risk of these events compared to the sulfinpyrazone and placebo groups.

Considering the "harder" endpoints of stroke or death, the risk in the aspirin group was reduced by approximately one-third ($p = 0.05$) compared to the placebo group. The difference between the sulfinpyrazone and placebo groups was not statistically significant.

When the patients were stratified by sex, the results were markedly different in men than in women. In men, aspirin reduced the risk of stroke and death by 50% ($p = 0.003$) compared to placebo (Figure). In women, who constituted about one-third of the study population, aspirin produced no significant reduction in risk.

In men, adding sulfinpyrazone to aspirin added no detectable benefit over aspirin alone, and giving sulfinpyrazone alone did not reduce the risk more than giving placebo (Figure).

The results indicate that in men threatened with a stroke in carotid or vertebral-basilar territory, the long-term use of aspirin, 1200 mg/day, is definitely effective in reducing the incidence of stroke and death, and also reduces the risk of recurrence of transient ischemic events. Aspirin does not reduce the risk substantially in women. Sulfinpyrazone is not effective in patients threatened with stroke.

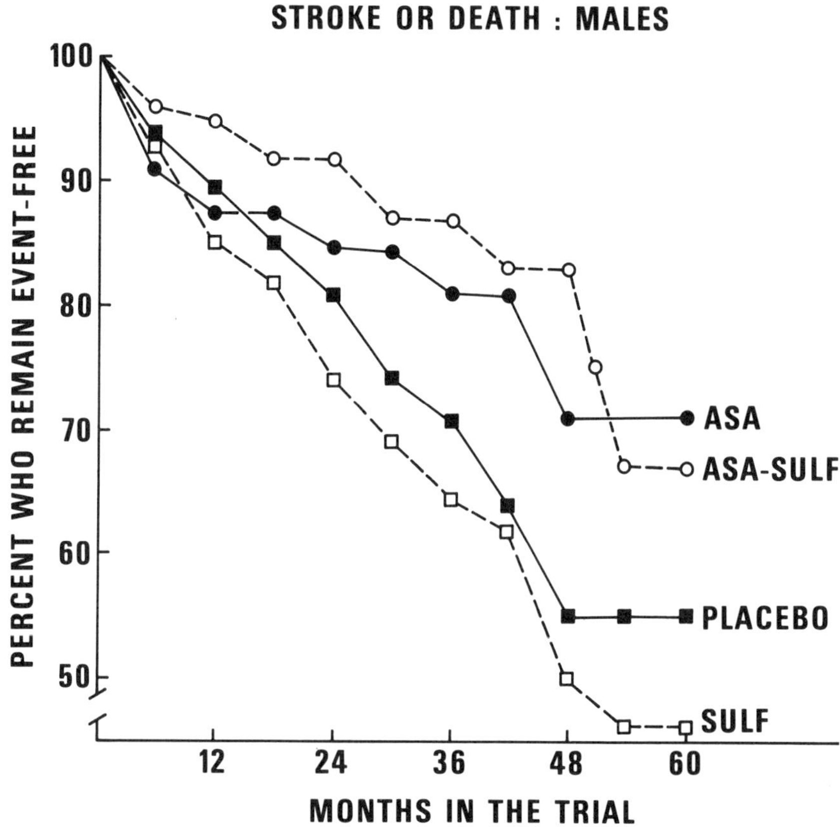

Figure. Results of life table analysis: comparison of event-free months in male patients over a 5-year period.

Side effects of the treatments were mostly gastrointestinal symptoms. The most common disturbing complication of therapy, as judged after 3 months of therapy, was upper abdominal pain. This occurred in all four treatment groups, being noted in 2.2% of the sulfinpyrazone group, 7.8% of the aspirin group, and 13% of those taking both active drugs, but also 3.4% of those taking only placebo. "Heartburn" was reported in 5.7% of the total patients and nausea in 5.3%. Both complaints were more frequent in patients taking combined therapy than in those taking aspirin alone. Hematemesis or melena occurred in 2.1% of the patients during the entire trial: 2.5% of the sulfinpyrazone group, 4.1% of the patients taking combined therapy, and 1.5% of the placebo group, but, surprisingly, in none of the patients taking aspirin alone.

REFERENCES

1. Fisher CM: Observations of the fundus oculi in transient monocular blindness. NEUROLOGY 9:333:347, 1959.

2. Russell RWR: Observations on the retinal blood vessels in monocular blindness. LANCET 2:1422-1428, 1961.

3. Smythe HA, Ogryzlo MA, Murphy EA, Mustard JF: The effect of sulfinpyrazone (Anturan) on platelet economy and blood coagulation in man. CAN MED ASSOC J 92:818-821, 1965.

4. Weiss HJ, Aledort LM: Impaired platelet connective-tissue reaction in man after aspirin ingestion. LANCET 2:495-497, 1967.

5. Zucker MB, Peterson J: Inhibition of adenosine diphosphate induced aggregation and other platelet functions by acetylsalicylic acid ingestion. PROC SOC EXP BIOL MED 127:547-551, 1968.

6. Barnett HJM: Transient cerebral ischemia: Pathogenesis, prognosis and management. ANN R COLL PHYSICIANS SURG CAN 7:153-173, 1974.

7. Gunning AJ, Pickering GW, Robb-Smith AHT, Russell, RR: Mural thrombosis of the internal carotid artery and subsequent embolism. Q J MED 33:155-195, 1964.

8. Barnett HJM: Pathogenesis of transient ischemic attacks. In: CEREBROVASCULAR DISEASES, edited by Scheinberg P. New York, Raven Press, 1976, pp. 1-21.

9. Warren BA, Vales O: Electron microscopy of the sequence of events in the atheroembolicocclusion of cerebral arteries in an animal model. BR J EXP PATHOL 56:205-215, 1975.

10. Whisnant JP, Matsumoto NM, Elseback LR: Transient cerebral ischemia attacks in a community. MAYO CLIN PROC 48:194-198, 1973.

11. Drake WE, Drake MAL: Clinical and angiographic correlates of cerebrovascular insufficiency. AM J MED 45:253-270, 1968.

12. Millikan CH: Treatment of occlusive cerebrovascular disease. In: CEREBROVASCULAR SURVEY REPORT FOR JOINT COUNCIL SUBCOMMITTEE ON CEREBROVASCULAR DISEASE, NATIONAL INSTITUTE OF NEUROLOGICAL AND COMMUNICATIVE DISORDERS AND STROKE AND NATIONAL HEART AND LUNG INSTITUTE (revised), edited by Siekert RG. Rochester, Whiting Press Inc., 1976, pp. 141-171.

13. Friedman GD, Wilson WS, Mosier JM, Colandrea MA, Nichaman MZ: Transient ischemic attacks in a community. JAMA 210:1428-1434, 1969.

14. Cartlidge NEF, Whisnant JP, Elveback LR: Carotid and vertebral-basilar transient cerebral ischemic attacks. MAYO CLIN PROC 54:117-120, 1977.

15. Marshall J: The natural history of transient ischemic cerebrovascular attacks. Q J MED 33:309-324, 1964.

16. Kishore PRS, Chase NE, Kricheff II: Ulcerated atheroma of carotid artery and cerebral embolism. In: ASPIRIN, PLATELETS AND STROKE, edited by Fields WS, Hass WR. St. Louis, Warren H. Green, 1971, pp. 13-27.

17. Eisenberg RL, Nemzek WR, Moore WE, Mani RL: Relationship of transient ischemic attacks and angiographically demonstrable lesions of carotid artery. STROKE 8:483-486, 1977.

18. Genton E, Barnett HJM, Fields WS, Gent M, Hoak JC: Cerebral ischemia: The role of thrombosis and of antithrombotic therapy. STROKE 8:147-175, 1977.

19. Fields WS, Lemak NA, Frankowski RF, Hardy RJ: Controlled trial of aspirin in cerebral ischemia. STROKE 3:301-316, 1977.

20. Barnett HJM: Platelets, drugs and cerebral ischemia. In: PLATELETS, DRUGS AND THROMBOSIS, edited by Hirsh J. Basel, S. Karger, 1975, pp. 232-252.

21. Gent M: Canadian cooperative study of recent recurrent presumed cerebral emboli (RRPCE). Design and organization of the study. In: PLATELETS, DRUGS AND THROMBOSIS, edited by Hirsh J. Basel, S. Karger, 1975, pp. 253-257.

22. Canadian Stroke Study Group: A randomized trial of aspirin and sulfinpyrazone in threatened stroke. I. Methods and neurological results. N ENGL J MED (In Press).

SUMMARY OF DISCUSSION BY PARTICIPANTS

Dr. Harker asked what was the distribution of hypertension among men and women in the study. Dr. Barnett replied that this is one question that they had not yet tackled in the analysis of the study. The only answer that he could give was that 28% of the total number of patients were hypertensive and that the ratio of men to women in the study was two men for each woman.

Dr. Genton then remarked that it was interesting that the only groups in which the sulfinpyrazone showed any trend (20% or so difference) were the patients in whom aspirin did nothing, namely women, hypertensive patients, and patients with single attacks. So again there may be a message in these data although the differences suggesting benefit did not reach significance.

Dr. Moore asked if there was anything in the clinical impression that hypertensives tend to have more severe hemorrhagic strokes. Dr. Barnett replied that judging from an initial inspection of the data, this won't be confirmed. Furthermore, in the study, more people died of heart disease than of stroke, as one might expect.

INFLUENCE OF ANTIPLATELET DRUGS ON PLATELET-SURFACE INTERACTIONS*

Edwin W. Salzman, M.D.

Department of Surgery, Harvard Medical School and Beth Israel Hospital, Boston, MA

ABSTRACT

Platelet aggregates are important in the thromboembolic complications of prosthetic devices, and drugs that alter platelet function have shown promise in clinical trials. Results with these drugs have increased insight into the interaction of platelets with artificial materials, particularly when the clinical experience has been correlated with the results of *in vitro* models.

In a bead column/surface contact model, the characteristic interactions of platelets with artificial surfaces resemble effects of adding thrombin or ADP to platelet-rich plasma. Anti-inflammatory agents and other antiplatelet drugs inhibit these reactions. Results in an *in vivo* model, survival of ^{51}Cr-labeled platelets in sheep bearing arteriovenous shunts of test materials, correlate well with results in the *in vitro* model. Findings in these model systems indicate that the initial events upon contact of a surface with plasma proteins persistently influence the long-term behavior of that surface toward blood.

A review of clinical studies discusses the effect of antiplatelet drugs on platelet survival and also on thrombotic complications of heart valve replacement and other conditions employing prosthetic devices.

*Supported by grants #HL14322, #HL20079 and #HL11414 from the National Heart, Lung and Blood Institute, National Institutes of Health. Original experiments reported here were performed in collaboration with J. N. Lindon and D. Brier.

INTRODUCTION

Thromboembolism accounts for much of the morbidity that attends the use of artificial organs and presents a difficult obstacle to the further development of prosthetic devices. Plasma coagulation with fibrin formation is the major problem when static blood stands in contact with artificial surfaces — for example, during storage in bags for transfusion or in reservoirs of extracorporeal circuits — but most clinical applications involve flowing blood, and aggregated platelets are more prominent.

Thromboembolic complications of artificial devices have been the subject of recent reviews (1-7). They range from gross thrombotic deposits with obstruction and failure of the device, or distal embolization with interruption of the circulation, to more subtle effects, such as diffuse microembolization, consumption and depletion of hemostatic elements, and disturbances in hemostatic function.

Intensive research has clarified many details in the mechanism of plasma coagulation and platelet physiology, but the earliest steps in activation of platelets by contact with foreign surfaces are not completely understood. Critical aspects of surface chemistry that dictate the reactivity of artificial materials with blood remain obscure. Even so, the demands of patient care have led to widespread use of prosthetic devices and *pari passu* to thromboembolism. No truly nonthrombogenic artificial material is at hand, but progress — largely empirical — has been made in fabrication of thromboresistant materials and in design of devices with improved rheologic properties. The use of anticoagulant drugs has been a valuable adjunct. More recently, drugs that alter platelet function have also shown promise in a limited number of clinical trials (1, 8-10). Their administration has increased insight into the interaction of platelets with artificial materials, particularly when the clinical experience has been correlated with the results of *in vitro* experiments in model systems.

IN VITRO BEAD COLUMN/SURFACE CONTACT MODEL

In most of our own studies of the response of platelets to foreign surface contact, we have relied upon an *in vitro* model in which whole blood anticoagulated with citrate is pumped from below at 37°C through a column of beads of the material to be assessed (11). Effluent blood is examined for evidence of retention of platelets within the column, release of platelet constituents, biochemical changes induced by platelet activation, and other effects. The method avoids an air-blood interface with its attendant problem of protein denaturation. The technique is simple, reproducible, inexpensive, versatile, and adaptable to study of any material that can be cast from solution as beads or coated on preformed beads of other composition. The surface/volume ratio can be varied and may be very high, e.g., up to 1600 cm^2 for 3 ml of blood, so the method is a severe test of blood-surface compatibility. The technique is useful for comparison of materials or for study of alterations in the blood induced by disease or by pharmacologic agents. Examination by scanning electron microscopy permits detailed analysis of the contribution made by platelet adhesion or aggregation to retention of platelets within the bead column.

When whole blood is passed through a column of beads of virtually all materials, single platelets adhere to the surface (Figure 1). Platelet aggregates develop subsequently by accretion on the platelets that first adhered to the polymer surface. When platelet aggregation is prominent, there is usually evidence of serotonin release. Less reactive surfaces do not induce demonstrable serotonin secretion. Reuptake of serotonin by platelets retained within the column occurs but can be minimized by addition of imipramine. Small platelet aggregates are sometimes seen in the absence of serotonin release.

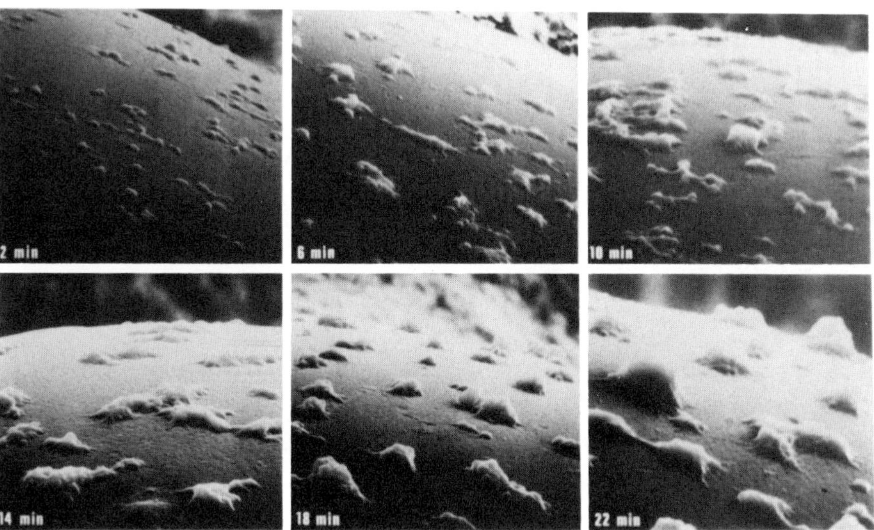

Figure 1. Sequence of events in platelet retention upon passage of whole blood through a column of polystyrene beads.

Mechanisms

Interaction of platelets with artificial surfaces sets off a series of reactions reminiscent of the effects of addition of thrombin or ADP to platelet-rich plasma. There is formation of prostaglandin endoperoxides and their products and reduction in the platelet content of cyclic AMP (12). The former effects can be totally blocked and the latter reduced by aspirin and other non-steroidal anti-inflammatory agents. Such drugs produce a dose dependent inhibition of platelet secretion and aggregation. They appear to have no effect on adhesion of platelets to polymer beads, even at 10^{-3} M concentration, in contrast to their reputed inhibition of platelet adhesion to collagen (13). This behavior is characteristic of aspirin, indomethacin, and sulfinpyrazone, the latter having been shown to inhibit arachidonic acid cyclo-oxygenation (14) although it is not, strictly speaking, an anti-inflammatory agent.

At concentrations of inhibitor which appear to eliminate serotonin release completely, there is still demonstrable formation of small aggregates of platelets (Figure 2). Since ADP release is thought to parallel serotonin release, these observations suggest the existence of some pathway to surface-induced platelet aggregation aside from the secretion of ADP from platelet storage granules.

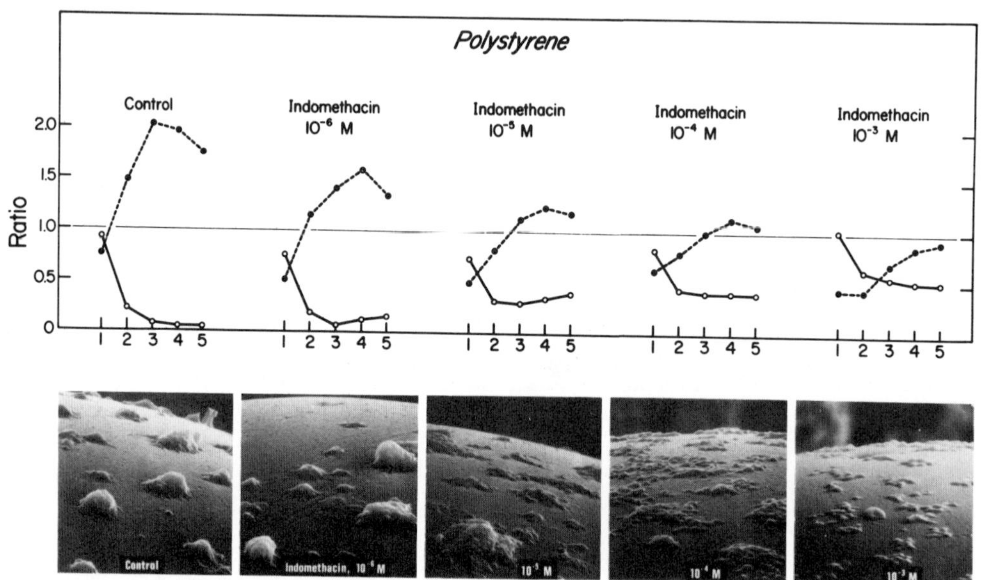

Figure 2. Addition of indomethacin 10^{-4} M before whole blood is passed through a column of beads reduces the size of platelet aggregates but does not totally prevent their formation, although serotonin release is completely eliminated. For details of methods, see reference 11.

Several forms of mechanical stimulation of platelets have been shown to lead to reduced levels of cyclic AMP (12), a result also seen in platelet suspensions upon addition of ADP or thrombin (15). Platelet cyclic AMP is reduced by centrifugation, stirring with kaolin powder, or agitation in the presence of latex particles. Conversely, an increase in cyclic AMP is a feature of the action of many drugs that inhibit platelet function (15). Prostaglandins PGE_1, PGD_2, PGE_2 (the latter only in high concentrations), and prostacyclin (PGI_2) reduce platelet secretion and aggregation by stimulating adenylate cyclase, while papaverine, dipridamole, and caffeine act by inhibiting phosphodiesterase. In contrast to the action of anti-inflammatory inhibitors of prostaglandin synthesis, substances that increase platelet cyclic AMP also inhibit adhesion of platelets to surfaces (11). When studied in a platelet suspension in an aggregometer, they block so-called "primary" or reversible aggregation as well (16). The adenylate cyclase stimulants are more potent in this respect than are the inhibitors of phosphodiesterase, probably because they produce a greater rise in the levels of cyclic AMP.

Limitations of *In Vitro* Models

An important limitation of *in vitro* methods such as the bead column technique is the fact that their use is restricted to acute experiments of relatively short duration. Although there is evidence (see below) that the long-term behavior of a surface may be influenced by the history of its first few seconds in contact with blood, a thromboresistant material suitable for clinical application may be required to remain free of thrombus for months or years.

A further problem of *in vitro* methods is the necessity for anticoagulation of the blood. Whether performed with citrate or heparin, anticoagulation largely eliminates the participation of thrombin in events associated with blood-surface contact. The proposition that thrombin is generated and makes a substantial contribution to the reactions induced by foreign surfaces *in vivo* is supported by identification of fibrinopeptide A in the blood of animals with intravascular catheters (17), and also by the clinical effectiveness, albeit imperfect, of heparin and oral anticoagulants in reducing thromboembolic complications of intravascular devices.

These criticisms are answered to some extent by supplementary use of *in vivo* techniques, which, although expensive and subject to many variables, have the advantage of a real-life situation. Extensive experience in patients (18-20) has confirmed determination of platelet lifespan as a sensitive indicator of platelet consumption in thrombotic events, whether induced by disease or by exposure of blood to artificial surfaces, e.g., prosthetic heart valves or Scribner shunts. It has not been proven that drugs that correct shortened platelet survival provide a guarantee of freedom from thrombosis in states with short platelet lifespan. This point should be kept in mind in interpretating the literature and in reading the later portion of this report dealing with clinical experience

^{51}Cr-LABELED PLATELET SURVIVAL MODEL

We have studied the survival of ^{51}Cr-labeled platelets in sheep bearing arteriovenous shunts of test materials (21). Short lengths of silicone rubber tubing implanted in the carotid artery and jugular vein provide access to the circulation. The material to be assessed is prepared as tubing 90-125 cm long and 2-3 mm internal diameter, and is interposed between the two silicone rubber ends. Platelet lifespan determined in these animals is highly reproducible and has been useful for comparison of thromboresistant materials. With very reactive materials, the shunt may become occluded by thrombus within the 5-day period of observation, whereas with more nearly bland materials, thrombotic occlusion is rare but shortened platelet survival is the rule. In a limited number of experiments in which comparisons with data from *in vitro* studies have been possible, a good correlation has been found.

Representative data obtained from study of a large number of materials are shown in Table 1, which does not include the results of experiments with more reactive materials that produced thrombotic occlusion of the shunts. Platelet lifespan appeared to be longer in the animals bearing only the 7-cm basic silicone shunt than in unoperated animals, probably because of greater platelet activation during venipuncture in unoperated sheep compared with blood collected directly from the arterial end of a shunt. Among the materials tested, only non-crosslinked, silica-filler-free polydimethyl siloxane, a polyether polyurethane, and polymethyl acrylate failed to shorten platelet survival. The first two of these materials have been among the best tolerated components in clinical applications as aortic balloons for circulatory assistance, membrane oxygenators, and angiographic catheters.

A film of adsorbed plasma proteins forms immediately upon exposure of a surface to blood (22-25). There is evidence that the nature of this coating dictates the reactivity of a surface with platelets. Precoating a surface with fibrinogen solution increases its reactivity toward platelets; for many surfaces, albumin has the opposite effect (26-28).

Some surfaces, e.g., polymethyl acrylate, appear passive when tested *in vitro* after preincubation with platelet-free plasma (11).

TABLE 1. ^{51}Cr PLATELET SURVIVAL IN SHEEP AFTER EXPOSURE TO ARTERIOVENOUS SHUNTS OF TEST MATERIALS

Material	No. of Sheep	Mean Half-life (hr) ± SD	P (compared to Shunt Control)
Unoperated control	21	63.1 ± 11.2	<0.001
Shunt control	18	78.3 ± 11.6	-----
Silastic	24	59.8 ± 9.1	<0.001
Polydimethyl siloxane	9	69.8 ± 13.9	NS
Polyvinyl chloride (Tygon)	5	48.6 ± 7.7	<0.001
Polyvinyl chloride (IV)	5	50.7 ± 13.9	<0.001
TFE	5	49.4 ± 10.9	<0.001
PMA/AN	5	57.9 ± 14.4	<0.001
Polystyrene	9	62.5 ± 14.4	<0.01
Polyvinyl acetate	6	69.1 ± 7.7	<0.04
Polymethyl acrylate	20	76.7 ± 9.4	NS
Polyethyl methacrylate	5	60.4 ± 11.4	<0.004
Polymethyl methacrylate	5	68.1 ± 8.5	<0.04
Polypropyl methacrylate	4	63.5 ± 10.0	<0.02
Polyurethane	18	72.8 ± 12.1	NS

Passivation requires 2-10 min and presumably involves progressive alterations in composition or configuration of adsorbed proteins. Other surfaces, e.g., polystyrene, polyvinyl acetate, are made more reactive or are unchanged by preincubation with plasma.

Preincubation (2-10 min) of polymethyl acrylate tubing with autologous platelet-free citrated plasma prolonged platelet life-span with this polymer in six of seven sheep (p=0.055) (21). Because determination of platelet survival requires several days, it appears that the initial events upon contact of a surface with plasma proteins have a persistent effect on long-term behavior of the surface toward the blood. This observation has important implications for development of nonthrombogenic materials and perhaps for the conditions of their implantations.

CLINICAL RESULTS

In considering the use of antithrombotic drugs to prevent thromboembolism induced by artificial surfaces, one must distinguish between evidence for an action on platelet function or other aspects of hemostasis tested *in vitro* and actual antithrombotic efficacy, which can only be treated in clinical trials in human patients. Even an effect on determinations of platelet lifespan, which appear to reflect consumption of platelets in thrombotic events or a predisposition to thrombosis or both, cannot be taken as the equivalent of thrombosis. Results of such assessments may be a useful and important guide to the organization of clinical trials but cannot be a substitute for the trials themselves.

Prosthetic Heart Valves

Insertion of prosthetic heart valves is now a standard form of management of advanced valvular heart disease. The principal complication in patients surviving operation is thromboembolism, which may occur in almost half of nonanticoagulated patients with aortic valve prostheses and even more often with mitral valves (1). Routine use of oral anticoagulants has significantly reduced the frequency of thromboembolism. The incidence varies with different valves and appears to be a function of the material from which the valve is constructed, the rheology of blood flow through the valve, the position of the valve within the heart, e.g., aortic vs. mitral, and perhaps the reactivity of the patient's blood (29). Peripheral emboli are reduced by valves whose static parts are totally covered with cloth, providing a surface on which the inevitable thrombus can be firmly anchored. In patients with cloth-covered valves in the aortic position, it has even been possible to discontinue anticoagulants after an initial conditioning period, although this practice is not universally approved. Mitral valves involve a greater hazard of late thromboembolism, and long-term anticoagulation is the rule.

Although the intensity of anticoagulation is inversely correlated with the frequency of postoperative thromboembolism (30), thromboembolic complications continue to plague patients even when the prothrombin time is greatly prolonged. Sullivan and associates (31,32) were the first to show that an agent altering platelet function, dipyridamole, reduced thromboembolism when given in conjunction with warfarin, in comparison with a control group who received warfarin alone. These results were supported by studies of platelet survival in patients with prosthetic valves, whose typically shortened platelet lifespan was increased to normal by dipyridamole, 400 mg daily, or by dipyridamole, 100 mg daily, in combination with aspirin. Aspirin alone had no effect on platelet survival in these patients, or in those of Stuart (33), but in a similar patient group, Dale (34) found that aspirin in combination with warfarin was superior to warfarin alone for prevention of thromboembolism. The combination of aspirin and warfarin was also reported to be effective by Altman (35). The antithrombotic efficacy of aspirin combined with dipyridamole was studied in nonrandomized trials by Taguchi (36), who found them effective, and by Bjork (37), who found them ineffective.

Genton and associates (38-40) have published several reports of prolongation of platelet survival and subsequently of a reduction in thromboembolic complications through the use of sulfinpyrazone. Less extensive data supporting the use of dipyridamole in conjunction with warfarin were also reported by Arrants (41), Meyer (42), and Rabello (43). Suloctidil has been found to correct shortened platelet survival due to prosthetic valves (44), but the number of patients in this study was too small to assess the antithrombotic action of the drug.

Accumulating evidence suggests that agents that alter platelet function are not sufficient by themselves to offer complete protection against thromboembolic complications after implantation of prosthetic heart valves, but in combination with oral anticoagulants they are highly effective. A hint that such combinations may introduce a substantial hazard of hemorrhagic side effects was contained in the report of Sullivan *et al.* (32); two patients receiving dipyridamole plus warfarin had fatal hemorrhagic complications. This prospect was not critically examined in subsequent reports of combined therapy and needs to be considered further.

An exciting development in valvular replacement was the introduction of glutaraldehyde-treated porcine valves, which have been virtually free of thromboembolism even without antithrombotic drugs (29). They have enjoyed increasing popularity at the expense of valves constructed of metal or polymers. The thromboresistance of porcine valves is customarily attributed to their "biologic" surface, but it is by no means proven that this is the reason they do not develop thromboembolic complications. A dead valve pickled in glutaraldehyde has little in common with natural endothelium. The rheologic properties of porcine valves are exceptionally favorable, since they are center-opening valves in which the cusps flatten out against the outflow tract during ejection, and cul-de-sacs are eliminated.

Intravascular Catheters

Insertion of catheters into blood vessels has become a common feature of modern diagnosis and therapy in applications ranging from angiography to intra-aortic balloon assistance of the failing heart. Thromboembolism is a frequent and serious complication, leading to significant symptoms in 1 to 2% of arteriographic procedures (1). The true incidence is probably much higher: studies using "pullout" techniques have found a 40% incidence of "sleeve thrombi" during arteriography (45). Transport of the thrombus to remote sites by successive introduction of other catheters may lead to embolization to the coronary arteries or the brain.

An improvement in thromboembolism rates has been achieved through the use of materials with improved thromboresistance, such as copolymers of polyurethane and silicone or catheters to which heparin has been bonded on the surface. Antithrombotic drugs are a useful adjunct. Systemic heparin is widely used during coronary angiography and appears to be effective (46,47). Since thrombi in these settings are principally composed of platelets rather than fibrin, the efficacy of heparin emphasizes the importance of thrombin in platelet reactions induced by artificial surfaces.

Patency of arm vessels used for angiography has not been improved by aspirin in two trials (48,49), but dextran, which alters platelet function and also interferes with polymerization of fibrin, appears to have some value (50).

Prosthetic Vascular Grafts

The late patency of artificial blood vessels implanted to bypass or replace diseased arteries is significantly inferior to the results obtained with autologous saphenous veins. Prosthetic grafts are not nonthrombogenic. They are constructed of woven or knitted dacron mesh, which upon implantation always acquires a coat of thrombus. The platelet-fibrin deposits eventually organize through the ingrowth of capillaries and fibrous connective tissue, and the fabric graft acquires a viable lining.

Trials of heparin or oral anticoagulants have failed to improve the long-term success of vascular grafts. Following the report of Evans and Irvine (51) that graft patency was inversely correlated with platelet adhesiveness, Slichter *et al.* (18,52) observed reduced platelet survival in patients and in baboons with prosthetic grafts, which could be corrected by large doses of dipyridamole or by smaller doses of dipyridamole in combination with aspirin, but not by aspirin alone. Platelet survival returned to normal after a number of months; the authors thought this reflected total endothelialization of the grafts. The effectiveness of sulfinpyrazone in prolonging graft patency was examined by Blakely (53), who found no reduction in closure rates through the use of this agent.

The possibility that other agents affecting platelet function may favorably influence the long-term course of patients bearing prosthetic blood vessels deserves further exploration.

Arteriovenous Shunts

Access to the circulation is frequently provided by chronic implantation of silicone rubber tubes of small diameter as arteriovenous shunts. The principal use of such devices has been as an adjunct to hemodialysis in patients with acute or chronic renal failure. Less frequent applications include parenteral alimentation and repeated transfusion. Thrombosis is a common problem and frequently leads to loss of function of the shunt. Infection and bleeding are encountered somewhat less often. The use of oral anticoagulants, at one time advocated as an aid to maintenance of shunt patency, is fraught with difficulties in the uremic patient, who is already at risk from defective hemostasis.

Following the demonstration that platelet survival was reduced in patients with arteriovenous shunts, it was shown that dipyridamole (18) was able to restore platelet survival to normal. A prospective controlled trial (54,55) has now achieved a significant reduction in shunt thrombosis through the use of sulfinpyrazone. Aspirin reduced the rate of occlusion of a surgically created arteriovenous fistula in patients with renal failure, but this was accomplished at the expense of an increased incidence of hemorrhagic complications (56).

Intravascular shunts placed between the lateral cerebral ventricles and jugular veins for the relief of hydrocephalus are frequently complicated by pulmonary embolization. Platelet lifespan was found to be short in these patients, and the abnormality has been corrected with dipyridamole or aspirin (57). Data concerning the effects of such drugs on thrombotic complications have not been reported.

Cardiopulmonary Bypass

Extracorporeal circulation of the blood for bypass of the heart and lungs during cardiac operations has profound effects on hemostasis, which have been extensively reviewed (58-61). Hemorrhage is a frequent and serious complication, resulting from a combination of heparin anticoagulation; consumption of platelets and thrombocytopenia developing despite the use of heparin; activation of fibrinolysis; inconstant reduction in levels of labile clotting factors; and a defect in platelet function that may result from incomplete induction of the platelet release reaction and acquisition of an acquired "storage pool disease" (62). Disseminated intravascular coagulation is a rare complication (63). Microembolization may contribute to the morbidity of cardiopulmonary bypass (64,65).

Dipyridamole has been administered to experimental animals to reduce the consumption of platelets associated with circulation through the pump oxygenator and to decrease microembolism, but the results have been inconclusive and sometimes contradictory (66-68). Dextran has also been employed for this purpose in man (69).

Data regarding the use of antiplatelet agents in cardiopulmonary bypass are sparse and equivocal. At present we can make no recommendation concerning their value. Further studies are in order.

When extracorporeal membrane oxygenation (ECMO) is employed for support of patients in respiratory failure, the problems of acute cardiopulmonary bypass are magnified. Systemic heparinization is required, and bleeding complications are common. Thrombocytopenia is a frequent problem. Bloom and associates (70) found no benefit from the use of dipyridamole or aspirin in sheep subjected to ECMO.

Hemodialysis

Circulation of the blood through an artificial kidney is less apt to induce a major hemostatic defect than is cardiopulmonary bypass, probably because of the slower rates of blood flow and the subnormal platelet reactivity in patients with uremia, but a significant reduction in circulating platelet numbers occurs. Heparin may be employed systemically or may be given only in the extracorporeal circuit and neutralized with a protamine infusion as the blood is returned to the patient ("regional heparinization"). Consumption of platelets during hemodialysis has been reduced by the use of aspirin (71-73), sulfinpyrazone (71), and RA233 (73), a drug resembling dipyridamole. There also appears to be some reduction in formation of thrombus within the dialyzer through the use of these agents in addition to routine heparin anticoagulation.

REFERENCES

1. Berger S, Salzman EW: Thromboembolic complications of prosthetic devices. In PROGRESS IN HEMOSTASIS AND THROMBOSIS, Vol. II, edited by Spaet TH. New York, Grune and Stratton, Inc., 1974, p. 273.

2. Salzman EW: Blood platelets: Their behavior with respect to extracorporeal membrane oxygenation. In ARTIFICIAL LUNGS FOR ACUTE RESPIRATORY FAILURE, edited by Zapol WM, Qvist J. Washington D.C., Hemisphere Corp., 1976, p. 105.

3. Salzman EW: Nonthrombogenic surfaces: Critical review. BLOOD 38:509-523, 1971.

4. Mason RG: The interaction of blood hemostatic elements with artificial surfaces. In PROGRESS IN HEMOSTASIS AND THROMBOSIS, Vol. 1, edited by Spaet TH. New York, Grune and Stratton, 1972, p. 141.

5. Scarborough DE: The pathogenesis of thrombosis in artificial organs and vessels. CURR TOP PATHOL 54:95, 1971.

6. Leonard EF, Friedman LI: Thrombogenesis on artificial surfaces: A flow reactor problem. CHEM ENG PROGR SYMP SER 66:59-71, 1970.

7. Bruck SD (Ed): BLOOD COMPATIBLE SYNTHETIC POLYMERS: AN INTRODUCTION. Springfield, Mo., Charles C Thomas Publishers, 1974.

8. Verstraete M: Are agents affecting platelet functions clinically useful? AM J MED 61:897-914, 1976.

9. Genton E, Gent M, Hirsh J, Harker LA: Platelet-inhibiting drugs in the prevention of clinical thrombotic disease. N ENGL J MED 293:1174-1178, 1236-1240, 1296-1300, 1975.

10. Weiss HJ: Antiplatelet drugs - A new pharmacologic approach to the prevention of thrombosis. AM HEART J 92:86-102, 1976.

11. Salzman EW, Lindon J, Brier D, Merrill EW: Surface induced platelet adhesion, aggregation, and release. PROC NY ACAD SCI 283:114-127, 1977.

12. Salzman EW, Lindon JN, Rodvien R: Cyclic AMP in human blood platelets. Relation to platelet prostaglandin synthesis induced by centrifugation or surface contact. J CYCLIC NUCLEOTIDE RES 2:25-37, 1976.

13. Cazenave J-P, Packham MA, Guccione MA, Mustard JF: Inhibition of platelet adherence to a collagen-coated surface by nonsteroidal anti-inflammatory drugs, pyrimido-pyrimidine and tricyclic compounds, and lidocaine. J LAB CLIN MED 83:797-806, 1974.

14. Ali M, McDonald JWD: Effects of sulfinpyrazone on platelet prostaglandin synthesis and platelet release of serotonin. J

LAB CLIN MED 89:868-875, 1977.

15. Salzman EW: Cyclic AMP and platelet function. N ENGL J MED 286:358-363, 1972.

16. Salzman EW, Levine L: Cyclic 3', 5'-adenosine monophosphate in human blood platelets: II. Effect of N^6-2'-O-dibutyryl cyclic 3', 5'-adenosine monophosphate on platelet function. J CLIN INVEST 50:131-141, 1971.

17. Wilner GD, Casarella WJ, Fenoglio C, Baier RE: *In vivo* fibrinopeptide a generation induced by angiographic catheters. THROMB HAEMOSTAS 38:73, 1977.

18. Harker LA, Slichter SJ: Platelet and fibrinogen consumption in man. N ENGL J MED 287:999-1005, 1972.

19. Steele PP, Weily HS, Davies H, Genton E: Platelet function studies in coronary artery disease. CIRCULATION 48:1194-1200, 1973.

20. Steele PP, Weily HS, Genton E: Platelet survival and adhesiveness in recurrent venous thrombosis. N ENGL J MED 288:1148-1152, 1973.

21. Coe N, Collins R, Jagoda A, Brier D, Lindon J, Merrill E, Cohen R, Salzman E: *In vivo* assessment of thromboresistant materials by determination of platelet survival. THROMB HAEMOSTAS 38:204, 1977.

22. Vroman L, Adams AL: Identification of rapid changes at plasma-solid interfaces. J BIOMED MATER RES 3:43-67, 1969.

23. Dutton RC, Webber AJ, Johnson SA, Baier RE: Microstructure of initial thrombus formation on foreign materials. J BIOMED MATER RES 3:13-23, 1969.

24. Lyman DJ, Brash JL, Chaikin SW, Klein KG, Carini M: Effect of chemical structure and surface properties of synthetic polymers on the coagulation of blood. II. Protein and platelet interaction with polymer surfaces. TRANS AM SOC ARTIF INTERN ORGANS 14:250-255, 1968.

25. Scarborough DE, Mason RG, Dalldorf FG, Brinkhous KM: Morphological manifestations of blood-solid interfacial reactions. LAB INVEST 20:164-169, 1969.

26. Packham MA, Evans G, Glynn MF, Mustard JF: Effect of plasma proteins on the interaction of platelets with glass surfaces.

J LAB CLIN MED 73:686-697, 1969.

27. Salzman EW, Merrill EW, Binder A, Wolf CF, Ashford TP, Austen WG: Protein-platelet interaction on heparinized surfaces. J BIOMED MATER RES 3:69-81, 1969.

28. Zucker MB, Vroman L: Platelet adhesion induced by fibrinogen adsorbed onto glass. PROC SOC EXP BIOL MED 131:318-320, 1969.

29. Salzman EW: Thromboembolic complications of cardiac and vascular prostheses. In SURGERY OF THE CHEST, edited by Sabiston DC, Spencer FG. Philadelphia, W.B. Saunders Co., 1974, p. 1220.

30. Duvoisin GE, Brandenburg RO, McGoon DC: Factors affecting thromboembolism associated with prosthetic heart valves. CIRCULATION 35 (Suppl 1):70-76, 1967.

31. Sullivan JM, Harken DE, Gorlin R: Pharmacologic control of thromboembolic complications of cardiac valve replacement. N ENGL J MED 279:576-580, 1968.

32. Sullivan JM, Harken DE, Gorlin R: Effect of dipyridamole on the incidence of arterial emboli after cardiac valve replacement. CIRCULATION 39 (Suppl 1):149, 1969.

33. Stuart RK, McDonald JW, Ahuja SP, Coles JC: Platelet survival in patients with prosthetic heart valves. AM J CARDIOL 33:840-844, 1974.

34. Dale J, Myhre E, Storstein O, Stormorken H, Efskind L: Prevention of arterial thromboembolism with acetylsalicyclic acid. AM HEART J 94:101-111, 1977.

35. Altman R, Boullon F, Rouvier J, Rada R, DeFuenta L, Favaloro R: Aspirin and prophylaxis of thromboembolic complications in patients with substitute heart valves. J THORAC CARDIOVASC SURG 72:127-129, 1976.

36. Taguchi K, Matsumura H, Washizu T, Hirao M, Kato K, Kato E, Mochizuki T, Takamura K, Mashimo I, Morifuji K, Nakagaki M, Suma T: Effect of athrombogenic therapy, especially high dose therapy dipyridamole, after prosthetic valve replacement. J CARDIOVASC SURG 16:8-15, 1975.

37. Björk V, Henz A: Management of thrombo-embolism after aortic valve replacement with the Bjork-Shiley tilting disc valve. Medicamental prevention with dicumarol in comparison with dipyridamole - acetylsalicyclic acid. Surgical treatment of prosthetic thrombosis. SCAND J THORAC CARDIOVASC SURG 9:183-

191, 1975.

38. Weily HS, Genton E: Altered platelet function in patients with prosthetic mitral valves. Effects of sulfinpyrazone therapy. CIRCULATION 42 (Suppl 3):205, 1970.

39. Weily HS, Steele PP, Davies H, Pappas G, Genton E: Platelet survival in patients with substitute heart valves. N ENGL J MED 290:534-537, 1974.

40. Steele P, Genton E: Thromboembolism and platelet survival time before and after valve surgery. ADV CARDIOL 17:189-198, 1976.

41. Arrants JE, Hariston P, Lee WH, Jr.: Use of dipyridamole (persantine) in preventing thromboembolism following valve replacement. CHEST 58:275, 1970.

42. Meyer JS, Charney JZ, Rivera VM, Mathew NT: Cerebral embolization: Prospective clinical analysis of 42 cases. STROKE 2:541-554, 1971.

43. Rabello C, Rivas JA, Rocha F *et al.*: Estudo da ação de Dipiridamol na evolução de pacientes submetiedos à substitui çao de prôteses valvares. REV BRAS CLIN TER 2:95, 1973.

44. Moriau M, Ferrant A, Beys C, Hurlet A, Chalant C, Ponlot R, Jaumain P, Goenen M, Masure R: Evaluation of the antithrombotic properties of suloctidil in patients with substitute heart valves. THROMB HAEMOSTAS 38:96, 1977.

45. Siegelman SS, Caplan LH, Annes GP: Complications of catheter angiography. Study with oscillometry and "pullout" angiograms. RADIOLOGY 91:251-253, 1968.

46. Walker WJ, Mundall SL, Broderick HG, Prasad B, Kim J, Ravi JM: Systemic heparinization for femoral percutaneous coronary arteriography. N ENGL J MED 288:826-828, 1973.

47. Eyer KM: Complications of transfemoral coronary arteriography and their prevention using heparin. AM HEART J 86:428, 1973.

48. Hynes KM, Gau GT, Rutherford BD, Kazmier FJ, Frye RL: Effect of aspirin on brachial artery occlusion following brachial arteriotomy for coronary arteriography. CIRCULATION 47:554-557, 1973.

49. Freed MD, Rosenthal A, Fyler D: Attempts to reduce arterial thrombosis after cardiac catheterization in children: Use of

percutaneous technique and aspirin. AM HEART J 87:283-286, 1974.

50. Jacobsson B: Use of dextran for prophylaxis against thromboembolic complication in arterial catheterization. ACTA CHIR SCAND (Suppl) 387:103, 1968.

51. Evans G, Irvine WT: Long-term arterial-graft patency in relation to platelet adhesiveness, biochemical factors and anticoagulant therapy. LANCET 2:353-355, 1966.

52. Slichter SJ, Harker L, Sauvage L: Platelet consumption as a measure of endothelialization of aorta-femoral grafts. PROC AM SOC HEMATOL, Florida, 1972, p. 46.

53. Blakely JA, Pogoriler G: A prospective trial of sulfinpyrazone after peripheral vascular surgery. THROMB HAEMOSTAS 38: 238, 1977.

54. Kaegi A, Pineo GF, Shimizu A, Trivedi H, Hirsh J, Gent M: Arteriovenous-shunt thrombosis: Prevention by sulfinpyrazone. N ENGL J MED 290:304-306, 1974.

55. Kaegi A, Pineo GF, Shimizu A, Trivedi H, Hirsh J, Gent M: The role of sulfinpyrazone in the prevention of arterio-venous shunt thrombosis. CIRCULATION 52:497-499, 1975.

56. Andrassy K, Ritz E, Schoeffner W, Hahn G, Walter K: The influence of acetylsalicyclic acid on platelet adhesiveness and thrombotic fistula complications in hemodialysed patients. KLIN WOCHENSCHR 49:166-167, 1971.

57. Stuart M, Stockman J, Murphy S, Schut L, Ames M, Urmson J, Oski F: Shortened platelet lifespan in patients with hydrocephalus and ventriculojugular shunts: Results of preliminary attempts at correction. J PEDIATR 80:21-25, 1972.

58. Gralnick HR, Fischer RD: The hemostatic response to open-heart operations. J THORAC CARDIOVASC SURG 61:909-915, 1971.

59. Heiden D, Mielke CH, Rodvien R, Hill JD: Platelets, hemostasis and thromboembolism during treatment of acute respiratory insufficiency with extracorporeal membrane oxygenation. J THORAC CARDIOVASC SURG 70:644-655, 1975.

60. Backmann F, McKenna R, Cole ER, Najafi H: The hemostatic mechanism after open-heart surgery. I. Studies on plasma coagulation factors and fibrinolysis in 512 patients after extracorporeal circulation. J THORAC CARDIOVASC SURG 70:76-85, 1975.

61. Bick RL: Alterations of hemostasis associated with cardiopulmonary bypass: Pathophysiology, prevention, diagnosis, and management. SEMIN THROMB HEMOSTAS 3:59-82, 1976.

62. Harbury CB, Galvan CA: A bleeding diathesis associated with a platelet storage pool deficiency acquired during cardiopulmonary bypass surgery. THROMB HAEMOSTAS 38:237, 1977.

63. Boyd AD, Engleman RM, Beaudet RL, Lackner H: Disseminated intravascular coagulation following extracorporeal circulation. J THORAC CARDIOVASC SURG 64:685-693, 1972.

64. Allardyce DB, Yoshida SH, Ashmore PG: The importance of microembolism in the pathogenesis of organ dysfunction caused by prolonged use of the pump oxygenator. J THORAC CARDIOVASC SURG 52:706-715, 1966.

65. Ashmore PG, Svitek V, Ambrose P: The incidence and effects of particulate aggregation and microembolism in pump-oxygenator systems. J THORAC CARDIOVASC SURG 55:691-697, 1968.

66. Rittenhouse EA, Hessel EA, Ito CS, Merendino KA: Use of Persantin to reduce microaggregation in the pump oxygenator. SURG FORUM 21:142-144, 1970.

67. Becker RM, Smith MR, Dobell ARC: Effect of dipyridamole on platelet function in cardiopulmonary bypass in pigs. SURG FORUM 23:169, 1972.

68. Mielke CH, Hill JD, Gerbode F: Drug influence on platelet loss during extracorporeal circulation. J THORAC CARDIOVASC SURG 66:845-854, 1973.

69. Long DM, Todd DB, Indeglia RA, Varco RL, Lillehei CW: Clinical use of dextra-40 in extracorporeal circulation - A summary of 5 years' experience. TRANSFUSION 6:401-403, 1966.

70. Bloom S, Zapol W, Wonders T, Berger S, Salzman E: Platelet destruction during 24 hour membrane lung perfusion. TRANS AM SOC ARTIF INTERN ORGANS 20-A:299-305, 1974.

71. Winchester JF, Forbes CD, Courtney JM, Prentice CRM: Effect of sulfinpyrazone and aspirin on platelet loss induced *in vitro* by activated charcoal hemoperfusion. THROMB HAEMOSTAS 38:93, 1977.

72. Lindsay RM, Prentice CRM, Kennedy AC, McNicol GP: Studies on thrombus formation and prevention within haemodialysers. BR J HAEMATOL 22:640-641, 1972.

73. Lindsay RM, Prentice CRM, Ferguson D, Burton JA, McNichol GP: Reduction of thrombus formation of dialyser membranes by aspirin and RA 233. LANCET 2:1287-1290, 1972.

SUMMARY OF DISCUSSION BY PARTICIPANTS

Dr. Brinkhous said he had always suspected (but was unable to prove) that the von Willebrand factor was very important in the thrombogenic nature of the protein layer that is adsorbed to the surface. When his group analyzed the levels of the von Willebrand factor, platelet aggregating type, among all the animals, they found that the sheep was near the top of the list; only the goat had higher levels. If one wants to get thrombosis via platelet adhesion and with this mechanism, the sheep should be a very good animal to use. Dr. Salzman replied that he was very pleased to hear about the sheep's von Willebrand factor level. But they actually selected the sheep initially because it was docile, large, easy to obtain blood samples from, and not too expensive. It turns out that the animals also are predisposed to thrombosis.

Dr. Brinkhous' second comment was about the precoating with albumin or other plasma proteins. His perception is that an adsorbed layer is not a static layer, and that dynamic exchange with the plasma proteins in the blood was going on. Therefore, while the coating procedure may seem useful for brief studies, he anticipates that in due course the layer would be remodeled to reflect what is in the plasma of the animals. Dr. Salzman responded that this emphasizes the importance of doing studies that go on over a period of time rather than only acute studies. And this is one of the shortcomings of *in vitro* methods. On the other hand the evidence that the early events when blood first contacts the surface may have a lasting effect implied that the turnover may not be the same for all surfaces. His group found, for example, that pre-exposure to platelet-free plasma is not able to passivate a lot of other polymers, whereas for polymethylacrylate his paper showed what happened. So it is likely that the establishment of an equilibrium with differences in the composition of the adsorbed protein coat or perhaps in the configuration of adsorbed protein molecular species may differ from material to material.

Dr. Gorman commented on some of his own work showing that if one uses a thromboxane synthetase inhibitor the aggregation due to either endoperoxide or arachidonic acid is blocked. But at the same time normal cyclo-oxygenase products are still produced, namely prostaglandin E_2 and D_2. Also, there probably isn't any inhibition of prostacyclin synthesis in endothelial cells. Dr. Gorman then asked what Dr. Salzman's impression would be of the advantage of a thromboxane synthetase inhibitor in this type of long-term chronic therapy. Dr. Salzman replied that theoretically, and from Moncada and Vane's first paper on prostacyclin, there would be some advantage to a thromboxane synthetase inhibitor which would not at the same time block prostacyclin production. The potential criticism of the use of aspirin as an antithrombotic agent is that theoretically it should block both thromboxane production and prostacyclin production, so that it might not tend to swing the balance much against thrombosis. In fact, all the studies that Dr. Salzman was aware of that have looked at aspirin as an antithrombotic agent have either shown that it is effective or not effective. He is not aware of any studies that have shown that the patient receiving aspirin has an increased incidence of thromboembolism, so it was not clear to him how synthesis of prostacyclin fits into the picture.

Dr. Didisheim remarked that it sounded as if Dr. Salzman's *in vivo* model in the sheep was, if not identical, at least very similar to Dr. Harker's baboon model and this afforded us a beautiful opportunity to study the role of species selection in these two models if the same biomaterials have been used. He wondered if perhaps he or Dr. Harker could comment on platelet survival and other measures of thrombogenicity of these materials in the two models. Dr. Harker replied that Dr. Salzman's lengths of tubing were at least twice as long as the ones they were studying, and Dr. Harker's group gets into the problem of occlusion with the repeated uses of those longer lengths. He asked Dr. Salzman what proportion of occlusion occurs in their animals when they use tubing of 120 cm. Dr. Salzman answered that it depends on the material. The more reactive the material, the more likely one is to get occlusion. The materials which he mentioned in the paper were all relatively unreactive compared with other materials that they have studied which have had a significant occlusion rate. Short lengths of Silastic tubing inserted into arteries and veins and simply connected by a short connector (when they are not testing animals) stay patent for a long period of time, and they have had AV shunts remain patent in sheep for as long as 9 months. But the long lengths of tubing that they study are only in place long enough to do platelet survival tests; after a week they are taken out. Dr. Harker concluded that in order to compare the models, they would have to exchange some tubing and also control other aspects of the experiment.

Session IV

DISCUSSIONS

H. J. Day, Chairman

A DISCUSSION OF THE POSSIBLE SIGNIFICANCE OF PGI_2 IN THROMBOSIS

J. Bryan Smith, Ph.D.

Cardeza Foundation and Department of Pharmacology

Thomas Jefferson University, Philadelphia, PA

Before discussing the significance of PGI_2 in thrombosis, it is appropriate to acknowledge that its discovery is due to the contributions of three groups. First, credit should be given to Pace-Asciak and Wolfe (1) who in 1971 were working together at McGill University in Montreal. They isolated, identified, and described the unique chemical properties of a noval compound, 6(9)-oxyprostaglandin $F_{2\alpha}$, which was produced from arachidonic acid by homogenates of rat stomach. Secondly, we would not even be discussing PGI_2 today were it not for the discoveries of Moncada, Gryglewski, Vane and others (2,3,4) at the Wellcome Research Laboratories in England. They showed that blood vessels make a prostaglandin, temporarily named PGX, with unique and potent biological properties. Finally, credit is due to Johnson, Morton, and others of The Upjohn Company (5) who collaborated with the Wellcome group and proved that the names 6(9)-oxyprostaglandin $F_{2\alpha}$ and PGX are synonymous. They suggested the use of the trivial name prostacyclin to describe PGX, and I suspect that PGI_2 will continue to be called prostacyclin henceforth.

It is well established that treating PGE with acid produces PGA and treating PGE with base produces PGB. Pace-Asciak and Wolfe (1) discovered that homogenates of rat stomach not only produced PGE_2 and $PGF_{2\alpha}$, but also converted arachidonic acid into two compounds which had the chromatographic properties of PGE but which were stable in basic solutions. The structures of these compounds were formulated after mass spectrometric analysis of suitable derivatives. One of these compounds is what we now call prostacyclin.

The discoveries of Moncada and coworkers (2) emanated from the isolation of the prostaglandin endoperoxides PGG_2 and PGH_2 in

1973 by Hamberg and Samuelsson (6) and Nugteren and Hazelhof (7), and the findings that these substances both cause platelet aggregation and contract strips of rabbit aorta (8). Moncada and associates found that microsomes prepared from pig or rabbit aortas contain an enzyme that transforms prostaglandin endoperoxides to an unstable principle which inhibits platelet aggregation and relaxes some blood vessels. This principle, which they called PGX, was estimated to be almost 30 times more potent than either PGE_1 or PGD_2 as an inhibitor of aggregation.

Johnson, Morton, and coworkers (5) incubated radioactive PGH_2 with pig aorta microsomes and allowed the reaction to proceed until biological activity was lost. The major product isolated from this incubation was identified as 6-keto-$PGF_{1\alpha}$. This compound had also been found by Pace-Asciak (9) in his studies with rat stomach, and therefore it appeared that the rational route from PGH_2 to 6-keto-$PGF_{1\alpha}$ was via prostacyclin. Prostacyclin was prepared by chemical synthesis and was shown to relax both the rabbit mesenteric and coeliac artery strips and to inhibit platelet aggregation. As a result of elegant radioactive dilution experiments, Johnson and associates were able to conclude that the PGX discovered by Moncada is identical to prostacyclin.

By 1975 the pathways for the oxygenation of arachidonic acid in platelets had been elucidated by Hamberg and coworkers (10,11). These studies indicated that the formation of thromboxane A_2 was obligatory for aggregation by the arachidonate pathway. Thus it has been postulated (2) that a balance between the amounts of thromboxane A_2 formed from PGH_2 by platelets and prostacyclin formed from PGH_2 by vessels might be critical for thrombus formation. How we can test this proposal is what we must discuss today.

Many questions can be asked concerning the significance of prostacyclin in thrombosis. Is the continuous generation of prostacyclin by vessel walls the biochemical mechanism underlying their ability to resist platelet adhesion? Is PGH_2 released from platelets attempting to stick to vessel walls used by the vessel to generate prostacyclin which prevents platelets from sticking? Does plaque formation on the arterial wall hinder access of the platelet endoperoxides to the prostacyclin generating system? Does the generation of prostacyclin in the arterial wall play a part in the local control of vascular tone? Is prostacyclin formation restricted to the vessel wall? How does prostacyclin work? And so on.

Some of these questions can be answered by *in vitro* experiments, and this is obviously a very active field of research at this time. Prostacyclin is the most potent stimulator of platelet adenylate cyclase ever discovered (12,13). There seems little question that it inhibits platelet aggregation by elevating platelet cyclic AMP. Subsequent to the discovery by Saba and Mason (14) that endothelial cells release an activity that inhibits platelet aggregation, Weksler and associates (15) and Harker and colleagues (16) have presented evidence that cultured endothelial cells derived from human umbilical veins or bovine aorta produce prostacyclin. Cultured fibroblasts, smooth muscle cells, or human blood leukocytes do not do so, but it would be wrong to assume that only endothelial cells can produce prostacyclin; for example, seminal vesicles from the bull are highly active in producing prostacyclin and 6-keto-$PGF_{1\alpha}$ (17).

Some questions concerning the significance of PGI_2 in thrombosis will only be answered by *in vivo* experiments. This is exemplified by aspirin. It is well established that aspirin inhibits platelet aggregation *in vitro*, and logically it was suggested that aspirin might be antithrombotic *in vivo* (18). We now know that this effect of aspirin on platelets is due to its ability to inhibit the formation of prostaglandin endoperoxides and consequently thromboxane A_2. We also know that this same property of aspirin will prevent the vessel wall from producing prostacyclin. Thus it is conceivable that under certain conditions aspirin might even prove to be prothrombotic *in vivo*.

What models are available for research on arterial thrombosis and how pertinent are they to the human situation? One point concerns sex. About 3 years ago, we reported that arachidonic acid causes sudden death in New Zealand rabbits and that these rabbits were protected from death if they were given aspirin (19). In view of Dr. Barnett's presentation at this Workshop showing that aspirin appears to be much more effective in men than women, it is worth noting that the rabbits we used were all males. Peter Ramwell and colleagues (20,21) recently reported experiments on the thrombotic effects of arachidonic acid in rats; they found a marked sex difference in the response.

Another point is, exactly what do we mean by "damage" to the endothelium? In many of the models, thrombosis is initiated by damaging the vessel wall electrically or mechanically, e.g., by ballooning or applying ultrasound. Does this stop or accelerate prostacyclin biosynthesis? In saying that damage initiates the process, do we mean simply that lysis of endothelial cells is the initiating factor in atherosclerosis — as it apparently can be — or that the human disease results from a more specific insult? Obviously, after lysis it is difficult to envisage increased prostacyclin formation. On the other hand, the interaction of some agent with a specific receptor on the endothelial cell might increase prostacyclin formation.

Now we will have discussion from the floor on some of these questions. I promised to give Dr. Hoak some time first.

REFERENCES

1. Pace-Asciak C, Wolfe LS: A novel prostaglandin derivative formed from arachidonic acid by rat stomach homogenates. BIOCHEMISTRY 10:3657-3664, 1971.

2. Moncada S, Gryglewski R, Bunting S, Vane JR: An enzyme isolated from arteries transforms prostaglandin endoperoxides to an unstable substance that inhibits platelet aggregation. NATURE 263:663-665, 1976.

3. Gryglewski RJ, Bunting S, Moncada S, Flower RJ, Vane JR: Arterial walls are protected against deposition of platelet thrombi by a substance (prostaglandin X) which they make from prostaglandin endoperoxides. PROSTAGLANDINS 12:685-713, 1976.

4. Moncada S, Gryglewski RJ, Bunting S, Vane JR: A lipid peroxide inhibits the enzyme in blood vessel microsomes that generates from prostaglandin endoperoxides the substance (prostaglandin X) which prevents platelet aggregation. PROSTAGLANDINS 12: 715-737, 1976.

5. Johnson RA, Morton DR, Kinner JH, Gorman RR, McGuire JC, Sun FF, Whittaker N, Bunting S, Salmon J, Moncada S, Vane JR: The chemical structure of prostaglandin X (prostacyclin). PROSTAGLANDINS 12:915-928, 1976.

6. Hamberg M, Samuelsson B: Detection and isolation of an endoperoxide intermediate in prostaglandin biosynthesis. PROC NATL ACAD SCI USA 70:899-903, 1973.

7. Nugteren DH, Hazelhof E: Isolation and properties of intermediates in prostaglandin biosynthesis. BIOCHIM BIOPHYS ACTA 326:448-461, 1973.

8. Hamberg M, Svensson J, Wakabayashi T, Samuelsson B: Isolation and structure of two prostaglandin endoperoxides that cause platelet aggregation. PROC NATL ACAD SCI USA 71:345-349, 1974.

9. Pace-Asciak C: A new prostaglandin metabolite of arachidonic acid. Formation of 6-keto-$PGF_{1\alpha}$ by the rat stomach. EXPERENTIA 32:291-292, 1976.

10. Hamberg M, Samuelsson B: Prostaglandin endoperoxides. Novel transformations of arachidonic acid in human platelets. PROC NATL ACAD SCI USA 71:3400-3404, 1974.

11. Hamberg M, Svensson J, Samuelsson B: Thromboxanes: A new group of biologically active compounds derived from prosta-

glandin endoperoxides. PROC NATL ACAD SCI USA 72:2994-2998, 1975.

12. Gorman RR, Bunting S, Miller OV: Modulation of human platelet adenylate cyclase by prostacyclin (PGX). PROSTAGLANDINS 13: 377-388, 1977.

13. Tateson JE, Moncada S, Vane JR: Effects of prostacyclin (PGX) on cyclic AMP concentrations in human platelets. PROSTAGLANDINS 13:389-397, 1977.

14. Saba SR, Mason RG: Studies of an activity from endothelial cells that inhibits platelet aggregation, serotonin release, and clot retraction. THROMB RES 5:747-757, 1974.

15. Weksler BB, Marcus AJ, Jaffe EA: Synthesis of PGI$_2$ (prostacyclin) by cultured human and bovine endothelial cells. PROC NATL ACAD SCI USA (In Press).

16. Harker LA, Joy N, Wall RT, Quadracci L, Striker G: Inhibition of platelet reactivity by endothelial cells (Abstract). THROMB HAEMOSTAS 38:137, 1977.

17. Wen-Chang C, Murota S: Identification of 6-ketoprostaglandin F$_{1\alpha}$ formed from arachidonic acid in bovine seminal vesicles. BIOCHIM BIOPHYS ACTA 486:136-144, 1977.

18. Weiss HJ, Aledort LM, Kochwa S: The effect of salicylates on the hemostatic properties of platelets in man. J CLIN INVEST 47:2169-2180, 1968.

19. Silver MJ, Hoch W, Kocsis JJ, Ingleman CM, Smith JB: Arachidonic acid causes sudden death in rabbits. SCIENCE 183:1085-1087, 1974.

20. Uzunova A, Ramey E, Ramwell PW: Effect of testosterone, sex and age on experimentally induced arterial thrombosis. NATURE 261:712-713, 1976.

21. Uzunova AD, Ramey ER, Ramwell PW: Arachidonate-induced thrombosis in mice: Effect of gender or testosterone and estradiol administration. PROSTAGLANDINS 13:995-1002, 1977.

DISCUSSION

HOAK: I would like to present very briefly some of our recent findings with cultured endothelial cells and their capacity to produce an inhibitor of platelet aggregation which can be modified by aspirin.

An *in vitro* method was employed using a monolayer of cultured human endothelial, fibroblast, or smooth muscle cells to detect adherence of ^{51}Cr-labeled platelets. One ml aspirin in incubation medium (IM) or 1 ml IM (control) was incubated with the monolayer for 30 min at 37°C with rocking. The preincubation solution was removed and the dish was washed twice. One ml 0.08 U/ml thrombin in IM or 1 ml IM (control) was added, followed immediately by 0.5 ml untreated ^{51}Cr-platelets in Tyrode's solution. The dish was then rocked 30 min at 37°C. No significant difference ($p > 0.10$) was observed when aspirin-treated platelets were employed (Table).

TABLE. BOVINE THROMBIN-INDUCED ADHERENCE OF PLATELETS TO ENDOTHELIUM TREATED WITH ASPIRIN AND UNTREATED SMOOTH MUSCLE CELLS

Monolayer	Aspirin (mM)	% Adherence* Control	Thrombin (0.8 U/ml)
Endothelium	0	1.7 ± 0.4	2.1 ± 0.4
Endothelium	0.5	1.6 ± 0.1	11.9 ± 5.0
Endothelium	1.0	1.4 ± 0.1	28.4 ± 4.7
Endothelium	2.0	2.0 ± 0.3	38.9 ± 5.4
Smooth muscle†	0	1.8	82.8 ± 1.8

*Percent adherence was calculated by dividing cpm of cells attached to the monolayer after incubation by total cpm in the dish, x 100.

†Percent adherence for smooth muscle cells = means ± SE from two experiments in duplicate (four dishes); other data from three experiments in duplicate (six dishes).

Note that washed platelets or aspirin-treated washed platelets did not adhere to either untreated monolayers or aspirin-treated endothelial monolayers in the absence of thrombin. In contrast, platelet adherence occurred when unaggregated platelets were incubated with cell monolayers, including endothelium which had been treated with thrombin, but adherence to endothelium was significantly less. Adherence was enhanced significantly by treatment of the endothelial cell monolayer with aspirin even when aspirin-treated platelets were used, and adherence values approached those seen with smooth muscle cells.

SPAET: What happened to the pH of your entire system when you added aspirin?

HOAK: The pH is buffered throughout; it's controlled.

GORMAN: I want to emphasize that controls are very important when you do endothelial cell experiments. When we first became aware of prostacyclin about 15 months ago, we already had the radioactive endoperoxide allowing us to do direct experiments and measure 6-keto $PGF_{1\alpha}$ production. We found that if you incubate radioactive endoperoxide with endothelial cells, you do indeed generate a substance that inhibits platelet aggregation. Now I've seen a lot in the literature about endothelial cells being incubated with arachidonic acid. Unfortunately, when I analyzed such extracts, there was almost no 6-keto $PGF_{1\alpha}$; the predominant products were PGD_2 and PGE_2. And if I boiled those extracts, I couldn't get rid of the anti-aggregating activity. So, as Dr. Salzman showed this morning, any agent that elevates cyclic AMP will tend to decrease platelet adhesiveness, and you could explain the data that we just saw by compromising PGD_2 or PGE_2 synthesis just as well as you could by inhibiting PGI_2. I think it's very important to characterize what our cells make before we start talking about prostacyclin. Now, endothelial cells do make prostacyclin, but it's in very, very small amounts, amounts difficult to demonstrate on an aggregometer.

HOAK: I agree. If you noticed, I didn't use the term "prostacyclin," but "inhibitor". There may be more than one protective mechanism provided by the endothelium.

HARKER: If you use a stirred plasma system to carry out your reaction and an inhibitor that is currently regarded as being specific for prostacyclin synthesis, namely, 15-hydroperoxy arachidonic acid, then the inclusion of that agent in your reaction mixture will allow the reaction between platelets and your inducing agent to proceed in the presence of endothelial cells that have been incubated with the inhibitor. In the absence of the inhibitor, then, of course, there is total inhibition of that reaction, suggesting that in that system the reaction is indeed dependent upon PGI_2 synthesis.

SMITH: I think that goes to another point. I know Vane suggested that the PGH_2 released from platelets can act as the precursor to the prostacyclin made by the endothelial cells. There is *in vitro* evidence with platelet aggregation that that is the case, but personally, I question whether it is possible.

HARKER: Well, certainly our evidence is that the platelet or an alternate source of the endoperoxides is not necessary, that endothelial cells in culture in the absence of any exogenous endoperoxide will synthesize PGI_2.

GORMAN: Just one thing along that line: Whether or not the platelet can feed the endothelium, I don't know. Theoretically, it is possible, because Dr. Fitzpatrick here at Upjohn has raised antibodies to endoperoxides, and we find that we can ablate much of the second wave of platelet aggregation with this antibody and can also ablate exogenous PGH_2. So it does appear that even in collagen-induced or the second wave of ADP- or epinephrine-induced aggregation, some of the endoperoxide does escape the platelet and is exteriorized, at least to an exterior receptor.

PACKHAM: Bryan, what's the current thinking about PGG_2 and H_2? Are they considered aggregating agents still or just precursors? Your slide is different this time.

SMITH: Well, I think there's some strong evidence from Bob Gorman that the formation of thromboxane is necessary for aggregation.

PACKHAM: So we should be talking about thromboxane A_2 and not about the three of them as aggregating agents?

SMITH: Yes, although I still have some reservations. I can tell you about some experiments that I've done, although they certainly don't prove the point: If you take rabbit platelets and challenge them with the azo analog of PGH_2, they will become refractory to this compound just as platelets challenged with ADP become refractory to ADP. If you then challenge these platelets with any of the other analogs of PGH_2, indeed azo-PGH_2 itself, the platelets do not aggregate. This is in keeping with some work of McIntyre and Gordon (personal communication). They found that N0164, sodium p-benzyl-4-[1-oxo-2-(4-chlorobenzyl)-3-phenyl-propyl]-phenyl phosphonate, inhibits the aggregation of platelets by PGG_2, PGH_2, and analogs of PGH_2 but does not inhibit aggregation induced by arachidonic acid. In other words, there is some evidence that there is a receptor for PGH_2 on the outside of the platelets. In contrast to these findings, Bob Gorman has worked with an azo analog of PGH_2 without a 15-hydroxyl group which is a very potent inhibitor of thromboxane synthetase. This compound inhibits aggregation by PGH_2 and at the same time blocks thromboxane function. So I would say at this time the weight of evidence is that thromboxane formation is necessary, but I don't think it's absolutely proven.

PACKHAM: Thanks. Jack, I had a question for you; when you said that treating the platelets with aspirin, you get exactly the same effect, did you mean treating both the endothelial cells and the platelets with aspirin at the same time?

HOAK: Yes, treating both.

PACKHAM: If you don't treat the endothelial cells in culture with aspirin but treat just the platelets, what do you get?

HOAK: Baseline values.

PACKHAM: The comment I wanted to make was this: If we're going to postulate that PGI_2 production prevents the vessel wall from being thrombogenic, and that platelets are supplying the precursors for PGI_2, you have to have some mechanism for stimulating the platelets to produce the precursors.

ROSS: Why do you have to postulate that? Why is it not possible to postulate that not only can the endothelial cells synthesize PGI_2 themselves, but perhaps could use an alternative pathway? But certainly one would not have to postulate that they're dependent upon the platelets for the synthesis of PGI_2. I didn't get that from any of the data I've heard.

SMITH: I think what Marian is implying is that when platelets are not activated, they are not releasing arachidonic acid or not releasing PGH_2, and therefore, only with activated platelets can you supply the PGH_2 for that pathway. In my introduction to this Discussion session I proposed that under certain conditions aspirin could be prothrombotic, and I would just like to examine in what situations that might be the case. For example, we heard this morning that aspirin was effective against thrombosis only in men. I was wondering if there was any data on the effects of aspirin on females who were on oral contraceptives. Is this a situation where aspirin might be prothrombotic? Does anyone know? [No answer.]

MOLONY: I want to ask a question of Dr. Salzman. Weren't the patients enrolled in the studies females beyond the menopausal years?

SALZMAN: Most, but not all.

MOLONY: So they should be lacking in estrogen, although perhaps not in FSH and LH.

KAPLAN: Coming back to Dr. Packham's question: If the endoperoxides don't directly aggregate platelets, then what is thought to be the mechanism of aggregation and release induced by some of the cyclic endoperoxide analogs? Are they thought to be converted to thromboxane analogs?

GORMAN: Well, actually, when we first started sending those compounds out, I wanted to call them thromboxane analogs rather than endoperoxide analogs. But we really don't know without equivocation the structure of thromboxane A_2; we only know indirectly what it should be. So it's probably begging the point to say that endoperoxide analogs are structurally similar or dissimilar to thromboxane A_2. Pharmacologically, Gordon Bundy's endoperoxide analogs and the Corey endoperoxide analog that Bryan showed you produce analogous thromboxane effects, not endoperoxide effects. And I think it will become clear that the thing that will govern which way the prostaglandin pathways will go once these phospholipases are activated is whether prostacyclin or thromboxane has been synthesized. Dr. Frank Sun at The Upjohn Company has done extensive studies in many kinds of cells and organs, and I don't think he's found any cell beside the macrophage that has both thromboxane synthetase and a prostacyclin synthetase that express simultaneously.

SMITH: Would anybody like to comment about the hypothesis of endothelial cell stimulation or endothelial cell lysis? We've done some very preliminary work on this, and there's also been some work done at Mayo with the spontaneously atherosclerotic pigeon. "Damage" has become a dirty word with platelets; should it also become a dirty word with endothelial cells?

ROSS: I have some sheer speculation. I think that you're quite right, that it does depend upon what one means by "damage". "Alteration" might be a better word, because, since we don't know what normal is, one can interpret as altered almost anything that's different from the norms that one accepts. I think that it's entirely conceivable that one can have alterations that cause no change in cell physiology, like insertions of different lipid molecules in the plasma membranes of cells, whereby cell function itself is not disturbed. On the other hand, I think it's also entirely conceivable that one can cause changes in the cells that are not toxic to the cells, but clearly change cellular function. So there is a broad spectrum of alterations and how they affect the cell's ability to make prostacyclin. I think one will have to ask more specific questions, such as, is prostacyclin synthetase in the cells altered under a given set of circumstances? And then work back to find out what the molecular mechanisms are. So I think you're quite right that the word "damage" probably is too harsh a word and that we have to think in much more subtle terms, in terms of cellular alterations.

HARKER: Some recent and preliminary data using homocystine as an injury indicate that PGI_2 synthesis is inhibited by that exposure. Whether or not a lesser concentration might have a phase of increased production, I think we have yet to determine. So I guess we're really talking about what a sublethal injury is, and whether that is stimulatory, and then what a lethal injury is; and *in vitro* some of those questions are approachable.

STEMERMAN: There are at least two other considerations that we have to bear in mind when we talk about endothelial damage. One is that if there is damage or loss of endothelial cells, there is regrowth; and in the regrowing cell there might be physiologic alterations. The other consideration is that endothelial cells are not all alike. A number of investigators have shown that endothelial cells in different sites differ morphologically. Capillary endothelium certainly differs from large vessel endothelium, and the endothelial cells that line the vessels of various hormonal organs, kidneys, etc., have different morphologic structures, and they may behave differently. I think that we should not just say "endothelial cells"; in the future we're going to have to be much more specific about the type and origin.

HOAK: I want to mention a modified endothelial cell which we have, namely, a transplanted hemangioma, a tumor of endothelium which we have cultured from the mouse. These cells are interesting from several aspects. First, they do not make prostacyclin. Second, they are thrombogenic. In the animal, thrombi form only in the vascular channels of the tumor and not in the normal vessels. Third, they show platelet adherence much like the fibroblasts or smooth muscle cells. But the most interesting thing is that they show evidence of the thrombin receptor mechanism which we find on normal endothelium but not on fibroblasts or smooth muscle.

SPAET: I'd like to add one additional dimension to the comments of Dr. Stemerman and Dr. Ross. Investigators have shown that endothelial cells can contract in response to histamine. And when they contract, apparently they create such a configuration that there is an area transiently exposed, not covered with endothelium. These cells round up, leaving subendothelial connective tissues exposed. This also creates areas of fantastically increased permeability to particles as large as carbon. So here is a form of transient damage; the situation is reversed when the pharmacological effect of histamine is withdrawn.

RELEVANCE OF *IN VITRO* AND ANIMAL MODELS TO CLINICAL THROMBOSIS

Paul Didisheim, M.D.

Thrombosis Research Laboratory, Department of Laboratory Medicine, Mayo Clinic, Rochester, MN

I have been thinking during this conference about the relevance to clinical thrombosis of the various experimental models that have been discussed. I now feel somewhat like the cartoon scientist sitting at the bench of his cluttered laboratory, gazing into space. In the background one colleague says to another: "Since he became an Aristotelian, he has stopped experimenting, and he now believes that all knowledge comes from thought alone." Perhaps it is unjustified to be *that* negative about the methods that have been described; yet it is vitally important to consider whether the experimental model which each of us doggedly espouses has any relevance to thrombosis in the human. This brings me to the definition of relevance. Dr. Spaet says what is relevant is the work being done in *his* laboratory.

The history of experimental models for the study of thrombosis has been reviewed (1). Over 300 years ago, Wiseman (2) published one of the earliest descriptions of the manner in which thrombi grow. Fifty years ago Rowntree and Shionoya (3) reported the first systematic study of factors influencing thrombus formation in an extracorporeal shunt. Most of the early observations were largely qualitative; recent emphasis has been placed on precise control of conditions and quantitation of results. The reports of Cazenave, Grabowski, and Harker at this Workshop exemplify this current approach.

To determine the relevance of a given model to clinical thrombosis, we must first define what that model actually measures. In reviewing the models discussed at this Workshop, it appears that very few of them actually measure thrombosis. In many instances phenomena are being observed, e.g., protein adsorption, platelet adhesion, or platelet aggregation, which are believed to be associated with thrombosis, but the dependence of thrombosis on these phenomena has not been unequivocally established in all instances.

I have attempted to classify these phenomena into 15 categories. I have listed them in the Table in the approximate sequence in which they are believed to occur, recognizing that there is considerable interplay among the various steps. We must ask with each one: What is the relevance to clinical thrombosis?

TABLE. PHENOMENA OBSERVED IN VARIOUS "THROMBOSIS" MODELS

	Phenomenon	Variables and Questions
1.	Protein adsorption	Adsorption to glass, synthetic polymers, subendothelium; use plasma or pure proteins?
2.	Platelet metabolism	Uptake of serotonin, adenosine, etc; synthesis of ADP, ATP, thromboxanes, etc.
3.	Platelet adhesion	Adhesion to glass, polymers, collagen, subendothelium; affected by anticoagulant and choice of anticoagulant.
4.	Platelet release	Release of ADP, ATP, serotonin, PF4, beta-thromboglobulin, mitogenic factor, etc.; affected by anticoagulant. Which release stimuli are relevant? At what concentrations?
5.	Platelet aggregation	Relevance of studies using PRP or washed platelets rather than whole blood; role of anticoagulant and flow conditions; relevance of aggregation threshold and inducers; spontaneous aggregation; role of circulating aggregates; *in vitro* vs. *in vivo* observations.
6.	Platelet disaggregation	Same variables and questions as in platelet aggregation.

	Phenomenon	Variables and Questions
7.	Clearance from circulation	Clearance of platelets (survival, turnover) in coronary artery disease, graft occlusion, prosthetic valves, etc. Where do platelets go? Clearance of proteins (fibrinogen, plasminogen), fibrinopeptide A, etc.; specificity for thrombosis.
8.	Fibrin formation	*In vitro* vs. *in vivo* correlation.
9.	Fibrin embolization	Same as in fibrin formation.
10.	Fibrinolysis	Same as in fibrin formation.
11.	Re-endothelialization	Affected by selection of species, techniques of de-endothelialization, and hemodynamic factors.
12.	Cellular proliferation	Tissue culture vs. *in vivo*; smooth muscle cells, endothelial cells, fibroblasts.
13.	Atherosclerosis	Spontaneous vs. induced by diet, balloon catheter, etc.; species selection.
14.	Homocystine-induced lesions	Quantitation of de-endothelialization, platelet adhesion, and platelet survival.
15.	Blood vessel metabolism	Synthesis of prostaglandins including prostacyclin (PGI_2); uptake and synthesis of other lipids.

The following observations may be made about these experimental approaches to the study of thrombosis:

1) Many of the above models are quite artificial, and often their relationship to clinical thrombosis is remote at best.

2) Many of them involve short-term experiments or acute induction of some process, in contrast to clinical thrombosis which usually results from relatively slower re-

actions.

3) The selection of the animal species to be used has frequently been based upon such factors as convenience and cost, rather than upon the demonstration of similarity of the species to the human with regard to the phenomenon to be studied.

4) Clinical thrombosis usually occurs in association with, and as a direct result of, some underlying disorder. Chief among these are atherosclerosis, myocardial infarction involving the endocardium, mitral stenosis with an enlarged ventricle, prosthetic heart valves, saphenous vein bypass grafts, and venous stasis. In contrast, most of the phenomena and experimental models listed above have not been observed or conducted in a setting which simulates the clinical conditions listed above.

Now I would like to proceed down the list of the 15 phenomena and call upon participants in the workshop who have had experience in investigating them. I would like each discussant to attempt to answer the question, What is the evidence that this phenomenon, when it occurs *in vivo*, is a prerequisite to clinical thrombosis?

REFERENCES

1. Didisheim P: Animal models useful in the study of thrombosis and antithrombotic agents. In PROGRESS IN HEMOSTASIS AND THROMBOSIS, Vol. 1, edited by Spaet TH. New York, Grune and Stratton, 1972, pp. 165-197.

2. Wiseman R: SEVERAL CHIRURGICAL TREATISES (ed. 2). Flesher and Macock for Royston, London, 1676, p. 4.

3. Rowntree LG, Shionoya T: Studies in experimental thrombosis. I. A method for the direct observation of extracorporeal thrombus formation. J EXP MED 46:7-12, 1927.

DISCUSSION

CHANDLER: One of the diseases in which thrombotic phenomena are very common is sickle cell anemia, a disease that is, of course, peculiar to man. Micro-infarcts are especially frequent in this disease and we wanted to devise a way to study the ischemic mechanisms in the microcirculation. It is traditionally held that microcirculatory ischemia in this disease is caused by packing of sickled red cells in the capillaries and precapillary arterioles. We made an extracorporeal unit[1] based on the experimental work of Paul Didisheim[2,3] and also on the experimental animal work of Evans and Gordon reported a few years ago. The device is a 27-gauge needle with the smallest available Silastic tubing attached to it. A brass clip creates a slot or slit in this tubing. We estimate the size of the slit to be about 15x500 micra, which in cross-sectional area would be about equivalent to a 100-micron arteriole. We used a certain angulation of the arm, and constant 30 mmHg pressure instead of the usual 40. After discharging some blood, we attached the unit. Immediately blood would begin to drop out at the end of the tubing at a rate such that we could collect the drops on filter paper in the usual way, at 0.2-min intervals. Immediately after the bleeding ceased, the Silastic was cut off, dropped into fixative within 30 sec, and fixed under vacuum for processing for electron microscopy. The platelets are extremely well preserved with this technique. A typical section through the slot shows that it is occluded by a plug composed almost exclusively of aggregated platelets, with only an occasional red cell or leukocyte.

When we began to study sickle cell anemia patients, we found two unexpected things. One was that only about half of them would occlude this Silastic unit. The other finding was that the plugs were always platelet plugs, never sickled red cells, despite oxygen saturation usually being between 50% and 60% so that there was ample opportunity for sickling.

HOAK: Dr. Chandler, how does this test correlate with the bleeding time?

CHANDLER: We've not compared our method with the bleeding time.

MOORE: Why do so few of the sicklers block the unit?

CHANDLER: I think this is probably related to the fact that these patients almost always have a hematocrit of about 25% and the blood is less viscous than normal. For example, SC patients, who usually occlude the unit, have a hematocrit of around 35%.

---

[1]Chandler AB, Hutson MS: Platelet plug formation in an extracorporeal unit. AM J CLIN PATHOL 64:101-107, 1975.
[2]Didisheim P: Microscopically typical thrombi and hemostatic plugs in Teflon arteriovenous shunts. In DYNAMICS OF THROMBUS FORMATION AND DISSOLUTION, edited by Johnson SA, Guest MM. Philadelphia, J. B. Lippincott, 1969, pp. 64-71.
[3]Didisheim P, Pavlosky M, Kobayashi I: Factors affecting hemostatic plug formation in an extracorporeal model. ANN NY ACAD SCI 201: 307-315, 1972.

Both they and sickle cell anemia patients have about the same elevated platelet count.

MOORE: I have difficulty understanding that, because what you showed in your slides was a plug that is solidly composed of platelets. That suggests to me that maybe sicklers are using up all their platelets elsewhere, so they don't have enough of them, or else theirs don't stick for some reason.

CHANDLER: I've never seen an ambulatory patient with sickle cell anemia who had thrombocytopenia. They usually have thrombocytosis. Maybe I didn't make it clear that 100% of the controls occluded the unit by platelet plugs. There was a *lack* of occlusion in sickle cell anemia patients, a decreased frequency of occlusion in comparison to control.

HARKER: In the ones that do not occlude, do you see a trellis of sickled red cells that tends to keep spaces open? Or do you see any potential explanation as to why there is not platelet occlusion there?

CHANDLER: That is a good question, and I really don't know the answer. Sometimes we would see that the blood coming out through the tube would be very dilute, almost like plasma. We run these tests only over 5 minutes. After 5 minutes we discontinue because the procedure gets too artificial.

DIDISHEIM: Going back to the list of 15 phenomena, Dr. Brinkhous, your laboratory has studied the early events of protein adsorption. Can you provide evidence not only for the event which we all accept occurs, but for the necessity of that event preceding thrombosis?

BRINKHOUS: In what situations can you get platelet thrombus without protein adsorption? I do not know of any but there may be. We worked intensively with biomaterials and tried to extrapolate this to the denuded de-endothelialized surface. We did some experiments with washed platelets and washed collagen, thinking that there certainly would be a cofactor needed if the protein adsorption occurred, but we couldn't verify this. I think that this is the mechanism with biomaterials, but whether this is the required mechanism with a vascular lesion, I do not know. By labeling the proteins you might get at this, but I do not know of anybody who has really looked at this critically.

The other thing that came up in the discussion this morning of Dr. Salzman's paper was the qualitative nature of this adsorbed membrane. We observed very early that if we used a well siliconized surface there was some protein adsorption, but that membrane was not very thrombogenic. So there must be a lot of different kinetics involved in the laying down of the protein and the resorption of the protein. I believe that this is a field that could be attacked by many people very profitably. Since we first published the model, there has been marked disinterest in this field, and I'm glad to see it brought up again. There are a lot of probes that can be used nowadays that couldn't be many years ago when we first did this. The first thing I would look at would be the von Willebrand factor composition of this protein.

DIDISHEIM: At any rate, there is a question mark about solid evidence for protein adsorption being critical to the process.

H. J. DAY: I'm not sure I agree there is a question mark. In the work that Harvey Weiss has done with Hans Baumgartner, von Willebrand factor really does seem to have some importance in adhesion of platelets to the vessel wall.

DIDISHEIM: Do platelets have anything to do with thrombosis?

DAY: Maybe John Colwell's information on von Willebrand factor levels in diabetics who have an increased tendency toward thrombosis is relevant here.

DIDISHEIM: There may be a correlation but is there evidence that it is solidly associated, that there is cause and effect?

SPAET: I think the discussion is getting a little far afield from the question of what first lays down on a surface that blood hasn't previously seen. There is a huge body of information on this. Ed Salzman and I were discussing who were the real pioneers in this field, and the name that came to both of us is Leo Vroman. Anybody who wants to see a whole series of references on this work can look at the two seminars from the bioengineering group, one published in 1977[4] and the other published in 1972[5].

One of the things I have been emphasizing is that this problem should get a much more interdisciplinary approach.

DIDISHEIM: I think most of us are familiar with Vroman's beautiful work on the process of protein adsorption on surfaces, but I'm asking the question whether there is proven relevance of this step to thrombosis. And I don't hear any evidence.

[4]Vroman L, Leonard EF (Eds): The behavior of blood and its components at interfaces. ANN NY ACAD SCI 283:1-560, 1977.

[5]Symposium on problems in evaluating the blood compatibility of biomaterials. BULL NY ACAD MED 48:211-493, 1972.

Maybe because of the long list of phenomena in the table, we should move on to the next one. Considering platelet metabolism, what is the significance of synthesis of ADP, ATP, prostaglandins and other materials within the platelet? How does this relate to thrombosis? Should we be measuring it?

H.J. DAY: The only bit of evidence I know is John Colwell's in the diabetics with thrombotic tendency. Now will you accept that some diabetics may have a thrombotic tendency? Possibly the reason is that these people have a turned-on arachidonic acid pathway. And if I were to put my money where I think it is going to pay off, this is one thing we should look at.

I think the fact that homocystine seems to turn off prostacyclin is very interesting. Maybe we should be looking at this rather than at platelet aggregation, platelet release, and so forth, which I don't think are going to pay off.

DIDISHEIM: Dr. Spittell, did you have some question about the relevance of these studies?

SPITTELL: I would like to know what the evidence is that there is an increased thrombotic tendency in the diabetic.

COLWELL: I think there is good evidence and literature on that, Dr. Spittell; I think that the atherosclerotic lesion of the diabetic tends to proceed at a more rapid rate. For example, more diabetics have gangrene. And the bulk of the patients who end up at autopsy with peripheral arterial disease and with thrombotic disease are diabetics. And on and on. I don't really think there is any problem.

SPITTELL: I know that data well because I have participated in developing some of it. The diabetic has four or five times the chance of losing a limb. But that's occlusive arterial disease, small vessel infarction. Thrombosis is another problem and I haven't been able to show it, and I don't know the data.

COLWELL: No, it's thrombosis as well.

DIDISHEIM: Moving right along — perhaps we could take the next four steps in the table together, since they are probably related: platelet adhesion, release, aggregation, and disaggregation. What is the significance of these and the importance of measuring these with regard to thrombosis?

PACKHAM: If you grant that platelets might be involved in arterial thrombosis, then obviously they adhere, release, and aggregate. There is good evidence that thrombi will break up under the force of flowing blood, and this is disaggregation. ADP-induced aggregates are not stable *in vivo*. ADP does not induce a second phase of platelet aggregation *in vivo* and so-called irreversible ADP-induced aggregation does not occur *in vivo*. The aggregates are quite unstable unless fibrin forms around them.

DIDISHEIM: What would you say about the relevance of *in vitro* platelet adhesion, aggregation, release, and disaggregation studies to *in vivo* events? I have in mind the role of the anticoagulant, flow conditions, surface selection, plasma protein adsorption, etc.

PACKHAM: The citrate anticoagulant has given us the artifact of the second phase aggregation, which of course is being used by all the investigators who are measuring the concentration of ADP required to cause biphasic responses. Whether this has any relevance or not to *in vivo* events, I don't know.

I think in many cases the so-called platelet hypersensitivity appears to be a hypersensitivity of the arachidonic pathway either to activation or to operation. The evidence is that the drugs which block the cyclo-oxygenase reduce the hypersensitivity. This isn't the case with all the tests measuring hypersensitive platelets. Certainly in the biphasic one it is the case, and probably the arachidonic pathway is the major one for this *in vitro* effect that we call "hypersensitive platelets."

DIDISHEIM: I think we will all grant that platelets do have a role in arterial thrombosis. From the standpoint of pathology, we see them there. The question is, can we draw inferences from the various *in vitro* studies? This is mostly what we are talking about in steps 3 through 6 in the table; what is the platelet's role? Is it really valuable to be measuring platelet adhesion, release, aggregation, and disaggregation *in vitro* as tests of the pre-thrombotic state? Yes or no? [No answer.] I take it by the silence that we don't really know.

COLWELL: There are two clinical states in which it seems these may be useful. Patients with type II hyperlipoproteinemias have hypersensitive platelets, and they have a high yield of atherosclerotic heart disease; I'm not sure which comes first, but that's the case. And they may be useful in diabetics, who have a high incidence of atherosclerotic heart disease.

Dr. Chandler's sickle cell story struck a chord in me. This is still unpublished, but Dr. Kay Sarji has been looking at platelet aggregation in sicklers, and she finds that they have inhibited aggregation. They also have a plasma factor which inhibits aggregation of normal platelets.

MOLONY: I've always wondered about the relevance of the aggregating agents in testing. Do you encounter these levels of aggregating agents normally in the body? And if so, why don't people aggregate all the time? Perhaps they do, and disaggregate. On the other hand, if the amounts required in tests are higher than the body ever encounters, why do the platelets aggregate in the body in the first place? I can see collagen perhaps, but what about epinephrine, thrombin, and so on?

DIDISHEIM: Dr. Packham, what is the relevance of the aggregating agents in the concentrations used *in vitro* to the clinical situation?

PACKHAM: Well, there's no problem about collagen. I think you have to consider local concentrations rather than bulk phase concentrations. Certainly around a platelet aggregate, for instance, where the coagulation system is activated, you might well build up sufficient thrombin to have quite an effect. Also, if there is disturbed flow with vortices, higher concentrations of aggregating agents would accumulate than would be present where flow is laminar, and they would be diluted quickly.

GORMAN: Thromboxanes and prostacyclin are made in very small amounts in the body and they are very potent. At a concentration of 50 ng/ml, thromboxane A_2 will cause aggregation that does not reverse on its own. However, if you add even 2.8 ng/ml of prostacyclin to that situation, then the aggregation immediately reverses. Thus even a so-called irreversible thromboxane A_2-induced aggregation is readily reversible by prostacyclin. It's immediate.

DIDISHEIM: Let's move on to some of the succeeding steps in the table - fibrin formation, embolization, and fibrinolysis. Would anyone like to speak in favor of or against the study of those phenomena as the endpoint in the experimental models? My own bias is that we should be looking more at models such as these in which we actually see thrombi occur.

MOORE: I'd like to comment on this at such length that I'll probably miss my plane! I really think that we are caught up in a historical problem when we talk about embolization. And it is largely due to the people like myself, pathologists who only believe what they see. They have to see a great big embolic thrombus with fibrin wrapped around it in a vessel before they believe that embolism exists.

Some years ago I got interested in the question of whether atherosclerotic aortas might cause damage to the kidneys. We engaged in some experiments in which we caused platelet aggregates to form in the aorta and embolize to the kidney vessels. One has to look with extreme care to actually find that happening as a morphological event; the problems of morphological sampling are fantastic. But we found that what happens is that after there is repeated embolization into the intrarenal vessels, there is loss of endothelium and smooth muscle cell proliferation - much like the events in the aorta we talked about yesterday, including deposition of lipid in the smooth muscle cells of those vessels.

Now what's happening in the brain? We heard this morning from Dr. Barnett about transient ischemic attacks, and that process in the brain is accepted. But people have a lot of difficulty accepting that it happens in the kidney, and I think that's because it's really hard to see, certainly in autopsy material.

It's very difficult to get people to accept that it happens in the heart, but it could be an important mechanism in mural thrombosis, nonocclusive thrombosis, and sudden death. It's intriguing that, as the Seattle group has demonstrated, among people who are resuscitated from ventricular fibrillation, those with a full thickness infarct (complete coronary occlusion) documented by enzyme changes and by ECG changes have better survival experience than those who don't. If you go a step further and say that at least some of those who don't have a full thickness infarct have a mural thrombus which is embolizing, which could set up all kinds of foci of arrythmia in the ventricular myocardium, those might be the people who could develop ventricular fibrillation and die suddenly. If you autopsy those people you really wouldn't find very much. You certainly wouldn't find an occlusive thrombus, and you would have to look hard to find the mural thrombus that was doing it.

So there's another level of debate here about what's happening in early thrombus and embolism. Particularly relevant to all that is the new knowledge about thromboxane A_2 and prostacyclin. If you have an early platelet aggregate, an early mural thrombus forming in a coronary vessel, that could put the coronary vessel into spasm; it could also put the embolized vessels into spasm, and could really set you up for some pretty dramatic ischemic change. Although that's all speculative, I don't think that it's too far-fetched. It really represents our difficulty in talking about thrombosis. With all our experimental designs and models, so much of what we do is inferential because it is very difficult, unless you've got a really good thrombus formed in the vessel and it blocks, to see what is going on either in man or an experimental animal.

CHANDLER: Just an extension of what Sean Moore said in relation to the pathogenesis of emboli in the circulation. We have to consider that there may be more than one way an embolus forms. One way an embolism forms is by breaking off from a mural thrombus. Another way is that an embolic thrombus might form in the bloodstream itself, in the flowing blood without first having formed on the wall and being dislodged. This can be nicely demonstrated experimentally and may indeed be relevant to some of these *in vitro* techniques.

DIDISHEIM: I would like to sum up now.

In the development of experimental models for the study of clinical thrombosis, it is recommended that in the future a greater attempt be made to simulate the conditions under which this occurs in patients. Particular emphasis should be placed upon the following features:

1) For *in vitro* studies, use of human blood; for *in vivo* studies, selection of an animal species whose blood-vessel or blood-biomaterial interactions have been shown to be similar to those in the human. Although the data are preliminary, they suggest that the dog and rabbit may be unsatisfactory and the baboon, macaque, and pig more satisfactory choices: see Dr. Grabowski's presentation in this Workshop.

2) Phenomena should be observed long enough to have relevance to the time sequence observed in clinical thrombosis.

3) Since thrombosis occurs in whole blood *in vivo*, models making use of whole blood are more likely to yield relevant data.

4) Since thrombosis occurs in the absence of added anticoagulant *in vivo*, models should be designed to avoid the use of anticoagulants; if this is impossible, the effect of the anticoagulant on the results should be determined by using suitable controls.

5) Since clinical thrombosis usually occurs as a consequence of atherosclerosis (the major etiologic factor in arterial thrombosis), myocardial infarction, mitral stenosis, prosthetic heart valves, saphenous bypass grafts, and/or venous stasis, more emphasis should be placed on the use of models which incorporate these major precursors of clinical thrombosis in the experimental design.

A DISCUSSION OF METHODS FOR PREDICTING PATIENTS WHO ARE PRONE TO PLATELET THROMBOEMBOLISM INCLUDING MEASUREMENTS OF BLOOD COMPONENTS*

J. C. Hoak, M.D.

Division of Hematology-Oncology, Department of Medicine and the Cardiovascular Center, University of Iowa, Iowa City, IA

The belief that aggregates of platelets may develop in the circulation and interfere with the vascular supply to vital organs is certainly not a new concept. It received further support from the observations of morphologists who found platelet aggregates as prominent components of thrombi and from studies in which the infusion of aggregating agents into local vascular beds caused organ injury or infarction in association with the formation of platelet aggregates. These lesions failed to develop if the animals were treated with inhibitors of platelet aggregation prior to the infusion of the aggregating agent.

More recently, there has been much interest in tests which can detect the participation of platelets in clinical thromboembolic events. Such tests are of obvious interest to the clinician who has little at hand to determine whether a given thrombotic event reflects the consequences of abnormal or aberrant platelet behavior. In general, these tests fall into four categories:

1) Hyperaggregability of platelets to standard aggregating agents.

2) Shortened platelet survival.

*This work was supported in part by the National Heart, Lung and Blood Institute through a Specialized Center of Research in Atherosclerosis, Grant 14230. Doctor Hoak was the recipient of Research Career Development Award K3-HL-19,370-10 from the National Heart and Lung Institute.

3) Development of increased platelet procoagulant activity.

4) Demonstration of platelet aggregates in blood samples from patients (fixation or filtration techniques) or a tendency for platelets to aggregate with stirring ("spontaneous aggregation").

It is difficult to provide an accurate appraisal of the comparative value of these tests because only rarely has a given laboratory been able to perform a complete battery of these tests in a given patient. This situation not only reflects the specialized nature of the tests, but the time and expense they require, and also the unfortunate tendency for a given laboratory to prefer a specific test, frequently one which it has developed. Consequently, one is left with the need to choose one or perhaps two of the tests which are available locally and hope that the results may provide some guidance toward a rational clinical decision.

Although a number of techniques have been employed to detect platelet aggregates in circulating blood, no one method can be considered satisfactory. A second and equally important problem is whether the platelet aggregates caused the lesion or developed as a secondary event without a cause and effect relationship.

The observation by Maca, Fry, and Hoak that a dilute solution of formalin would fix platelet aggregates in whole blood samples led to a simpler method for detecting platelet aggregates (1). In the original method, blood samples were drawn into a buffered EDTA-formalin fixative which prevented dissociation of the platelet aggregates. The erythrocytes were then lysed with 1% ammonium oxalate and the platelet aggregates were sized and counted using a hemocytometer chamber and phase-contrast microscopy. Although this procedure did not involve centrifugation, it had other disadvantages, including the necessity to lyse the red cells and the time required to perform the test.

The simpler method developed in our laboratory also employed formalin for the fixation of platelet aggregates in whole blood, but the Coulter counter was used to count platelets (2). Free-flowing venous blood (0.5 ml) was drawn directly into two separate syringes through a 19-gauge siliconized needle. One syringe contained 2 ml buffered formalin-EDTA solution and the other, buffered EDTA solution without formalin. After thorough mixing, they were transferred into siliconized glass tubes and kept at room temperature for 15 min. They were mixed again and centrifuged at 22°C at 200 x *g* for 8 min. Platelet counts were then determined on the supernatant platelet-rich plasma (PRP) samples. The result was expressed as the ratio of the platelet count in the formalin-EDTA PRP to that of the EDTA PRP. This method was based upon the concept that formalin would fix existing platelet aggregates which then would be centrifuged out, causing the platelet count to be decreased in the formalin-EDTA sample. The concept also involves the ability of EDTA to deaggregate the non-fixed platelet aggregates in the EDTA sample; although platelet aggregation is calcium dependent, irreversible platelet aggregates would not be detected by this method. The greater the number of platelet aggregates in a given sample, the lower the ratio. We have found normal values to be 0.8 to 1.

To date, our laboratory and many others have found the test useful in detecting patients who appear to have platelet aggregates playing a primary or secondary role in their clinical thromboembolic problem. In patients with transient cerebral ischemic attacks (TIAs) who had blood drawn within 48 hours of an attack, 44 of 66 patients had ratios below 0.8; see Figure 1 (3). Dougherty, Levy, and Weksler made similar observations and found a significant increase in the percentage of aggregated platelets in 53 patients with completed stroke and in 29 patients with transient ischemic attacks who were studied within 10 days of the acute event (4).

Of additional interest in their report was a series of observations in a patient with TIA who was followed up for 3 weeks

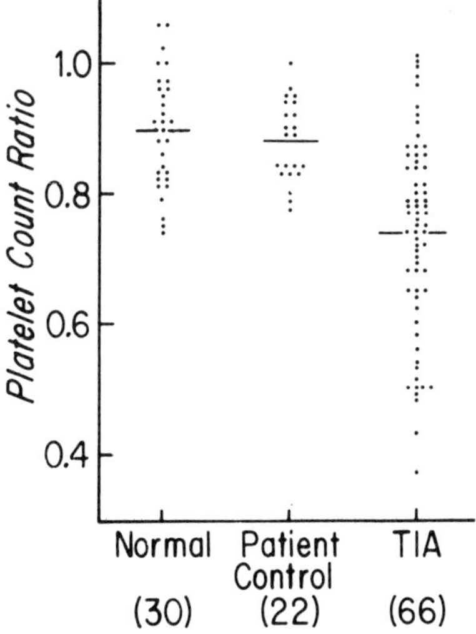

Figure 1. Platelet aggregate ratio values in patients with TIAs, normal subjects and patients without thromboembolic disorders. (From Wu and Hoak [3], reprinted with permission from STROKE.)

(Figure 2). The percentage of aggregated platelets was high at the time of the original episode. After the original episode, the patient was symptom-free and the aggregates fell nearly to normal by the 7th post-ischemic day. However, 19 days after the original episode, the patient experienced a recurrent TIA while receiving aspirin and dipyridamole. The percentage of aggregated platelets rose again; when symptoms stopped, the aggregates returned toward normal.

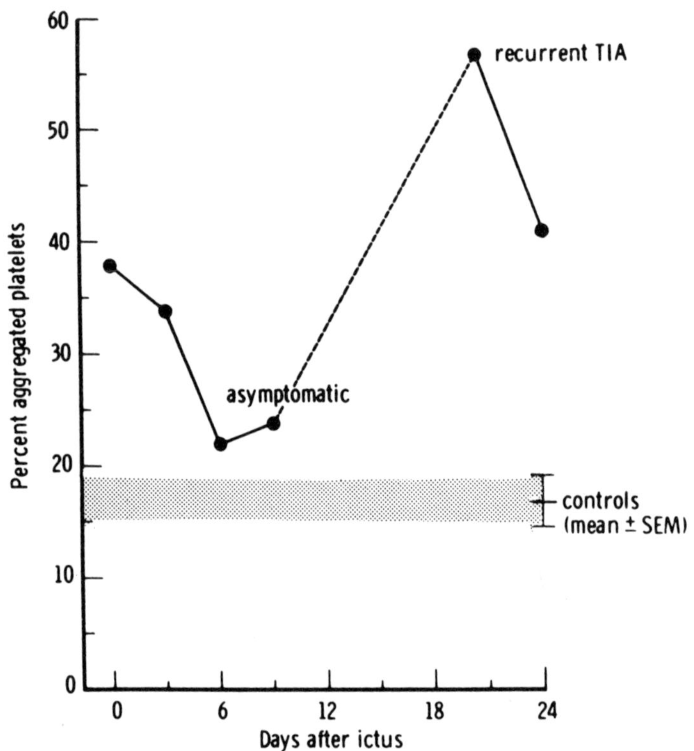

Figure 2. Percentage aggregated platelets in patient with recurrent TIA. (From Dougherty, Levy, Weksler [4], reprinted with permission from authors and LANCET.)

Progress has been made in the development of methods for the detection of platelet aggregates in whole blood. Significant questions remain, however, as to whether the detected aggregates are clearly circulating aggregates or whether the techniques select out a population of abnormal platelets which behave differently upon exposure to formalin than do normal platelets. It has been suggested that using the formalin fixation technique, aggregates might form *in vitro* as a result of centrifugation after contact with the formalin and would not reflect the *in vivo* situation. To evaluate this possibility, whole blood samples were studied from a patient known to have a low circulating platelet aggregate (CPA) ratio. One sample was drawn into formalin and allowed to sediment for 2 hours at 1 *g*. At this point a sample was obtained at the red cell interface and smears were prepared and stained. Numerous platelet aggregates were found (Figure 3). Similar results were obtained

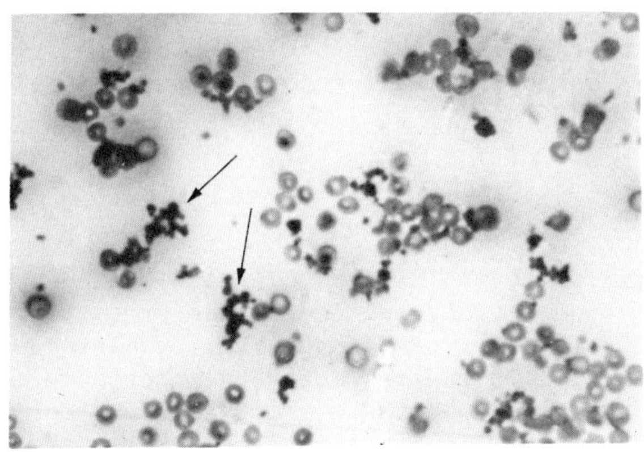

Figure 3. Platelet aggregates from a sedimented blood sample after fixation in formalin. The patient had recurrent TIA and an abnormal CPA ratio. Arrows point to examples of the aggregates. X92.

when blood was drawn into glutaraldehyde and also allowed to sediment without centrifugation. An example of the type of aggregate found in this preparation is shown in Figure 4.

Important questions remain concerning the mechanism of platelet aggregate formation in the various patient groups. Inherent in the formalin-EDTA method is the requirement that the platelet aggregates be reversible in the presence of EDTA. Therefore, it might be expected that irreversible platelet aggregation would not be detected by this method. Recently, we had the opportunity to perform special studies in three patients with acute cerebral

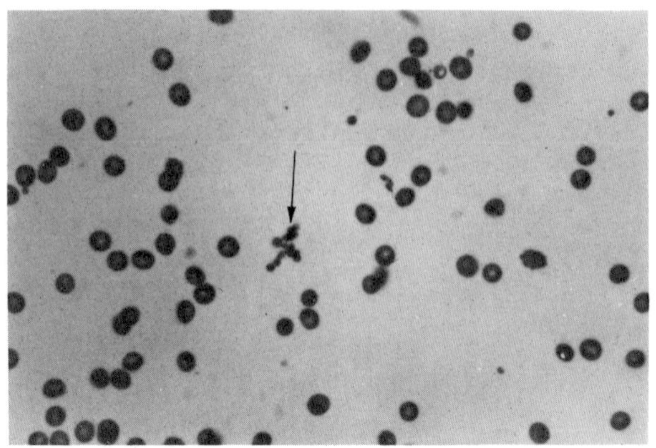

Figure 4. Platelet aggregate from a sedimented blood sample after fixation in glutaraldehyde. The patient had cerebral ischemia and an abnormal CPA ratio. The arrow points to an example of the type of aggregates found in this patient's sample. X92.

vascular insufficiency who had low CPA ratio values. Blood was collected in sodium citrate and then transferred to tubes containing one of the following: EDTA, heparin, 2-chloroadenosine, prostaglandin E_1, or saline. The respective samples were then agitated for 4 minutes and blood was taken from each tube for a CPA determination. In addition, peripheral blood smears were prepared and stained from samples without anticoagulant and from samples containing EDTA. The results are shown in the Table.

TABLE. EFFECTS OF INHIBITORS *IN VITRO* IN THREE PATIENTS WITH LOW BASELINE VALUES

Inhibitor	CPA Ratio Mean ± SE
None (baseline)	0.61 ± 0.02
EDTA	0.98 ± 0.02
2-chloroadenosine	1.02 ± 0.04
Prostaglandin E_1	0.93 ± 0.02
Saline-citrate	0.95 ± 0.02
Heparin	0.37 ± 0.03

It can be seen that all of the inhibitory agents except heparin caused the aggregates to disappear with a return of the CPA ratio to normal. In these three patients, aggregates of platelets (containing their granules) were seen on the smears from unanticoagulated blood (Figure 5) and heparinized samples, but not in smears from blood anticoagulated with EDTA. These results suggest that it is unlikely that thrombin was the mediator of platelet aggregate formation in this group of patients, and calcium appeared essential.

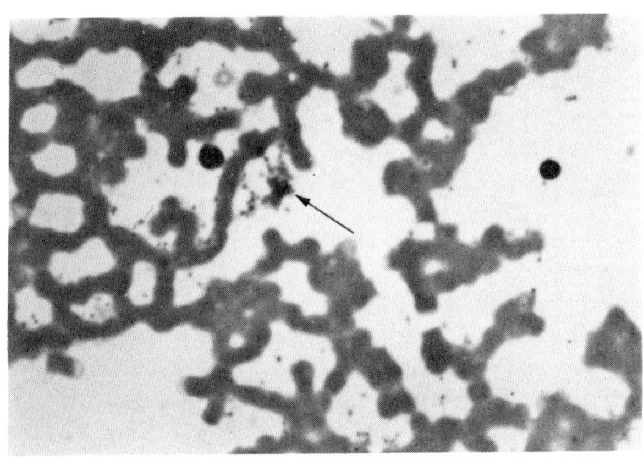

Figure 5. Platelet aggregate in an unfixed blood smear from a patient with acute cerebral ischemia and an abnormal CPA ratio. X92.

In summary, in recent years a number of approaches have been employed to determine the role of platelet aggregates in patients with thromboembolic disease. These include aggregability of platelets to standard stimuli, measurements of platelet survival, determinations of platelet procoagulant activity, and methods to detect platelet aggregates by fixation of whole blood samples. The formalin-EDTA method has proven useful in delineating groups of patients in whom platelet aggregates may be playing a primary or secondary role. The methods do not provide the complete answer, however, and I hope the discussion will offer some suggestions as to how to improve the situation.

ACKNOWLEDGEMENT

The valuable technical assistance of Ms. Donna Haycraft was greatly appreciated.

REFERENCES

1. Maca RD, Fry GL, Hoak JC: New method for detection and quantitation of circulating platelet aggregates. MICROVASC RES 4: 453-456, 1972.

2. Wu KK, Hoak JC: A new method for the quantitative detection of platelet aggregates in patients with arterial insufficiency. LANCET 2:924-926, 1974.

3. Wu KK, Hoak JC: Increased platelet aggregates in patients with transient ischemic attacks. STROKE 6:521-524, 1975.

4. Dougherty JH, Jr, Levy DE, Weksler BB: Platelet activation in acute cerebral ischaemia. LANCET 1:821-825, 1977.

DISCUSSION

BARNETT: Since this is really not a discussion of platelet function tests, but a method of predicting which patients are prone to platelet thromboembolism, I dare to mention that you should really include platelet count. After all, this gives me as a neurologist an easy way of telling whether the patient who has polycythemia or thrombocytosis is going to have amaurosus fugax, or transient ischemic attacks, or that other thing that turns up in neurology practice, the painful fingers and toes syndrome.

HOAK: Not all people with high counts will have aggregate formation and not all of them have symptoms. I think it is very difficult to make a decision about treatment in somebody who has a platelet count of 1 million and who is asymptomatic. We prefer to individualize the management of such patients rather than to establish a value for the platelet count which would indicate a need for treatment.

HARKER: We have had trouble getting a reproducible aggregate test on repeated sampling, on restudying patients day after day. For whatever it means, the observations of those tests have not concurred with platelet survival. I'm not implying that they have to correlate in order to be useful, but just that in our hands there is not a concordance. Even more troublesome has been the documentation that patients whose blood samples have been drawn in EDTA may have a significant disparity between the whole blood count of platelets versus what one determines in that EDTA sample. Also, some patients, who represent as many as 10% of the samples drawn, will have a higher platelet count when the blood is passed through a physically disrupting process, for example, when blood is forced through a 25-gauge needle. As you pointed out, EDTA does not ensure disggregation of any aggregates that may form *in vitro*. We have been troubled by the potential for artifact and the difficulty of reproducibility in our hands. Therefore we have been trying to determine aggregation formation *in vivo* using such procedures as laser beam light scattering. Those techniques show some promise, but they certainly have a way to go in order to be readily available for clinical purposes. But as to the aggregate test you described, we have mixed emotions.

HOAK: This has been true of a few groups. In most instances the workers have modified the techniques, have used different counting equipment, or have needed instruction in the technical details of the procedure. In regard to comparing the test with platelet survival, the only results we have are in patients with recurrent deep vein thrombosis, in which Dr. Wu found a relatively good correlation between ^{51}Cr-platelet survival and the CPA ratio.[1]

KAPLAN: I have a question about those last three patients that you discussed and the lack of inhibition by heparin of the platelet aggregates. Did heparin cause a lack of inhibition of aggregate formation or actually cause formation of aggregates? The ratio was considerably lower with the heparin than it was in the control state. What happens with platelets from normals in heparin?

HOAK: Yes, we also wanted to know that. We collected blood from normals into heparin, and the heparin did not cause changes in the CPA ratio.

H.J. DAY: Jack, in your prospective studies and in some of the work that you did originally setting up the tests, did you find some patients who did not have arterial thrombosis but had positive aggregate tests?

HOAK: You mean control patients who did not have thromboembolic disease but had abnormal values? The mean CPA ratio of the patient control group was a little lower than that of the normals; but it was still within the normal range.

DAY: Then the basic question under those circumstances would be, what action would you undertake if you found "normal" individuals who had positive aggregate ratio tests? Would you then suggest that these people go on any type of interrupted therapy?

HOAK: Let me give an illustration of what happened on one occasion. The young man who was working in the lab doing the CPA

[1]Wu KK, Barnes RW, Hoak JC: Platelet hyperaggregability in idiopathic recurrent deep vein thrombosis. CIRCULATION 53:687-691, 1976.

test came in one day and said, "What does it mean to have an abnormal value in this test? I happen to have an abnormal one." The test was repeated and it was still abnormal, and he said, "What should we do?" And I said, "I don't think we should do anything, we should just observe you." He came in about 3 days later and said, "I went down to give blood at the Blood Bank, and they wouldn't take my blood because they told me I am Australian antigen positive." Within a week he was jaundiced. This abnormal value was the forerunner at least in association with his acute serum hepatitis. I don't know how many viral infections influence this test but I suspect they may cause some changes.

Some of the people with autoimmune disease and people with chronic hepatitis have had abnormal values. You may have seen a report of one patient, age 21, who had a myocardial infarction and chronic hepatitis and had evidence of abnormal platelet aggregates.[2] They also had another woman patient, also 21, who had a stroke and also had chronic hepatitis, who had abnormal values. Now whether these aggregates are related to an autoimmune vasculitis or the presence of antigen-antibody complexes, I don't know. We have not seen abnormal values in normal people.

Perhaps we should change direction to talk about some tests or procoagulant effects such as Dr. Walsh uses. We have not used this test but perhaps others in the audience have - or used some other tests for procoagulant activity from platelets in people with thrombotic disease.

H. J. DAY: I'll talk about Peter Walsh's data. Peter studied two large groups of patients. He studied venous thrombosis patients[3] and was able to predict which patients would develop deep vein thrombosis sooner with his test than with ^{125}I fibrinogen, and then he was able to confirm the condition with ^{125}I fibrinogen and also with venography. He recently studied another group of patients who have had retinal vein thrombosis.[4] In this double-blind study the patients were referred to him by the ophthalmology department and he didn't know who had retinal vein thrombosis and who had not ever had retinal vein thrombosis. With his test, he was able to detect patients with the retinal vein thrombosis. I've forgotten

---

[2]Yon JL, Anuras S, Wu K, Forker EL: Granulomatous hepatitis, increased platelet aggregation and hypercholesterolemia. ANN INT MED 84:148-156, 1976.
[3]Walsh PN, Rogers PH, Marder VJ, *et al.*: The relationship of platelet coagulant activities to venous thrombosis following hip surgery. BRIT J HAEMATOL 32:421-437, 1976.
[4]Walsh PN, Pareti FI, Corvett J: Platelet coagulant activities and serum lipids in transient cerebral ischemia. N ENGL J MED 295:854-858, 1976.

what his correlation coefficient was, but it was rather high.

As you are probably all aware, there is a lot of controversy now as to exactly what Peter Walsh is measuring, and what is the significance of platelet coagulant activities. Is this indeed an effect of factor XI or factor Xa on platelets? There is some interesting and perhaps convincing work now coming out of several centers indicating that what he is measuring is probably factor V. I believe even Peter Walsh is beginning to believe that what he is measuring as platelet coagulant activity is a test tube variation, whereas others who are using radioimmune assay tests can actually measure factor V and therefore rule out factor Xa. He has been correlating the platelet coagulant activities with circulating platelet aggregates. He is able to make the test work. But I don't know his correlation.

HOAK: We haven't touched directly on the implications of finding so-called spontaneous platelet aggregation. This does not occur too often in normals except in women who are taking oral contraceptives. In that group it's a fairly common finding; but we do not find evidence of an abnormal CPA ratio in that group of women. Does anyone care to comment on spontaneous platelet aggregation? [No answer.]

DAY: It would seem that the techniques now available for predicting thromboembolism are preliminary.

PARTICIPANTS IN THE WORKSHOP

The editors:

H. James Day, M.D.
Department of Medicine
Section of Hematology
Temple University
Health Sciences Center
Philadelphia, PA 19140

Basil A. Molony, M.D.
Diabetes and Atherosclerosis Research
The Upjohn Company
Kalamazoo, MI 49001

Edward E. Nishizawa, Ph.D.
Diabetes and Atherosclerosis Research
The Upjohn Company
Kalamazoo, MI 49001

Ronald H. Rynbrandt, Ph.D.
Diabetes and Atherosclerosis Research
The Upjohn Company
Kalamazoo, MI 49001

Authors who presented papers:

H. J. M. Barnett, M.D.
Dept. of Clinical Neurological Sciences
University of Western Ontario
London, Ontario, Canada
N6A 5A5

K. M. Brinkhous, M.D.
Department of Pathology
University of North Carolina
Chapel Hill, NC 27514

Jean-Pierre Cazenave, M.D., Ph.D.
Department of Pathology
McMaster University
Hamilton, Ontario, Canada
L8S 4J9

John A. Colwell, M.D., Ph.D.
Department of Medicine
Endocrinology-Metabolism-Nutrition Division
Medical University of South Carolina
Charleston, SC 29403

Paul Didisheim, M.D.
Thrombosis Research Laboratory
Dept. of Laboratory Medicine
Mayo Clinic
Rochester, MN 55901

V. D. Fuster, M.D.
Dept. of Cardiovascular Diseases and Internal Medicine
Mayo Clinic
Rochester, MN 55901

Eric F. Grabowski, Ph.D.
Dept. of Laboratory Medicine
Mayo Clinic
Rochester, MN 55901

Edward Genton, M.D.
McMaster University
Hamilton, Ontario, Canada
L8S 4J9

Laurence A. Harker, M.D.
Harborview Medical Center
325 9th Avenue
Seattle, WA 98104

J. C. Hoak, M.D.
Division of Hematology-Oncology
Department of Medicine and the Cardiovascular Center
University of Iowa
Iowa City, IA 52242

Michael Hume, M.D.
Tufts University School of Medicine and Lemuel Shattuck Hospital
Boston, MA 02130

Karen L. Kaplan, M.D., Ph.D.
Dept. of Medicine
Columbia University
College of Physicians and Surgeons
New York, NY 10032

Sean Moore, M.D.
Department of Pathology
McMaster University
Hamilton, Ontario, Canada
L8S 4J9

J. F. Mustard, M.D., Ph.D.
Department of Pathology
McMaster University
Hamilton, Ontario, Canada
L8S 4J9

Marian A. Packham, Ph.D.
Department of Biochemistry
University of Toronto
Toronto, Ontario, Canada
M5S 1A8

Russell Ross, Ph.D.
Depts. of Pathology and Medicine
University of Washington
Seattle, WA 98195

Edwin W. Salzman, M.D.
Dept. of Surgery
Harvard Medical School and Beth Israel Hospital
Boston, MA 02215

J. Bryan Smith, Ph.D.
Cardeza Foundation and Dept. of Pharmacology
Thomas Jefferson University
Philadelphia, PA 19107

Theodore H. Spaet, M.D.
Hematology Division
Department of Medicine
Montefiore Hospital and Medical Center
Bronx, NY 10467

Michael B. Stemerman, M.D.
Beth Israel Hospital
Boston, MA 02215

Participants who did not present papers but contributed to the discussions:

Frank P. Bell, Ph.D.
Diabetes and Atherosclerosis Research
The Upjohn Company
Kalamazoo, MI 49001

A. B. Chandler, M.D.
Dept. of Pathology
School of Medicine
Medical College of Georgia
Augusta, GA 30901

Charles E. Day, Ph.D.
Diabetes and Atherosclerosis Research
The Upjohn Company
Kalamazoo, MI 49001

William E. Dulin, Ph.D.
Diabetes and Atherosclerosis Research
The Upjohn Company
Kalamazoo, MI 49001

Robert Gorman, Ph.D.
Experimental Biology Research
The Upjohn Company
Kalamazoo, MI 49001

Thomas Honohan, Ph.D.
Diabetes and Atherosclerosis
Research
The Upjohn Company
Kalamazoo, MI 49001

J. A. Spittell, Jr., M.D.
Dept. of Cardiovascular
Diseases and Internal Medicine
Mayo Clinic
Rochester, MN 55901

INDEX

Errata sheet (IFAVL 96):

In the course of the technical process three images were not printed on page 34.

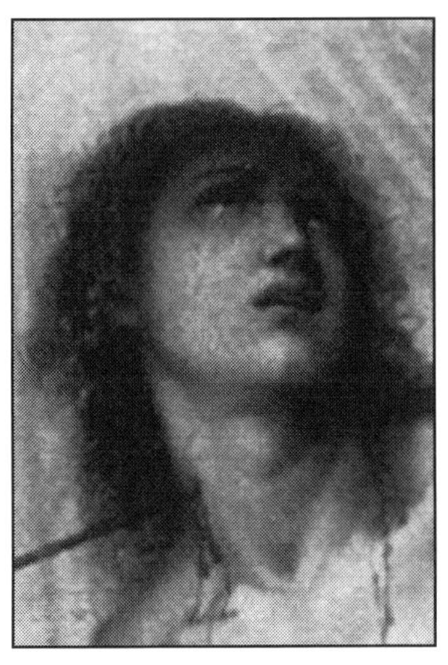

St. Sebastian of Sodoma, detail

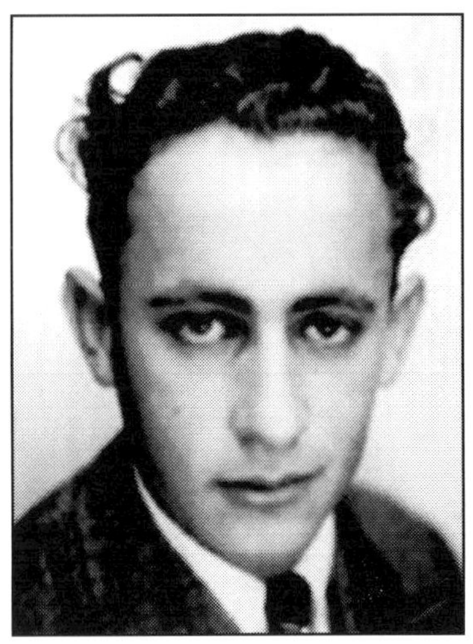

Henry

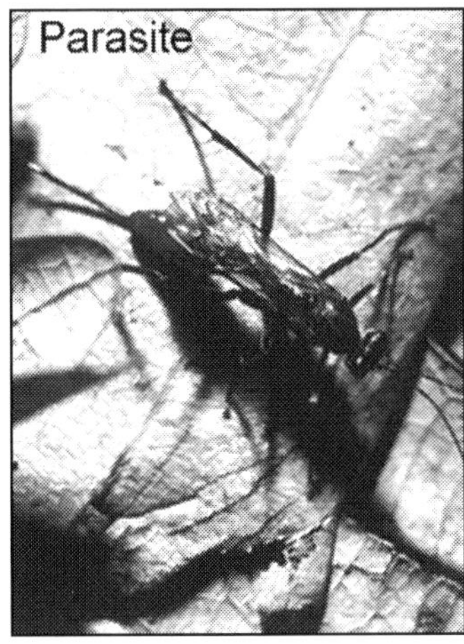

Ichneumon